MW01166189

More to Consider in the Battle Against Ulcerative Colitis

By Eugene L. Heyden, RN

Impact Health Publishing

Spokane, WA, USA

Impact Health Publishing
Spokane, WA USA

ISBN: 978-0-9828276-5-9

Printed in the United States of America

To those personally engaged in the battle against ulcerative colitis

Disclaimer: This book is presented solely for informational purposes. The information contained herein should be evaluated for accuracy and validity in the context of opposing data, new information, and the views and recommendations of a qualified health care professional, and not to be substituted for professional judgment and guidance or to provide reason to neglect or delay appropriate medical care. It is the reader and reader only who bears the responsibility for any actions that could be construed as being a response to the information contained herein. The statements and opinions expressed by the author have not been reviewed or approved by the FDA or by any other authoritative body, nor is the author endorsing any product, specific therapy, or any clinician mentioned within the pages of this book. This book is offered to the reader to broaden his or her understanding of the issues discussed and to help identify options that may be suitable for the individual to pursue, on behalf of self or others, under approval and direction of a qualified physician or medical team member. The reader is hereby on notice that educational material offered by the websites listed within this book may at some future time be modified or may no longer be provided. The author and publisher offer no guarantees of the accuracy or validity of the quotations incorporated into this presentation or the accuracy or validity of the information presented by the resources that are herein recommended.

~ *Preface* ~

S ince its first description by Wilks in 1859 (Leenen and Dieleman, 2007), ulcerative colitis has progressively claimed more and more victims. Today, approximately 1 million individuals in North America have the disease. (Or, it has them.) Worldwide, its incidence is on the rise. Ulcerative colitis is no small thing. It is a big deal! It is a disease that damages a life. Sometimes destroys a life. It must be stopped. Perhaps I can help.

In this book you will learn what ulcerative colitis is all about, how it arrives and strategies to make it go away. It also offers an in-depth look at how this disease can be treated more effectively than by drug therapy and little else. Don't get me wrong, we do need drugs in the battle against ulcerative colitis, but drug therapy alone does not seem to be the answer. There are problems.

> *Unfortunately, all these medicines have side effects. People have to suffer from severe effects and the course of UC [ulcerative colitis] is still characterized by periods of remission interspersed with exacerbations.* (Zhang et al., 2013)

Here you will discover a wide variety of actions an individual can take that may offer an advantage and increase the chances of achieving remission and limiting or eliminating the need for drug therapy.

Assuming you are the typical ulcerative colitis patient, it is likely you know little about the disease that you have, except for the suffering part. No doubt, you know *this* all too well, but know little else about the disease that is dominating your life. We'll work on the "little else" in the pages of this book.

Clearly, reading a book will not lead to remission . . . in any disease! But knowledge is power. This book will lay out many paths to consider, paths found in the medical literature and waiting for a motivated patient <u>in concert with a physician</u> who is willing to think outside of the box and guide the patient in the path of his or her choosing. Remission is possible! Always keep this in mind. And always keep in mind, remission in ulcerative colitis has been achieved by many, many individuals using alternative and complementary therapies. So why not you? No guarantees here, but in the pages of this book I will share with you story after story of remission in ulcerative colitis achieved by a variety of unconventional measures, sometimes occurring promptly and sometimes at a time when it seemed there was no end in sight.

So, let's dive right in, setting aside the notion that there is no way out of all the madness. Although the disease is serious business, that doesn't mean we can't have a little fun along the way as we journey together in the pages of this book.

~Eugene L. Heyden, RN

~References~

Leenen CH, Dieleman LA. **Inulin and oligofructose in chronic inflammatory bowel disease.** The Journal of Nutrition. 2007 Nov 1;137(11):2572S-5S.

Zhang DQ, Zhu JH, Chen WC. **Acarbose: a new option in the treatment of ulcerative colitis by increasing hydrogen production.** African Journal of Traditional, Complementary and Alternative Medicines. 2013;10(1):166-9.

~ x ~

~ *Contents* ~

Introduction

*In the past few years, we have gained considerable evidence that it is an abnormal mucosal immune reactivity, against enteric [gut] bacteria, that is **the key event** leading to intestinal injury in patients with IBD.* **~Lukas et al., 2006, emphasis added**

Conventional treatments for UC [ulcerative colitis] usually involves suppression or modulation of the host inflammatory response using corticosteroids, aminosalicylates or immunomodulatory agents, depending on the severity and localization of the disease. However, some individuals cannot tolerate these treatments, and they have various debilitating side-effects. **~Macfarlane et al., 2005**

Here in the pages of this book, I have an opportunity to share with you a story. It is a story about a very complex disease called ulcerative colitis. But I'll make it simple! And in this simple story about a very complex disease, I will include the stories of individuals who have achieved and maintained remission by the use of alternative and complementary measures. Of course, I'm assuming you would like to learn from the success of others.

Perhaps you know the disease all too well, and your life is so vastly different from anything you had in mind. Perhaps you would like to better understand the disease that you have. And perhaps you would like a change in the circumstances you are in. Have I got a book for you!

I suppose you would like to know why I spent several years of my life writing this book. It might be because the word is out: You have a disease that you know so little about, one that is out to destroy. (Did I just hear your cry for help?) Perhaps it is because knowing what I know, carries with it a certain degree of responsibility. It could be because I want you to keep your colon and not have it surgically taken away. And it might be that I think I'll scream the next time I hear someone say, "Ulcerative colitis is an autoimmune disease." (It is not.)

In any case, what I offer is a unique opportunity. I offer you the opportunity to learn what this disease is all about and how this disease can be managed differently—perhaps more effectively—than standard drug therapy (and little else).

So, automatically, I am a little at odds with conventional wisdom and medical practice. I don't mean to be. I don't want to be. But, whenever new ideas are discussed, and unconventional insights are shared, eyebrows are typically raised. Just keep that in mind. Also keep in mind, although I speak of alternative and complementary therapies, I am a big believer in the use of drugs. Being a Registered Nurse, I am certainly no stranger to the use and value of drug therapy. Drugs can be <u>very</u> skillfully and <u>very</u> effectively used in the battle against disease, ulcerative colitis included. Actually, I favor their use in the management of this disease. But so often they fail and so often they harm (and fail). Our physicians know this all too well. And most would agree: The use of drugs should be limited when there is a clear opportunity to do so. **I believe we should carve out opportunities to limit their use and perhaps achieve better outcomes, one motivated individual at a time.**

So, in my view, drugs are warranted if needed to quickly get on top of a situation, if they are safely succeeding, and particularly so if that's all the patient has an interest in. But drug therapy should not be the only game in town in the treatment of ulcerative colitis. I can safely say this, in as much as the medical literature offers many alternative and complementary therapies to manage this disease.

Here I will do most of the work, but you will need to pitch in. **First**, you will need to set aside any notion that, given a little help and with adequate motivation on your part, you cannot understand what the science is saying. Practically anything can be brought down to layperson level. You can do this! You *can* understand what this disease is all about and the reasons why the use of alternative and commentary measures can be effective tools in the battle against ulcerative colitis. **Second**, a personal comment is required. You want your life back, right? Commitment implies persistence. You get others to listen to you. You get someone (a physician) to respond and guide you in your efforts. You develop a winning attitude. There is no quit left in you! You realize you are at war.

But before we get started, I must issue this **warning:** Ulcerative colitis is just too complex, and the risks are too great, for you to attempt to manage this disease without the guidance of a physician. **I really mean this!** And perhaps most physicians want their patients to learn all they can, consider new ideas, offer suggestions, and adopt favorable lifestyle changes. But it is doubtful that your physician will want you to go out on your own or go against his or her advice. This seems reasonable. Always discuss with your physician any option you have an interest in perusing. *Always!* You can make mistakes, even with so called "natural therapies," and cause harm. I can give you example after example. And I will. So, promise me you will run things by a physician before you act on your own behalf or on the behalf of others.

There is one more thing we need to discuss before we continue. **Very important!** Be aware that there are divergent views on what ulcerative colitis actually is. Not everyone is on the same page. What I am leading up to is this: **I want you to be aware, right from the start, I view this disease differently than do others.** Again, consider the first quotation at the beginning of this *Introduction*. I'll repeat it here for your convenience.

> In the past few years, we have gained considerable evidence that it is <u>an abnormal mucosal immune reactivity</u>, against enteric [gut] bacteria, that is **the key event** leading to intestinal injury in patients with IBD. (Lukas et al., 2006, emphasis added)

I do not believe this concept at all. Not at all. I believe something else. **I believe ulcerative colitis is war.** *War!* **And I believe <u>this war is a war of necessity</u>.** Furthermore, I believe if you remove the reason(s) why this war is necessary, rather than simply manipulating the inflammatory response, a better outcome may be achieved. Let me explain.

The prevailing view, represented in part by the above quotation, goes something like this: IBD, ulcerative colitis included, is a disease caused by an abnormal immune response to normal, usual bacteria, and a loss of tolerance to the microbes within ensues. Inflammation follows. And, in as much as inflammation itself persists due to a complicated series of events—a response maintained by certain signaling molecules (cytokines) and activated proinflammatory pathways—suppressing these cytokines and modulating these pathways seems warranted and appears to be the key to success. And this might work, actually does work, but not as well or as often as we would like to see. The suffering of many, many individuals continues even under the best of medical care. Oftentimes, this disease is *so* resistant to our efforts. Perhaps we could use a few fresh, new ideas. Perhaps we should make it easier for the drugs to succeed and, hopefully, limit their need.

So why do I view ulcerative colitis as war, indeed, a war of necessity? It is because of this:

> *Normally, luminal bacteria in the gut are withheld from contact with the epithelium by an adherent mucus layer, but* **in UC the bacteria reside on the luminal surface where they probably induce and maintain the inflammatory process.** (Schneider et al., 2010, emphasis added)

Bacteria should *not* be living and replicating on the surface of the bowel. *Never* should this occur! A layer of mucus normally prevents relevant contact between the luminal surface of the bowel and bacteria. But in ulcerative colitis, the unthinkable occurs. There is a catastrophic loss of the protective mucous layer. This turn of events requires a deliberate inflammatory response. Bacteria, normally well tolerated, normally held at arm's length, are now a serious threat. They are now living and replicating on the surface of the rectum and likely the colon. And an invasion must be prevented.

It is signaling molecules (cytokines and others) and activated proinflammatory pathways, indeed it is inflammation itself that the body uses to deal with threats. **Bacteria living on the surface of the bowel is unquestionably a threat, one most serious, and an inflammatory reaction <u>must</u> follow and <u>must</u> continue.** The immune system—whether its response is normal, excessive, awkwardly expressed or impaired—is *compelled* to act. ***<u>This</u>* is the disease that you have.** The immune system is out to save your . . . well, you know.

Yet, inflammation is meant to be of short duration and to quickly solve a problem. When inflammation does not resolve in a timely, orderly fashion, for whatever reason, I see nothing but trouble ahead. Inflammation itself inflects damage to the very tissues it is trying to protect, so we do need to take measures, even by the use of potentially dangerous anti-inflammatory drugs, to control all the madness, dial things back, turn things around, and head the patient in the right direction. But we also need to address the underlying problem. Furthermore, we need to limit the use of potentially harmful drugs whenever possible. All would agree with this (I hope). And how this can be done, and done more effectively and safely, will be the focus of this presentation.

In *Chapter 1* you will learn a little more about the inflammatory response, what it is, what it does, why it persists, and why it seems to hate your guts. But before we continue, please read the following quotations very carefully:

> *A disturbed mucosal barrier is thought to be an <u>initiating</u> factor of the disease* and subsequent attacks from colonic commensal [normal, typical] bacterial flora result in inflammation of the mucosa. (Stremmel et al., 2010, emphasis added)

*Although <u>loss of tolerance</u> to the gut microbiota [microbes] is demonstrated in animal models of inflammatory bowel disease, there is only limited evidence for this finding in patients with Crohn's disease and **<u>none</u>** in those with ulcerative colitis.* (Danese and Fiocchi, 2011, emphasis added)

And, of course, one thing leads to another . . .

Once damaged, the barrier is unable to exclude highly immunogenic fecal bacterial antigens [immune stimulating bacterial components] from invading the normally sterile submucosa. (Pravda, 2005)

Samples from both CD [Crohn's Disease] and UC [ulcerative colitis] subjects contained significantly more bacteria when compared to normal control tissue, and a gradual increase was observed from noninflamed to inflamed biopsy material. (Sasaki and Klapproth, 2012)

So, in view of the quotation directly above, can you see why an aggressive inflammatory response is necessary? It is necessary to deal with all the bacteria that have breached the mucous layer of protection and have achieved relevant contact with the intestinal cells below. Bacteria, living where they should not be, is a recipe for disaster. Ulcerative colitis is a disaster.

Behold the gray box!

I love these gray boxes! Each one that I add to the end of a chapter gives me an additional opportunity to share with you other things that I believe may contribute significantly to the subject matter at hand. The gray box will become particularly useful should one want to study a particular subject in depth. But they also give me an opportunity to have a little more fun. We all know how boring medically related books and papers can be, so I will change this, one gray box at a time. I *will* be famous for my gray boxes; I just know it. The gray boxes are part of the experience of *More to Consider in the Battle Against Ulcerative Colitis.* Don't miss out!

On finding papers and videos on the web

That's easy! Go to Google (by way of example). Then, in the search box, type in the last name of the lead author and the title of the paper you wish to read. A list of candidate papers will appear. Just click on the one of interest, and it should appear in the blink of an eye. For videos, you need to first click the Video button at the top of the Google home page. Then type in the title of the video in the search box. Presto! You have a video to watch. (While on Google Video, try not to be distracted by videos of cute little kittens. Stay on track! You have a disease to fight! Cute little kittens can wait. Warning: Puppy dogs can be quite distracting, too. ... Now, where were we? Oh!) One other thing: Sometimes a paper or a video will be withdrawn from a particular website. But chances are someone else will have it, so keep searching. Finally, some sources charge a fee for their research papers, but if you keep looking you may be able to locate a website that will provide it free of charge. Here's a tip: Try clicking on "Related articles" or "All versions"—usually placed somewhere in the article listing—and you may find a source that will provide the paper free (while others want to charge you an arm and a leg).

Basic terms and concepts

Obviously, there are a few terms and concepts that you will need to become familiar with as we continue. For starters:

Inflammation—a cell or tissue response to a threat (e.g., injury or bacterial invasion), generally characterized by redness, pain, swelling, and sometimes ugliness. It involves changes in metabolism and cellular behavior, as well as the production of specific molecules (particularly complex proteins called cytokines) used to orchestrate the inflammatory response, a response that should defeat the enemy and lead to resolution (healing).

Cytokine—a regulatory protein produced by a cell for the purpose of promoting or decreasing an inflammatory response or other cellular activity. For example, **TNF-α** and **IL-10** are cytokines that act to increase the inflammatory response or decrease the inflammatory response, respectively. A cytokine produced by one cell may act locally, regionally, systemically, or even act on the cell of origin. Recently, the term cytokine has been expanded to include various regulatory peptides and growth factors that exert an influence on tissues and cells (Sturm and Dignass, 2008).

Inflammatory pathway—a series of cellular mechanisms that coordinate with each other to initiate and sustain a particular aspect of the inflammatory response. The inflammatory response is highly regulated. This requires cellular mechanisms that both activate or restrain a particular series of events that will increase or decrease inflammatory activity. An example of a proinflammatory pathway is **NF-κB**. The NF-κB is intimately involved in the pathogenesis and perpetuation of ulcerative colitis.

Epithelium—a group of cells positioned at a tissue surface. The intestinal epithelial cell lines the intestinal tract and is the interface between the external environment and the internal cells, tissues, and structures. The surface of the epithelial cells that line the gut are covered by a layer of mucus, giving rise to another term, *intestinal mucosa*, referring to both as one.

~References~

Danese S, Fiocchi C. **Ulcerative Colitis.** N Engl J Med. 2011 November 3;365(18): 1713–1725.

Lukas M, Bortlik M, Maratka Z. **What is the origin of ulcerative colitis? Still more questions than answers.** Postgraduate medical journal. 2006 Oct 1;82(972):620-5.

Macfarlane S, Furrie E, Kennedy A, Cummings JH, Macfarlane GT. **Mucosal bacteria in ulcerative colitis.** British Journal of Nutrition. 2005 Apr;93(S1):S67-72.

Pravda J. **Radical induction theory of ulcerative colitis.** World journal of gastroenterology: WJG. 2005 Apr 28;11(16):2371.

Sasaki M, Klapproth JM. **The role of bacteria in the pathogenesis of ulcerative colitis.** Journal of signal transduction. 2012;2012.

Schneider H, Braun A, Füllekrug J, Stremmel W, Ehehalt R. **Lipid based therapy for ulcerative colitis—modulation of intestinal mucus membrane phospholipids as a tool to influence inflammation.** International journal of molecular sciences. 2010 Oct;11(10):4149-64.

Stremmel W, Hanemann A, Ehehalt R, Karner M, Braun A. **Phosphatidylcholine (lecithin) and the mucus layer: Evidence of therapeutic efficacy in ulcerative colitis?.** Digestive diseases. 2010;28(3):490-6.

Sturm A, Dignass AU. **Epithelial restitution and wound healing in inflammatory bowel disease.** World journal of gastroenterology: WJG. 2008 Jan 21;14(3):348.

~ xxx ~

Chapter 1
Nonresolving inflammation

When a pathogen comes into contact with the host, a struggle [war]
between the pathogen and the local innate host defense systems ensues.
The resolution of this encounter is a critical determinant of whether the
interaction leads to infection and overt disease. **~Lu and Walker, 2001**

Inflammation is a normal and vital protective response *to the harmful*
stimuli such as infectious agents, antigen-antibody reactions, thermal,
chemical, physical agents, and ischemia [injury from low blood flow].
~Kulkarni et al., 2006, emphasis added

The **usual result of inflammation is protection** *from the spread of*
infection, followed by resolution—the restoration of affected tissues to
their normal structural and functional state.

The problem with inflammation is not how often it starts, but how
often it fails to subside. *Perhaps no single phenomenon contributes more*
to the medical burden in industrialized societies than nonresolving
inflammation. **~Nathan and Ding, 2010, emphasis added**

It appears that a central factor in virtually all inflammatory
modulatory genes is NF-κB. **~Neish, 2002**

I n the *Introduction* we learned that in ulcerative colitis, bacteria reside
<u>directly</u> on the surface of the bowel, more specifically the colon
and/or the rectum. And we learned that this situation should not be
taking place. Actually, this should <u>*never*</u> be taking place. We also learned
that inflammation occurs in response.   Inflammation is directed at
threats. It is purposeful. It is ***war!***

Normally, the physical layer of protection called the mucus layer prevents any contact between bacteria and the cellular lining of the gut. And, as you will later come to understand, it is one very sophisticated defensive barrier. But in ulcerative colitis this layer of protection is disturbed, compromised, progressively lost, and all hell breaks loose. The inflammation that follows fails to resolve . . . ***because it is necessary!*** Inflammation is occurring at a potential site for bacteria to enter (you), to advance (within you), and to destroy (you). And we just cannot let bacteria succeed in this effort. (We'd like to keep you around.) The immune system understands exactly what is going on, and inflammation is how it deals with the situation at hand. Inflammation stops bacteria in their tracks (or tries to), it controls their numbers, it deliberately tries to prevent their advance, but it's not a pretty sight and not always successful. **If unresolved, a disease process takes hold and takes on a life of its own.**

Inflammation, whether of short-term duration or whether it is persistent, is maintained by cellular mechanisms that become active in order to orchestrate the inflammatory response. One such mechanism, hidden deep with the cell—including both the intestinal epithelial cell and the immune cell—is a molecule called NF-κB. **When unleashed, NF-κB leads to the production of cytokines and other signaling molecules that compel other immune cells to act.** Some immune cells produce toxic chemicals in response. Some immune cells become more aggressive killers in response. Some immune cells respond by sending out molecular signals that invite (compel) other immune cells to join in the battle. And some immune cells tell other immune cells to immediately stop what they are doing, change into other forms, and play new roles. All the above is just a part of a bewilderingly complex network of actions that initiate, perpetuate, and control the inflammatory response, a response tailored to a particular threat. The immune system means business.

Since I want to keep the initial chapters relatively short, I will not go in great detail now on all the proinflammatory pathways, cell types, and cytokines involved. I wouldn't get very far anyway—even the physician is barely hanging on here, as things are incredibly complex! I simply want to tell you a story, a simple story. But do not despair, you will learn more concepts and terms—even the names of more cytokines and pathways—as we continue through the pages of this book, all brought down to earth so that even I can understand.

Let's wrap things up here and move on. I have so much to share.

In summary: I believe ulcerative colitis is war. It is a war of necessity, a campaign conducted for very good reasons. **Ulcerative colitis develops as an attempt to resolve or at least to decisively deal with one very serious problem, the problem of bacteria living where they should not be (and constantly threating invasion).** In ulcerative colitis, bacteria—even "normal" bacteria—are living and replicating directly on the surface of the rectum, and, if they are lucky and able to advance, they are living and replicating directly on the surface of the colon, as well. And they are on the move. Territorial expansion, the objective. This situation is *so* unacceptable. We should do something about this and do so without delay. The immune system has already gone to work and is trying to deal with the situation. However, and for a variety of reasons, with ulcerative colitis the immune system is struggling. But do not despair. I have some good news to share:

> *The mucosa of the colon is more likely to heal in patients with ulcerative colitis than in those with Crohn's disease.* (de Chambrun et al., 2010)

More good news:

> *The prognosis for patients with ulcerative colitis is generally good during the first decade after diagnosis, with a low rate of colectomy; over time, remission occurs in most patients.* (Danese and Fiocchi, 2011)

So you're in luck! (If you call ulcerative colitis luck.) But, wouldn't you know, I have some bad news to share:

> As the medical professionals taking care of patients with UC [ulcerative colitis], we have to admit that our treatment concepts have not been very successful. Ongoing disease activity is present in ~ 50% of all patients with UC, colectomy rates remain high, and impaired quality of life, sick leave and disability pensions are higher in patients with UC than in the general population. (Ochsenkühn and D'Haens, 2011)

More bad news:

> The most potent anti-inflammatory agent currently available, infliximab [Remicade], brought only one out of three patients into remission, not taking into consideration that one third of these patients were still receiving steroids in addition.

> In summary, the perception that UC is a benign disease is not justified. UC is a disease that leads to organ loss in **5–25%** of cases, is associated with increased mortality and has a negative impact on daily life. The drugs that we use and the way in which we use them do not bring the majority of affected patients into "remission," which is the most desirable outcome. UC is a potentially aggressive, most undertreated and sometimes lethal chronic disease. Only a minority of patients experience a disease course that can be called "benign." (Ochsenkühn and D'Haens, 2011, emphasis added)

Yes, you have a very tough disease to deal with, one that can be *so* resistant to our efforts. We could use some new ideas. Perhaps I can help.

More on ulcerative colitis

To get you off to a good start, I have selected the following videos to help broaden your understanding of the disease in question. Please take a few minutes to watch the following:

—**Ulcerative colitis – short animation from sixpartswater.org**
www.youtube.com/watch?v=FjUke8TMwhU

—**What is Ulcerative Colitis?**
www.youtube.com/watch?v=JMApMBY0CfQ

More on Crohn's disease

Some individuals are under the impression that ulcerative colitis and Crohn's disease are similar diseases or, perhaps, different forms of the same disease. So not the case! Although there are some similarities, there are many differences that set them apart. If you'd like, I can take you on a journey into the world of Crohn's disease. I have written a most informative book on the subject, entitled *More to Consider in the Battle Against Crohn's*. In the book I tell a different story than is typically being told. (Of course, you'd expect this.) I tell the story of the intense battle between pathogen and host over, of all things, iron. *Iron!* I also showcase alternative and complementary therapies that are suitable for use in the treatment of this disease. And you're in luck! The book includes a great deal of information relevant to the patient who suffers from ulcerative colitis—same immune system, different circumstances, different expression, different disease, but generally responsive to the same therapies. If interested, go to **www.impactofvitamind.com** to purchase a copy. And if you know an individual who suffers from Crohn's, promise me you will tell them about the book. And promise me you will do so without delay.

~References~

Danese S, Fiocchi C. **Ulcerative Colitis.** N Engl J Med. 2011 November 3;365(18): 1713–1725.

de Chambrun GP, Peyrin-Biroulet L, Lémann M, Colombel JF. **Clinical implications of mucosal healing for the management of IBD.** Nature reviews Gastroenterology & hepatology. 2010 Jan;7(1):15.

Kulkarni RG, Achaiah G, Narahari Sastry G. **Novel targets for antiinflammatory and antiarthritic agents.** Current pharmaceutical design. 2006 Jul 1;12(19):2437-54.

Lu L, Walker WA. **Pathologic and physiologic interactions of bacteria with the gastrointestinal epithelium.** The American journal of clinical nutrition. 2001 Jun 1;73(6):1124S-30S.

Nathan C, Ding A. **Nonresolving inflammation.** Cell. 2010 Mar 19;140(6):871-82.

Neish AS. **The gut microflora and intestinal epithelial cells: a continuing dialogue.** Microbes and Infection. 2002 Mar 1;4(3):309-17.

Ochsenkühn T, D'Haens G. **Current misunderstandings in the management of ulcerative colitis.** Gut. 2011 Sep 1;60(9):1294-9.

Chapter 2
What should and should not be

Health depends on a beneficial host-microbe interaction. This is
certainly true for intestinal health, particularly in the colon, which harbors a
greater and more diverse number of microorganisms than any other organ.
~Danese and Fiocchi, 2011, emphasis added

*A disturbed mucosal barrier is <u>thought to be an initiating factor</u> of
the disease and subsequent attacks from colonic commensal [normal,
typical] bacterial flora result in inflammation of the mucosa.* **~Stremmel
et al., 2010, emphasis added**

*The large bowel mucus layer effectively prevents contact between the
highly concentrated luminal bacteria and the epithelial cells <u>in all parts of
the normal colon</u>.* **Colonic inflammation is <u>always</u> accompanied by breaks
in the mucus barrier.** ~Swidsinski et al., 2007, emphasis added

*The main cytokine that seems to drive these changes is tumor necrosis
factor alpha [Tnf-α] in CD [Crohn's disease], whereas interleukin (IL-12)
may be more important in UC [ulcerative colitis].* **Therapeutic restoration
of the mucosal barrier would provide protection and prevent antigenic
overload due to intestinal "leakiness."** ~Salim and Söderholm, 2011,
emphasis added

Higher bacterial load has been reported in the mucus of IBD patients.
~Steidler, 2001

I suppose you would like to know how you contracted ulcerative
colitis in the first place. While there is still much yet to be discovered,
we now have a fairly good idea what is going on in this disease and why

it occurs. And, I suppose, I will need to document things more carefully from now on so you will not think that I pulled any of this out of thin air. Here I will share with you what can <u>easily</u> be found in the research and medical literature. That being said, in all likelihood you have probably heard little of what I am about share. The focus of others has been on how to manage this disease with medications (and little else). Unfortunately, because of this, so much is being ignored and so much is not being shared. With that out of the way, let's take a look at how the disease in question gets its start.

Ulcerative colitis is said to begin in the rectum and, as it progresses, moves upstream to include a part of, or perhaps the entire colon. And there seems to be a good reason why it starts in the rectum and why it progresses "upward" from there. The reason: The rectum is exposed to a greater magnitude of bacteria and irritating substances than is the colon, in as much as the rectum is a reservoir for stool that will later be eliminated at the proper time and the proper place (at least that's the plan). In addition, the rectum is, for some reason, less capable of neutralizing harmful byproducts of cellular metabolism (Pravda, 2005). One such byproduct is nitric oxide, a molecule that if not properly dealt with is capable of breaking down the mucosal barrier and allowing bacteria to reach the cells that line rectum and colon (Pravda, 2005; Roediger, 2008).

And so, we see, the rectum is a site most vulnerable. It could use our prayers. As the disease progresses, it expands to involve the colon. (More prayers needed.) But none of this should be happening. No, not at all.

To help protect the rectum—actually, to protect the entire intestinal tract (with some exceptions)—we create and continually renew a moving layer of mucus that intimately covers it all. The mucus layer may be considered the first <u>structural</u> layer of protection that defends the surface of the bowel from harm. And, boy, what a layer of protection it is!

Behold the mucus layer

The first layer of defense that pathogens encounter deals with manipulation of the nutrients available for the pathogens. The microbiota [gut bacteria] is able to either consume nutrients that are necessary for the pathogens to propagate or can produce products that may inhibit pathogen growth. **~Gill et al., 2011**

From studies investigating mucus in UC we know that there is a reduction of mucus thickness in active disease together with the presence of completely denuded areas with unprotected exposition of the submucosa to enteric bacteria. **~Fries and Comunale, 2011**

Affected mucus barrier increases permeability for bacteria, microbial products, and toxins that lead to damage of epithelial cells and result in systemic inflammatory process evident in patients with ulcerative colitis. **~Dorofeyev et al., 2013**

Before bacteria can adhere and invade the mucosa, they must first traverse the mucus barrier. The inflammation takes place <u>only</u> after the mucus barrier is broken and the defense is overwhelmed. ***UC is caused by a weakening in gut barrier, mainly due to increased infiltration of gut bacteria*** *and the resultant recruitment of neutrophils and formation of crypt abscess.* **~Chen et al., 2014, emphasis added**

The mucus layer is an essential layer of defense. First and foremost, it is a structural barrier. If intact, it keeps bacteria and the like from physically contacting the cell lining below. Must be important. Let's go into greater detail.

A mucus layer lines both rectum and colon, and is composed of two layers, an outer mucus layer and an inner mucus layer (Johansson et al., 2011). The outer mucus layer is rather loose, particularly its outer region, where it is colonized by most of the bacteria that reside within the bowel (McGuckin et al., 2011). And, by the way, this community of bacteria that live <u>near</u> the surface of this outer layer, is, itself, a formidable layer of defense (Gill et al., 2011). The typical organisms (collectively called commensals) that establish themselves in the outer layer of mucus, continually replicate and, by so doing, act to crowd out pathogenic bacteria that also wish to establish a foothold. In as much as there is always "someone" around willing to do us harm, this mucus layer, along with the dominant colonization by "friendly" bacteria, is so very important. They crowd out those that are evil. The "good" organisms aggressively compete for space and nutrients and secrete chemicals that kill off their competitors (Gill et al., 2011). Some even encourage you to do the killing for them, by stimulating the production of natural antimicrobial molecules directed at their enemies (Sleator, 2010; Gill et al., 2011). And since there is strength in numbers, the good bacteria generally prevail. It is called health. All this drama transpires in the looser regions of the outer mucus layer. A lot of trouble can occur following the loss or disruption, or dysfunction, of this complex layer of defense. For some reason, the disease ulcerative colitis readily comes to mind. And we're talking trouble!

The mucus layer is also a reservoir of molecules created by cells of the immune system (including the intestinal epithelial cell) that want nothing more than to kill specific bacteria, the ones that need to be held in check. These antibacterial molecules have names like cathelicidins, and defensins, and include immunoglobulins such as IgA (Salim et al., 2011). Yes, it is a killing field, this outer mucus layer of defense, just as it should be. Having this barrier, a barrier colonized by friendly bacteria, "seeded" with endogenous (made within) antimicrobials—and having it remain intact—is indispensable to the health of the bowel and the health of the individual involved. But there is a lot more going on here, more than meets the eye.

The bacteria that colonize the outer mucus layer also become a working partner with the underlying epithelial (surface) cell and with the immune cells that live and move beneath this one-cell-thick epithelial layer. They talk (molecularly) on a regular basis (Gill et al., 2011). They speak about the killing of others, other pressing issues, and the news of the day. Furthermore, bacteria are constantly being sampled (abducted), dissected alive, and analyzed by an immune cell called a dendritic cell. And from the information obtained, immune responses are adjusted to **1)** help maintain an acceptable diversity between the types of bacteria that the body will allow to colonize, or **2)** to organize a response to counter a new threat, should it present itself (Salim and Söderholm, 2011). Of course, there is always more to the story.

The bacteria that colonize the outer mucus layer are not just a bunch of freeloaders. They earn their keep. Besides crowding out the evildoers simply by existing and replicating at an incredible rate, they help break down food components that fuel the cells that line the colon. They manufacture vital vitamins for us. And they also help us make entertaining sounds—could come in handy when things get a little too boring or we simply want to impress others.

Importantly, the friendly bacteria that call the colon "home sweet home" help regulate host inflammatory responses and do so in many, many ways. Ingenious ways! This community of tiny little buddies—with perhaps a few bad guys thrown in here and there to keep us on our toes— is so indispensable. Because of all of its duties, and the sheer number of cells involved (10 trillion more of "them" than there are of "you")—and the fact that they have a dynamic effect on the host organism (you)—the bacterial contents of the bowel are regarded as an actual endocrine organ (O'Hara and Shanahan, 2006; Bevins and Salzman, 2011). Besides regulating the regional immune system, the substances produced by this "organ" can be absorbed, act locally, or can travel to distant places and create special effects. This endocrine organ is, basically, the colonized outer mucus layer. The inner mucus is not particularly involved here because it is or should be devoid of bacteria. It is just there to serve.

The inner mucus layer is similar yet quite different from the outer mucus layer. Rather than being mobile across the surface of the intestinal epithelial layer, the inner mucus layer is firmly attached to the intestinal epithelial cells below (Johansson et al., 2011). This key layer of protection is constantly renewed, too, and over time transitions to become the outer mucus layer (Johansson et al., 2010). In fact, *"Mucus production and secretion is a continuously ongoing process with a renewal of the inner protective mucus in the distal colon within an hour."* (Chen et al., 2014) And unlike the outer mucus layer, which is loose and constantly being degraded, the inner mucus layer is tightly organized and is net- or mesh-like in character (Johansson et al., 2011). It is so tightly organized that it serves as a formidable physical barrier so that bacteria simply cannot pass (Johansson et at., 2010), yet not so tightly organized as to prevent fluids, nutrients, and certain molecules from crossing (McGuckin et al., 2011). This inner mucus layer is one very important defense mechanism, one that helps prevent bacterial contact with the underlying intestinal epithelial cell and helps prevent excessive immune system activation (Gill et al., 2011). But what if it is damaged, degraded, or lost? I don't even want to think of all the problems this turn of events could create.

> *Once present on the colonic mucosal surface, exposure to high concentrations of fecal bacterial antigens [immune system-activating bacterial components] stimulates neutrophils to secrete their own tissue damaging oxygen radicals. Neutrophil mediated damage attracts additional neutrophils from the subjacent intravascular compartment to the mucosal surface.* (Pravda, 2005)

So, we see, bacteria living on the surface of the cells that line the rectum and colon are met with an immune response that is clearly purposeful yet so very, very damaging. And, of course, one thing leads to another.

> ***Infection and inflammation in the intestine alters the commensal microbiota*** *[bacterial community] in response to the changed mucosal microenvironment. Similarly, non-infectious damage to the gastrointestinal epithelium can change the microbial*

populations and facilitate enteric infections by compromising mucosal barrier function. (McGuckin et al., 2011, emphasis added)

Sounds like "we" have a big problem on our hands. Sounds like "we" have our work cut out for us. Sounds like "we" are about to meet a nice new doctor. Sounds like "we" need to focus on repairing the mucus layer and reestablishing within the outer mucus layer a normal bacterial community. Of course, "we" could place our focus on something else, like manipulating the inflammatory response. But then, you want to get to the bottom of things, right? Certainly, as long as it doesn't drastically alter host defense, there is a place for manipulating the inflammatory response, but there is also a place for focusing on repairing (healing) the various barriers of defense—the mucus layer and its resident bacterial community, included. But all this can wait. We have another layer of defense to discuss.

Behold the intestinal epithelial cell

It may be interesting here to bear in mind that intestinal epithelial cells (IEC), which are in close contact with the bacterial antigens [immune system activating bacterial components] present in the intestinal lumen, may act as antigen presenting cells. ~**Steidler, 2001**

Epithelial cells are also capable of communicating and modulating underlying immune cells, thus being essential in maintaining mucosal and commensal homeostasis. ~**Salim and Söderholm, 2011**

What is clear from animal studies is that the integrity of the colonic epithelial surface barrier is paramount in maintaining immune quiescence within the colonic tissues and preventing the colonic immune system from mounting an immune response to the high concentrations of bacterial antigen that is poised to invade the normally sterile subepithelial environment. ~**Pravda, 2005**

The intestinal epithelial cell is not your ordinary cell, not even your ordinary "surface" cell. ***The intestinal epithelial cell is an immune cell!***

> *The intestinal epithelial cell has moved to the forefront of these studies where it has been shown to be an <u>active participant</u> in mucosal immunoregulation and inflammation."* (Mayer, 2000, emphasis added)

Because of so many of its behaviors, we should regard the intestinal epithelial cell as an immune cell in its own right. *"Enterocytes can and do manifest the full spectrum of the inflammatory process."* (Neish, 2002) Furthermore, *"epithelial cells secrete cytokines and chemokines, which not only regulate mucosal immune responses but also regulate inflammatory responses."* (Mayer, 2000) Fortunately, should the mucus barrier be disturbed or absent, there is an immune cell already in place, ready to respond. The cell? The intestinal epithelial cell. The Response? ***War!***

When conditions allow bacteria to reach the epithelial layer and colonize, they could not have chosen a worse place to try to establish a home. Did no one tell them that *they are living directly on top of an immune cell?!!* And this epithelial cell—this immune cell—<u>will</u> swing into action. It is angry, too angry for words.

The intestinal epithelial cell will now act in concert with its neighboring intestinal epithelial cells—along with the immune cells that infiltrate this barrier (e.g., neutrophil)—to orchestrate an immune response . . . but only for about 3 to 5 days. In 3 days or so, the individual intestinal epithelial cell will vanish! *Vanish!* Astonishingly, the natural life span of this cell is only 3 to 5 days, then it will be replaced (Sharma et al., 2010). At the end of its natural life span, the intestinal epithelial cell will commit suicide and will do so without hesitation. It is programmed to do this. This normal action, suicide, too, acts as a layer of defense. By dying intentionally at the ripe old age of 3 to 5 days, it will make room for a younger, more effective and vigorous replacement. And by dying purposefully, and vanishing from the scene of the battle, it will take along with it any bacteria that have invaded or have firmly attached (Vossenkämper et al., 2011). This intestinal epithelial cell is quite a cell. Its ways are most fascinating.

Epithelial cell behavior

The epithelium cells provide a structural barrier, manufacture most, but not all, components of the secreted barrier, are sensors of the external environment, and emit signals regulating underlying innate and adaptive immunity. ~**McGuckin et al., 2009**

This seems a little odd—cellular behavior as a defense barrier? But this is a valid concept. When forced to do so, the intestinal epithelial cell will take on a pathogen directly—actually phagocytose or "swallow up" the little guy (McGuckin et al., 2009). Even though the epithelial cell appears at times to be a victim, it is really a hero, reminiscent of one of those all-too-frequent "taking a bullet for someone else" movie scenes, as it encounters an assault from a pathogen. Accordingly, the epithelial cell will take on the pathogen directly, more interested in saving you than in saving itself. Now the following is most unexpected: The intestinal epithelial cell can actually reorganize and transform its physical self, as needed, to form accessory structures that allow it to engulf (phagocytose) bacteria (Neal et al., 2006). This is quite a cell, this intestinal epithelial cell.

We used to think that this community of epithelial cells was simply a physical barrier, allowing nutrients to pass but keeping bacteria out— that's it! But now we know so much more. As previously mentioned, the epithelial cell has the tools to take on, kill, or otherwise deal with an intruder, one that has made the big mistake of challenging this barrier of angry immune cells. Of course, this response will be an inflammatory response. And, of course, NF-κB will sustain the inflammatory response. That's its job.

And so, we see **the first immune cell a bacterium will face will be, most likely, the intestinal epithelial cell**. Boy, I hope someone doesn't come along and interfere with the ability of this cell to perform its duties as an immune cell and a true killer, and restrict its many protective actions. Remember, overall, the actions of the immune system are purposeful! Accordingly,

> *Together, these observations highlight the importance of NF-κB signaling networks within the intestinal epithelium in sustaining normal mucosal homeostasis and in mediating pathogen-specific responses. These studies point to substantial challenges in the development and use of inhibitors of **NF-κB signaling pathways** in intestinal inflammation as **these pathways have protective as well as deleterious effects**.* (Xavier and Podolsky, 2007, emphasis added)

Let's continue. The intestinal epithelial cell is *so* fascinating.

The intestinal epithelial "immune" cell has more than an inflammatory response to throw at bacteria that have arrived on the scene and threaten an invasion. It can eat the damn thing! (Sorry for such language, but the threat of bacterial invasion brings out the worst in me.) But before it devours and destroys threatening bacteria, it is all into signaling.

Before "eating" the first bacterium of many, the intestinal epithelial cell will sense the presence of the enemy and signal to the immune cells in the neighborhood, by chemokine creation and release, that the enemy has arrived at the gates (Blikslager et al., 2007; Neish, 2002). There is a profound sense of urgency, who knows what will happen next? The entire planet is at risk! And the intestinal epithelial cell will continually signal, perhaps frantically, to alert the immune cells in the region of the danger (Neish, 2002).

So, in the event of threatened bacterial invasion, the intestinal epithelial cell will send out a message conveying its concern. But once the enemy is close enough, there is more to do than just sit around and send out signals. It is now time to "eat" the enemy. And eat the enemy it does. It devours the enemy, and it does so as a defensive measure.

Now, having devoured the enemy, the intestinal epithelial cell has some important decisions to make. It can internally wrap it in a "blanket" (autophagosome) to isolate it, then kill the enemy before it itself dies. Or, the intestinal epithelial cell can pass the invader right on through and out the back door (Schoultz et al., 2011), if you will, and right into the hands of a professional immune cell, one that is lying in wait and ready for dinner. You should see the surprised look on the invader's face. The bacterium thinks it has arrived in a new home, only to get the boot and face a fate worse than death, plus death. *"Once translocated, bacteria must survive attack by macrophages."* (Cossart and Sansonetti, 2004) Ordinarily, this means certain death. The bad news: Many bacteria *can* survive the attack of the killer cell we call the macrophage. More bad news: Some bacteria actually want to be eaten (Cossart and Sansonetti, 2004), somehow knowing that they possess the ability to survive what's in store. And if they can survive being eaten alive, they have a greater chance of being successful later in life (and will have one *great* story to tell to their grandchildren).

From the pathogen's perspective, after it infects the epithelial cell, it knows that it has little time to waste. It only has 3 to 5 days, or less, to get used to its new home and to create an army of clones with which to launch an invasion. The epithelial cell will die shortly, this I know. And this invader and its family will go down, one way or another, unless it or a family member can escape destruction, prolong the life of the cell, or plan a cunning and effective exit strategy—not a very stable environment to raise a family, but a pathogen's gotta do what a pathogen's gotta do.

Before the epithelial cell commits "programmed suicide"—a normal process, but now a process with more urgency and purpose—the cell has another clever little trick up its sleeve. This brave little cell (a cell so small you cannot see it with the naked eye) recognizes that it is infected and will unleash a platoon of "walking" proteins (Jahreiss et al., 2008; Blander, 2007) that will seek out and find the little "blanket-wrapped weasel" (the scientists make these words up, not I) that has dared to enter. Having found the blanket-wrapped weasel (BWW) in what is called a "phagosome," a "walking" protein will now drag the BWW over to a digestive organelle (small organ within the cell) called the lysosome (Jahreiss et al., 2008). The phagosome will then fuse with the lysosome, and the BWW will die a grizzly death. That sounds good to me! But the story doesn't end there.

The lifeless body of the invader will provide nutrients for the cell, or a dismembered part thereof will be "presented" to internal sensors that will recognize the invader and secrete cytokines to help orchestrate an inflammatory response, one that is directed against this particular, unique brand of pathogen. Gotta love the epithelial cell! Your very existence depends on this level of sophistication. (You didn't know any of this stuff, did you?)

When an epithelial cell dies a day or two before its time, something needs to be done, and done quickly! A hole or "gap" in the barrier has been created. And the neighboring epithelial cells will know precisely what to do. They will now flatten out to close the gap created by the cell that has passed away and has fallen by the wayside (Iizuka and Konno, 2011). They will also create and extend little arm projections toward each other to bridge the gap (Blikslager et al., 2007). The larger the gap (wound), the greater number of surrounding epithelial cells will need to be frantically involved in spreading out and closing up the gap. Of course, they are all dead in a few days, so these cells will eventually be replaced by brand new epithelial cells that, too, get the chance to live the life of an epithelial cell and die the death of an epithelial cell.

My, oh, my! What a story! It took me months of study and effort to write these few pages on epithelial cell behavior. And what a layer of protection it is! But there is more. This cell has a special talent to deploy.

This cell, this intestinal epithelial cell, *this immune cell*, is what we call an antigen-presenting cell. Accordingly, it takes tiny pieces of the dead (bacteria) and passes them on to the network of immune cells below that have already been alerted that something is up and are eagerly waiting for up-to-date information. "What is this thing?" "What does it do?" "Who does it belong to?" "How should we respond?" These are the questions the immune cells below are eager to find answers to so they can formulate the appropriate response. And what is the response? **War is the response!** We also call it an inflammatory response. We call it inflammation. And it is a war that is being fought not only on the surface of the intestinal epithelial cell but has also extended to the tissue regions below. But, although necessary, this war should *never* have occurred. And it should be brought to an end. Its resolution will undoubtedly involve healing of what is called the mucus membrane, a term used here that includes the mucus layer, both the outer and inner mucus layer, and, of course, the associated layer of intestinal epithelial cells.

It's time for a direct quote. Please read carefully.

> The management of UC is undergoing significant changes. One aspect that has received more attention lately is the importance of mucosal healing. Already in 1923, however, Sir Arthur F Hurst, one of the first authors to describe UC, concluded in an article that "no case of UC can be regarded as cured until the sigmoidoscope shows that the mucus membrane is perfectly healthy." <u>This treatment goal got lost or seems to have been ignored</u> in the meantime by several generations of physicians. A century later, the role of mucosal integrity has again moved into the center of interest.
>
> Mucosal healing as a therapeutic target has not been widely accepted. (Ochsenkühn and D'Haens, 2011, emphasis added)

Hard for me to believe that the goal of mucosal healing was ever lost sight of or was ever ignored by those trying their best to make people well. But it was. Unfortunately, the focus in ulcerative colitis has been primarily on suppressing the immune response rather than addressing the underlying cause. Perhaps thinking that the immune response is the disease, the true nature of the battle was misunderstood. Perhaps, it still is.

Ulcerative colitis in an instant!

One "health" practice in the past—and I certainly hope is not in use today—was the use of hydrogen peroxide as an enema. It was used for nearly 100 years as a treatment for both constipation and fecal impaction (Mandzhieva et al., 2019; Lee and Yoo, 2017). Only problem: It resulted in ulcerative colitis. Not every time, but many times. It did this by degrading and penetrating the mucus layer (of protection) and dislodging the intestinal epithelial cells below. This creates an immediate inflammatory response, mounted to control the situation. It creates war!

> *Even small amounts of hydrogen peroxide could cause human UC as was reported by Bilotta and Waye in 1989 after experiencing an epidemic of hydrogen peroxide-induced colitis in the GI endoscopy unit at their institution due to the inadvertent installation of hydrogen peroxide during colonoscopy.* (Pravda, 2005)

Aside from the above, hydrogen peroxide is ordinarily a problem for the intestinal epithelial cell. This cell generates hydrogen peroxide as a byproduct of cellular metabolism. Aberrant cellular metabolism, producing excess hydrogen peroxide and/or ineffective neutralization of this damaging compound, can lead to injury of the colonic epithelial barrier. *"Once damaged, the barrier is unable to exclude highly immunogenic fecal bacterial antigens from invading the normal sterile submucosa."* (Pravda, 2005)

I suspect many ulcerative colitis patients in the past never knew it was a hydrogen peroxide enema that enslaved them to a lifelong burden of disease.

Autoimmunity in ulcerative colitis?

Autoimmunity is typically defined as an attack by an individual's immune system directed at what should have been recognized as a normal component of the individual. Apparently, in ulcerative colitis, some autoimmunity may occur, as the immune system can produce damaging antibodies against the mucus-producing goblet cells (Fries and Comunale, 2011).

Autoimmunity may also be directed at components of the epithelial cell as well as components of a certain immune cell, the neutrophil (Danese and Fiocchi, 2011). All this seems to be a result and not the cause of the inflammatory disease we recognize as ulcerative colitis (see Wen and Fiocchi, 2004). Indeed, *"a variety of infectious agents have been demonstrated to possess the ability to induce or activate autoreactive immune cells."* (Wen and Fiocchi, 2004)

Some bacteria seem to trigger autoimmunity by what is called "molecular mimicry"—a situation wherein certain bacterial components resemble part of the human, and attention by the immune cells is directed at both. All of this is fascinating to someone, but not to me. (I just said this for effect. I really am interested and engaged.) But regardless of the occurrence of autoimmunity and molecular mimicry, ulcerative colitis can and does go into remission.

Genetic predisposition

You often hear that ulcerative colitis occurs *"in genetic predisposed individuals."* Certainly, this can be the case, but not always. Apparently, *"no genetic associations can be confirmed in 84% of ulcerative colitis patients."* (Kaunitz and

Nayyar, 2015, emphasis added) So you can blame your genetics if you want, but at one point in time you didn't have ulcerative colitis even though your genetic makeup did not fundamentally change. I'll give you other things to blame, in the following chapter.

~References~

Bevins CL, Salzman NH. **The potter's wheel: the host's role in sculpting its microbiota.** Cellular and Molecular Life Sciences. 2011 Nov 1;68(22):3675.

Blander JM. **Signalling and phagocytosis in the orchestration of host defence.** Cellular microbiology. 2007 Feb;9(2):290-9.

Blikslager AT, Moeser AJ, Gookin JL, Jones SL, Odle J. **Restoration of barrier function in injured intestinal mucosa.** Physiological reviews. 2007 Apr;87(2):545-64.

Chen SJ, Liu XW, Liu JP, Yang XY, Lu FG. **Ulcerative colitis as a polymicrobial infection characterized by sustained broken mucus barrier.** World Journal of Gastroenterology: WJG. 2014 Jul 28;20(28):9468.

Cossart P, Sansonetti PJ. **Bacterial invasion: the paradigms of enteroinvasive pathogens.** Science. 2004 Apr 9;304(5668):242-8.

Danese S, Fiocchi C. **Ulcerative Colitis.** N Engl J Med. 2011 November 3;365(18): 1713–1725.

Dorofeyev AE, Vasilenko IV, Rassokhina OA, Kondratiuk RB. **Mucosal barrier in ulcerative colitis and Crohn's disease.** Gastroenterology research and practice. 2013 May 7;2013.

Fries W, Comunale S. **Ulcerative colitis: pathogenesis.** Current drug targets. 2011 Sep 1;12(10):1373-82.

Gill N, Wlodarska M, Finlay BB. **Roadblocks in the gut: barriers to enteric infection.** Cellular microbiology. 2011 May;13(5):660-9.

Iizuka M, Konno S. **Wound healing of intestinal epithelial cells.** World journal of gastroenterology: WJG. 2011 May 7;17(17):2161.

Jahreiss L, Menzies FM, Rubinsztein DC. **The itinerary of autophagosomes: from peripheral formation to kiss-and-run fusion with lysosomes.** Traffic. 2008 Apr;9(4):574-87.

Johansson ME, Gustafsson JK, Sjöberg KE, Petersson J, Holm L, Sjövall H, Hansson GC. **Bacteria penetrate the inner mucus layer before inflammation in the dextran sulfate colitis model.** PloS one. 2010 Aug 18;5(8):e12238.

Johansson ME, Larsson JM, Hansson GC. **The two mucus layers of colon are organized by the MUC2 mucin, whereas the outer layer is a legislator of host–microbial interactions.** Proceedings of the national academy of sciences. 2011 Mar 15;108(Supplement 1):4659-65.

Kaunitz J, Nayyar P. **Bugs, genes, fatty acids, and serotonin: Unraveling inflammatory bowel disease?.** F1000Research. 2015;4.

Lee JS, Yoo JK. **Chemical colitis caused by hydrogen peroxide enema in a child: case report and literature review.** Environmental health and toxicology. 2017;32.

Lu L, Walker WA. **Pathologic and physiologic interactions of bacteria with the gastrointestinal epithelium.** The American journal of clinical nutrition. 2001 Jun 1;73(6):1124S-30S.

Mandzhieva B, Khan M, Rashid MU, Shobar R, Khan AH. **Hydrogen Peroxide Enema-induced Proctitis in a Young Female: A Case Report.** Cureus. 2019 Dec;11(12).

Mayer L. **Epithelial cell antigen presentation.** Current opinion in gastroenterology. 2000 Nov 1;16(6):531-5.

McGuckin MA, Eri R, Simms LA, Florin TH, Radford-Smith G. **Intestinal barrier dysfunction in inflammatory bowel diseases.** Inflammatory bowel diseases. 2009 Jan 1;15(1):100-13.

McGuckin MA, Lindén SK, Sutton P, Florin TH. **Mucin dynamics and enteric pathogens.** Nature Reviews Microbiology. 2011 Apr;9(4):265.

Neal MD, Leaphart C, Levy R, Prince J, Billiar TR, Watkins S, Li J, Cetin S, Ford H, Schreiber A, Hackam DJ. **Enterocyte TLR4 mediates phagocytosis and translocation of bacteria across the intestinal barrier.** The Journal of Immunology. 2006 Mar 1;176(5):3070-9.

Neish AS. **The gut microflora and intestinal epithelial cells: a continuing dialogue.** Microbes and Infection. 2002 Mar 1;4(3):309-17.

Ochsenkühn T, D'Haens G. **Current misunderstandings in the management of ulcerative colitis.** Gut. 2011 Sep 1;60(9):1294-9.

O'Hara AM, Shanahan F. **The gut flora as a forgotten organ.** EMBO reports. 2006 Jul 1;7(7):688-93.

Pravda J. **Radical induction theory of ulcerative colitis.** World journal of gastroenterology: WJG. 2005 Apr 28;11(16):2371.

Roediger WE. **Nitric oxide from dysbiotic bacterial respiration of nitrate in the pathogenesis and as a target for therapy of ulcerative colitis.** Alimentary pharmacology & therapeutics. 2008 Apr;27(7):531-41.

Salim SA, Söderholm JD. **Importance of disrupted intestinal barrier in inflammatory bowel diseases.** Inflammatory bowel diseases. 2011 Jan 1;17(1):362-81.

Schoultz I, Söderholm JD, McKay DM. **Is metabolic stress a common denominator in inflammatory bowel disease?.** Inflammatory bowel diseases. 2011 Sep 1;17(9):2008-18.

Sharma R, Young C, Neu J. **Molecular modulation of intestinal epithelial barrier: contribution of microbiota.** BioMed Research International. 2010 Jan 31;2010.

Sleator RD. **Probiotic therapy-recruiting old friends to fight new foes. Gut pathogens.** 2010 Dec;2(1):5.

Steidler L. **Microbiological and immunological strategies for treatment of inflammatory bowel disease.** Microbes and infection. 2001 Nov 1;3(13):1157-66.

Stremmel W, Hanemann A, Ehehalt R, Karner M, Braun A. **Phosphatidylcholine (lecithin) and the mucus layer: Evidence of therapeutic efficacy in ulcerative colitis?.** Digestive diseases. 2010;28(3):490-6.

Swidsinski A, Loening-Baucke V, Theissig F, Engelhardt H, Bengmark S, Koch S, Lochs H, Dörffel Y. **Comparative study of the intestinal mucus barrier in normal and inflamed colon.** Gut. 2007 Mar 1;56(3):343-50.

Vossenkämper A, MacDonald TT, Marchès O. **Always one step ahead: how pathogenic bacteria use the type III secretion system to manipulate the intestinal mucosal immune system.** Journal of Inflammation. 2011 Dec;8(1):11.

Wen Z, Fiocchi C. **Inflammatory bowel disease: autoimmune or immune-mediated pathogenesis?.** Journal of Immunology Research. 2004;11(3-4):195-204.

Xavier RJ, Podolsky DK. **Unravelling the pathogenesis of inflammatory bowel disease.** Nature. 2007 Jul;448(7152):427.

Chapter 3

Enemies of the state
(you were in)

The importance of the mucus layer as a barrier to enteric [within the gut] pathogens is emphasized by the fact that many pathogens have acquired virulence factors to overcome and penetrate the intestinal mucus barrier . . .. [Certain pathogens] can secrete proteases [enzymes] that can degrade the mucus layer. **~Gill et al., 2011**

In IBD, disruptions of essential elements of the intestinal barrier lead to permeability defects. These barrier defects exacerbate the underlying immune system, subsequently resulting in tissue damage.

Therapeutic restoration of the mucosal barrier would provide protection and prevent antigentic overload due to intestinal "leakiness." **~Salim and Söderholm, 2011**

I can't emphasize this enough (but I'll try): ***"Normally, luminal bacteria in the gut are withheld from contact with the epithelium by an adherent mucus layer."*** (Schneider et al., 2010, emphasis added)

And when the unthinkable happens, that is, relevant bacterial contact with intestinal epithelial cells, the immune system will respond. ***This is the disease that you have!*** The inflammation that follows, occurs out of necessity—an immune response initiated on order to deal with one very serious problem. However, it is the character, complexity, or perhaps the dysfunctionality of the response that grabs all the attention. But regardless of where the emphasis is placed, what you have is one very hideous disease. As if I need to remind you of the following:

The symptoms [of ulcerative colitis] are extremely unpleasant and impact all aspects of life. They include diarrhea, abdominal pain, rectal bleeding, fever, weight loss, lethargy and loss of appetite. If left untreated, malnutrition dehydration and anemia follow, which, in extreme cases, can even lead to death. (Steidler, 2001)

So, as you can see, we have a hideous disease on our hands. And if you have fallen prey to this hideous disease, you have probably asked yourself this question a time or two: "Why me?" In this chapter I will try my best to answer the question. Here, I will identify a number of enemies of the state you were in before you contracted this hideous disease. Each topic of discussion that follows deserves an entire chapter, but it won't happen here! I need to keep things brief and right to the point, so we don't get too bogged down (or lost in the weeds). Let's get started and do so without delay.

Threats to our mucosal layer of defense

From the studies investigating mucus in UC we know that there is a reduction of mucus thickness in active disease together with the presence of <u>completely denuded areas</u> with unprotected exposition of the submucosa to enteric bacteria. **~Fries and Comunale, 2011**

Some bacteria can dissolve the protective inner mucus layer. Defects in renewal and formation of the inner mucus layer allow bacteria to reach the epithelium, and have implications for the cause of colitis. **~Chen et al., 2014**

The first physical layer of protection, the mucus layer, is a layer of protection against *ever* experiencing ulcerative colitis. And since it is so intimately associated with the intestinal epithelial cell, I can refer to both by use of the term ***intestinal mucosa***.

Fortunately, there are no genetic abnormalities that prevent the creation of the mucus part of this critical layer of defense (Salim and Söderholm, 2011), although some genetic abnormalities may alter its character and reduce its effectiveness (Fries and Comunale, 2011). That being said, one key feature in ulcerative colitis is a reduction in the numbers of mucus-producing goblet cells (Fries and Comunale, 2011). This, of course, is bad news, and would only serve to complicate matters. Yet, there are forces in play that act to increase mucus production, ostensibly to compensate for a reduction in goblet cell numbers—not working out too well! But once upon a time, and for a long period of time, things were going quite well regardless of your genetics. At one point in time, you did not have ulcerative colitis, so genetic predisposition was not an issue. You were happy then. But you had enemies of the state you were in, enemies that wanted to end all this happiness. It is apparent, now, that the enemies of the mucus layer have achieved success. (And nobody wants to be you, including you.)

Here, we will take notice of a few enemies of the mucus layer, enemies that made you more vulnerable to the disease that you have. We will start with what I consider to be one of the biggest threats to whom you were and whom you now are.

Dysbiosis

Although commensal [normally present] microorganisms do not generally cause disease, this is context dependent: <u>when the mucosal surface is damaged, the **commensal microorganisms can become opportunistic pathogens**</u> and contribute to pathology. ~McGuckin et al., 2011, emphasis added

Microbial flora in patients with ulcerative colitis differs considerably from that in controls, in both composition and spatial distribution (mucosal invasion). ~Lukas et al., 2006

Loss of natural intestinal diversity and a shift of bacterial composition towards a more deleterious profile might reflect the net effect of environmental influences over the past few decades leading to the dramatic increase of IBD. **~Rehman et al., 2010**

Infection and inflammation in the intestine alters the commensal microbiota in response to the changed mucosal microenvironment. **Microbial flora in patients with ulcerative colitis differs considerably from that in controls,** *in both composition and spatial distribution (mucosal invasion).* **~McGuckin et al., 2011. Emphasis added**

Evidence also supports that defects in mucosal immunity can result in profoundly altered commensal colonization of the intestine, termed dysbiosis. However, **even a __normal__ immune response to infectious challenge can induce dysbiosis.** *Typically, the disruption is transient, and with resolution of the infection, the changed microbiota returns to base line. However,* **in some cases the changes in the microbiota can favor the survival of the invading pathogen** . . .. **~Bevins and Salzman, 2011, emphasis added**

Others may not place dysbiosis, defined as an abnormal bacterial composition in the gut, on the top of the list of risk factors for ulcerative colitis, but that won't stop me! Clearly, dysbiosis is a major contributing factor, perhaps #1. When factors in play expose the epithelial layer that resides below the mucus layer of defense, even the "good" bacteria will go over to the dark side (Ohkusa et al., 2009; McGuckin et al., 2011; Bevins and Salzman, 2011). *Everyone* is now a suspect! And we all know bacteria cannot be trusted. No, not in the least.

Dysbiosis can be considered an important pathogenetic factor with advancement of growth of invasive bacteria. *It can also facilitate bacterial translocation through the mucosal barrier to the mesenteric lymph nodes.* (Comito and Romano, 2012, emphasis added)

Dysbiosis predisposes to ulcerative colitis in multiple ways. **First**, in dysbiosis, the colonies of "good bacteria" are disadvantaged, not by more "good bacteria," but by bacteria bent on evil, bacteria that have somehow been able to increase in numbers. Colonization resistance has taken a hit! I sure hope the mucus layer of protection can withstand such a negative turn of events. But watch out! Some of these guys eat mucus for lunch! (McGuckin et al., 2011; Gill et al., 2011, de Groot et al., 2017) **Second**—there is no second. The first was bad enough! Now it's a waiting game to see if something will happen in favor of the pathogens and assist them in their efforts to reach the epithelial lining of the bowel. The "good bacteria" are not as strong of a force as they once were. And now what I call "reverse colonization resistance" occurs: "the bad" start crowding out "the good" and do so on an ongoing basis. Dysbiosis favors the colonization of bad bacteria and the crowding out of good bacteria, and at the expense of you. But regardless of "who" has reached the epithelial surface of the bowel, whether they are "good" or whether they are "bad," I see trouble ahead.

> *The surface epithelial cell layer can probably withstand and handle some bacteria, but will probably have difficulty withstanding substantial direct bacterial contact for a long period. Excessive bacterial contact will cause bacterial leakage into the tissue, something that could trigger the subepithelial adaptive immune system.* (Johansson et al., 2014)

Apparently, there is a **second** after all. Dysbiosis represents a shift in concentrations of "good" bacteria, little creatures that just want to graze, produce beneficial byproducts for their host, and sneakily kill off their competitors and enemies of the state. But dysbiosis increases the concentrations of "bad" bacteria that live to create havoc. And one way to create havoc is to produce a gas called nitric oxide (NO).

Bacteria less favorable to bowel health collectively produce large amounts of NO. The more NO, the more the mucus layer is under threat. NO can promote the breakdown of the mucus layer and allow the exposure of bacteria to the cells below (Roediger, 2008) Not surprisingly, *"luminal bacteria in UC produced more nitric oxide than a control population."* (Roediger, 2008) And increased NO production along with another metabolic byproduct, sulphide, and I see trouble ahead.

> *The prolonged production of bacterial NO with sulphide can explain the initiation of barrier breakdown, which is <u>central</u> to the pathogenesis of UC.* (Roediger, 2008, emphasis added)

I'm sure there is a **third**, a **fourth**, and no doubt many, many other reasons why dysbiosis predisposes to ulcerative colitis, but we need to move on. We don't have all day. We have a disease to defeat. Time is of the essence.

Next, we'll examine the reasons why dysbiosis is so common in our society. There are common environmental threats to bacterial diversity and the healthy balance between good and bad bacteria.

Environmental threats favoring dysbiosis

> *Unnecessary use of antibiotics and excessive hygienic precautions (e.g. natural versus chlorinated drinking water) together with the Western diet further contribute to a decreased microbial diversity in the adult gut.*
> **~Van den Abbeele et al., 2013**

> *The authors [investigating the association between iron in municipal water supplies and the incidence of IBD] found that [the] risk of developing inflammatory bowel disease was associated with high iron content.* ***The relative risk of developing inflammatory bowel disease, including <u>ulcerative colitis</u> and Crohn's disease increased by 21% . . . when the iron content in drinking water increased by 0.1 mg/l.*** *~Aamodt et al., 2008,* **emphasis added)**

There are several environmental factors that predispose to the development of ulcerative colitis. I'll mention three.

The emergence of IBD in the early years of the last century has coincided with an increased use of water purification programs, namely chlorination. A coincidence? Maybe. The problem with chlorination is that, while it kills off bad bacteria, its ingestion kills off good bacteria, too. Chlorination has been recognized as a predisposing factor to developing dysbiosis (Van der Abbeele et al., 2013). And as we have learned in the previous section, dysbiosis predisposes to ulcerative colitis. Turning our attention elsewhere . . .

Perhaps quite surprisingly, drinking water high in iron can predispose to ulcerative colitis. It does this by unbalancing the microbiome in the gut by selectively feeding bacteria that require iron for their persistence.

That iron exposure could promote dysbiosis and can lead to harm, may come as a surprise to you. Go ahead, be surprised, but consider this:

> Accumulating evidence indicates that excess of unabsorbed iron that enters the colon lumen causes unwanted side effects at the intestinal host–microbiota interface.

> Notably, accumulating evidence suggests that unabsorbed iron can stimulate growth and virulence of bacterial pathogens in the intestinal environment.

> Besides the effects of iron on the gut microbiota, which may cause a _shift towards a more pathogenic profile_ and an increase in virulence of enteric pathogens, _iron may also directly exert unfavorable effects on the gut epithelium_ most likely by the promotion of redox stress. (Kortman et al., 2014, emphasis added)

Iron, in excess of individual need, is a potent driver of dysbiosis. Diets high in iron, iron supplements, and now recently recognized, water high in iron, are implicated in favoring dysbiosis and are associated with the risk of ulcerative colitis. No one else is telling you any of this, are they? And I don't know why.

Another environmental risk predisposing to dysbiosis is birth by C-section. The baby born under this circumstance, is not first exposed to the environment of the vagina. In the vagina there are teeming multitudes of healthy bacteria that are available on a moment's notice to inoculate the baby during his or her journey through the birth canal and into the world at large. Instead, a C-section birth first exposes the baby to skin bacteria. This mode of delivery inoculates the baby's gut with a less diverse and more pathogenic microbiome profile. There is controversy whether C-section does or does not increase the risk of ulcerative colitis, but it does lead to dysbiosis at the very beginning of life outside the womb (where most of us live). So, when all is said and done, C-section is undoubtedly a risk factor for ulcerative colitis. Indeed, one study of over 2 million individuals found 4,318 cases of ulcerative colitis; and concluded that C-section increased the risk of IBD (both Crohn's and ulcerative colitis) by **14%** before age 36 (Bager et al., 2012). However, this finding may be confounded in that C-section babies may be nearly twice as likely not to be breast-fed (Bager et al., 2012). Which leads us to this:

The lack of breast feeding, and whatever substitutes for breast milk (dairy or formula), at the very beginnings of life on the outside, is an environmental risk factor for the development of ulcerative colitis (Xu et al., 2017). It is the protective effects of components in breast milk, and the friendly bacteria transferred from breast to baby during nursing, that offers both immediate and extended protection against the development of ulcerative colitis and other diseases as well, diseases that occur later in life. It does this by positively influencing the integrity of the intestinal layer of defense, in addition to preventing dysbiosis by promoting the growth of good bacteria (Xu et al., 2017). These initial protections against disease appear to continue to offer a degree of protection throughout life. But things don't always go as planned.

Antibiotics

Early and frequent antibiotic treatment in childhood increases the risk for ulcerative colitis. **~Lukas et al., 2006**

Depletion of commensal microbes and changing the microbiota composition by antibiotic administration affects intestinal immune defenses.

Thinning of the mucus layer [by Flagyl] may increase contact between epithelial cells and the microbiota, thereby enhancing innate immune stimulation and elevating the inflammatory tone of the intestine. **~Ubeda and Pamer, 2012**

Antibiotic use has been shown to alter gut flora, at both a general level and specific to certain microbes; moreover, alterations have been shown to be long-lasting. Thus, there is evidence suggesting an association between antibiotic usage and both pediatric and adult-onset IBD.

We were able to demonstrate a significant dose-dependent association between antibiotic use and adult-onset IBD. This relationship exists irrespective of the disease type (i.e., CD vs. UC), and was still present at 5 years before an individual's first recorded IBD diagnosis. **~Shaw et al., 2011**

Short-term treatment in humans with a single dose of oral antibiotics affects the gut microbiota for as long as 4 weeks before it then tends to revert to its original composition. **~Vrieze et al., 2010**

Disconcertingly, antibiotics appear to have a long-lasting effect implied by the association of IBD with exposure up to 5 years before diagnosis. There is evidence that antibiotics may impact the diversity of certain bacterial groups for at least 2 years. **~Nguyen, 2011**

Clearly, antibiotics are nothing to play around with. Antibiotic use, while <u>necessary</u> (so the patient can live to later come down with IBD?), appears to be a significant risk factor for both adult- and child-onset IBD, ulcerative colitis included. Antibiotics do this by disrupting the balance between "good" and "bad" bacteria, a balance that once offered so much protection. **Antibiotic use is the gift of dysbiosis**!

Antibiotics are highly effective in suppressing bacterial flora at the site of inflammation but are accompanied by extreme rebound effects and increase of mucosal bacterial concentrations far above levels observed prior to therapy. It is also alarming that this rebound effect seems to selectively enhance groups of bacteria that are the primary targets of antibiotic therapy such as Bacteroids (targeted by metronidazol), and Enterobacteriaceac (targeted by ciprofloxacin).

The suppressive effects of antibiotics on the mucosal flora are accompanied by <u>massive</u> rebound effects. *The concentration of mucosal bacteria are dramatically increased as soon as 1 week after cessation of antibiotic therapy, remaining at a high level that is at least one power higher over a period of 5 months as compared to the group without antibiotic treatment.* (Swidsinski et al., 2008, emphasis added)

I hope the above reference will serve as a warning to you against <u>unnecessary</u> antibiotic exposure. I paid close attention. And I have made myself this promise: Personally, I will take an antibiotic <u>only</u> if clearly needed and no other options appear reasonable. Then, following a course of "needed" antibiotics, I will read up on the use of pre- and pro-biotics to counter the negative effects of antibiotic therapy, then take action. As for you, the past use of antibiotics—due to its negative effects on the balance between good and evil bacteria—may have tipped the scales in the direction of ulcerative colitis. Not so fun, is it? Ironically, you now have a disease that may require antibiotics from time to time to keep you going. I believe, in ulcerative colitis, antibiotics can be strategically used and a particular issue can be resolved. But I also believe antibiotic use may make matters worse. I know I will get in trouble for saying this: Just because your physician can do it, doesn't mean a physician should do it. Be careful here! Consider the following:

Controlled trials with narrow spectrum antibiotics in ulcerative colitis have not demonstrated a consistent benefit. Thus, they have little, if any, role in the treatment of active disease except in patients with septic complications related to fulminate colitis in whom they may help avert a life-threatening infection. However, limited studies raise the possibility of an effect of broad spectrum antibiotic therapy. (Sartor, 2013)

All I ask is that you (and the physician) be careful with antibiotics. Very careful. Very, very careful. Avoid their use whenever possible. Although they are an indispensable tool in medicine, **and absolutely necessary under many, many circumstances**, they *can* increase one's risk of ulcerative colitis, or for those with this disease they can make matters worse.

But antibiotic use does not only come from medical decision-making. You are likely on antibiotics now! There are literally "tons" of antibiotics used in agriculture, and they just may be having a significant impact on human health (Kaur et al., 2011). Agricultural antibiotics may be playing a subtle role in increasing our risk of IBD by promoting dysbiosis (Willing et al., 2011; Kaur et al., 2011; Looft and Allen, 2012). Antibiotics are given to farm animals, not only to treat them when they are sick (and might die before they can be slaughtered) but also to make them fat. *Fat!* The agribusiness people discovered over 60 years ago that if you give a cow (or a chicken) dysbiosis, via antibiotics, it will gain weight. (This happens to people, too.) It is possible that agricultural antibiotics plays at least some role in the pathogenesis of ulcerative colitis in the carnivores within our midst. One more antibiotic issue to discuss then we will move on.

The use of antibiotics for children is quite high. One might say "alarmingly high." But when a society, like, almost totally ignores vitamin D, what do you expect? Vitamin D deficiency is widespread in children and reduces a child's resistance to infection. And "Mom" wants that damn runny nose treated (or else!), so little Charlie will receive a round of antibiotics he probably did not need in the first place. But it does not take a round of antibiotics to cause problems. It only takes one oral dose to greatly disturb his bacterial flora and for weeks, perhaps much longer

(Swidsinski et al., 2008). Charlie's risk of ulcerative colitis will now be elevated. Something Charlie did not need.

Now was that a clever way to interject the subject of vitamin D into our conversation, or what? I needed to! There is truth here! Many individuals require antibiotics for infections that they would not have acquired were it not for their embarrassingly (and tragically) low vitamin D status. Which leads us to . . .

Vitamin D deficiency

> *Vitamin D deficiency has been linked to several different diseases, including the immune-system diseases ulcerative colitis and Crohn's disease.* **~Cantorna et al., 2004**

> *Patients with a defect in the mucosa may experience a higher risk of microbial infection, for example, which may trigger the onset of IBD in patients who are predisposed. Our study showed that vitamin D is able to strengthen the mucosal barrier by upregulating some of the key tight junction proteins.* ***In a vitamin D-deficient state, mucosal barriers are more susceptible to injury that leads to infection and IBD.*** **~Li, 2008, emphasis added**

> *One popular nutrient that is used frequently as an immune modulator in autoimmune conditions is vitamin D. However, **<u>most clinicians are not aware of the role vitamin D plays directly in intestinal permeability</u>**.* **~Brady, 2013, emphasis added**

Vitamin D is a fascinating topic to me. So much so, I wrote a book on the subject entitled ***The Impact of Vitamin D Deficiency***. And I wouldn't mind selling you one. (Makes a good gift, too.) You can find it on Amazon, on BookDepository.com or on my website, www.impactofvitamind.com. Be that as it may, what is important to the conversation at this point in time is the role vitamin D plays in the prevention of ulcerative colitis.

Somehow, low vitamin D or altered signaling at the level of the VDR [vitamin D receptor], is important to the pathogenesis of ulcerative colitis (Wang et al., 2010).

And there is more to the story.

> We report that probiotics increase the expression of intestinal VDR [vitamin D receptor] and enhance the number of Paneth cells, thus inhibiting pathogenic bacterial invasion and inflammation. (Wu et al., 2015)

A Paneth cell is a specialized immune cell imbedded within the layer of intestinal epithelial cells, the function of which is to produce antimicrobial molecules. Found primarily in the small intestine, in ulcerative colitis Paneth cells can also be found in the colon (Tanaka, et al., 2001). Apparently, good bacteria can influence the ability of vitamin D to stimulate the production of antimicrobials by these specialized cells, antimicrobials directed against pathogens, produced to control their growth and to inhibit invasion (Wu et al., 2015). *This could come in handy!* And there is more.

Vitamin D, via its receptor, favorably regulates intestinal epithelial cell permeability—protecting against an influx of *"harmful substances such a microorganisms, toxins, and antigens from the body, and thus [vitamin D] plays a critical role in mucosal homeostasis. Impaired barrier function can lead to gut hyperpermeability and trigger inflammation."* (Du et al., 2015) Is it any wonder, vitamin D deficiency is on the list of enemies of the state you were in?

Cytokine dysregulation

> *Any combination of such factors [genetic susceptibility, exposure to environmental pathogens or toxins, etc.] can contribute to dysregulated immunity and **aberrant cytokine production, which has been shown to compromise the structural integrity of the intestinal epithelium.*** ~Detzel et al., 2015, emphasis added

The large bowel mucus layer effectively prevents contact between the highly concentrated luminal bacteria and the epithelial cells in all parts of the normal colon. <u>*Colonic inflammation is always accompanied by breaks in the mucus barrier.*</u> **~Swidsinski et al., 2007, emphasis added**

Vitamin D has also been shown to regulate cytokine pathways. . . . *vitamin D induced a dose-dependent down regulation of proinflammatory cytokines IL-6, TNF-α, IL-17, and IFN-γ, while increasing the anti-inflammatory cytokine IL-10.* **~Gubatan et al., 2018, emphasis added**

The cells of the immune system, along with the molecules they produce, control practically everything in this life—inflammation for defense, healing, and orderly growth. With respect to the gut, immune cells secrete cytokines (like IL-10) that continually act to restrain inflammation and maintain a healthy, steady state of affairs. Problems with immune cells, as well as problems with the inappropriate overproduction or under-production of key cytokines, can have a negative effect on the mucus layer of defense (Gubatan et al., 2018).

And wouldn't you know, vitamin D deficiency can unbalance the cytokines that are produced by the immune cells of the gut (Gubatan et al., 2018)—one more reason why vitamin D sufficiency is protective against ulcerative colitis. It is also protective against its relapse.

. . . higher serum vitamin D correlates with greater serum anti-inflammatory to proinflammatory cytokine ratios, and these anti-inflammatory cytokine phenotypes are associated with increased presence of histologic mucosal healing and decreased risk of clinical relapse. (Gubatan et al., 2018)

And so we see, cytokine dysregulation is a powerful thing. Some believe it *is* the disease we call ulcerative colitis; and, accordingly, their job is to battle cytokine dysregulation by manipulating things to produce a more favorable cytokine profile or to neutralize an offending cytokine— not a bad idea! Biologics do this. The success of infliximab (Remicade) is credited to its ability to alter cytokine profiles and promote the demise of a specific immune cell called a T cell, a cell that often has inflammation in mind (Xu et al., 2014; Neurath and Travis, 2012). These and other actions of infliximab can lead to healing (Neurath and Travis, 2012). And listen to this:

> *Because chronic inflammatory diseases depend on the recruitment of inflammatory cells, **<u>any approach</u> that reduces the number of inflammatory cells in the site of disease may be of benefit.*** (Feldmann and Steinman, 2005, emphasis added)

Of course, infliximab and other biologics can fail to deliver on their promises and can produce severe side effects. So, we could use an alternative or two in our bag of tricks, particularly so for those who cannot tolerate this form of therapy or who are no longer willing to take the risk or unwilling to deal with the side effects.

That being said, the success of biologics in promoting mucosal healing underscores the powerful effect cytokine dysregulation can exert on the intestinal epithelial lining. Cytokine dysregulation may have led to the disease you are not particularly pleased with at the moment. Clearly, cytokine dysregulation is another enemy of the state you were in.

Alcohol

> *In a prospective cohort study, Jowett found that individuals who consumed the most alcohol **tripled their risk of UC relapse** compared to those who drank the least.* **~Pravda, 2005, emphasis added**

> *A high alcohol intake was associated with an increased risk of relapse and many alcoholic drinks contain large amounts of sulfates as additives. A high sulphur diet, either from sulfur amino acids or sulfate additives, results in the generation of hydrogen sulfide and mucosal damage in the colon.* **~Jowett et al., 2004**

Sulfates in alcohol may be enough to tip the scales against you, favoring the pathogenesis of ulcerative colitis. Alcohol consumption is an added burden to ~~beer~~ bear for both rectum and colon. Sulfates in its various forms can be very damaging, not only to the mucus membrane (Jowett et al., 2004), but also to the DNA of the intestinal epithelial cell (Attene-Ramos et al., 2007). Among other things, sulfates are carcinogenic! (Attene-Ramos et al., 2007). And anything that increases the risk of ulcerative colitis relapse threefold should probably be looked at in a review of the factors that lead to ulcerative colitis and lead to relapse following remission. Alcohol does this. Sorry! And you thought a ruined life, damaged personal relationships, accidental death, and a liver an individual can no longer feel comfortable with were the primary problems associated with alcohol use. You were wrong.

It appears that alcohol can damage in a couple of different ways. Alcohol disturbs the metabolism of the rectum and colon by creating toxic metabolites that will need to be neutralized (good luck here!). This business places a great burden on our antioxidant defenses, making life more challenging at the cellular level (Pravda, 2005). Furthermore, alcohol perturbs the balance between the various members of the gut flora. So, like many other things in our society, alcohol is the gift of dysbiosis (Mutlu et al., 2012).

Alcohol exposure can promote the growth of Gram negative bacteria in the intestine which may result in accumulation of endotoxin. In addition, alcohol metabolism by Gram negative bacteria and intestinal epithelial cells can result in accumulation of acetaldehyde, which in turn can increase intestinal permeability to endotoxin . . .. Alcohol-induced generation of nitric oxide may also contribute to increased permeability to endotoxin . . .. (Purohit et al., 2008)

Based on the above quotation, we know a little more of the dangers posed by alcohol consumption. It predisposes to ulcerative colitis for multiple reasons. It promotes the growth of harmful bacteria. It allows harmful bacterial components, like endotoxin, to sneak past the normally tight junctions between epithelial cells, tight junctions that were loosened by alcohol. And alcohol consumption increases the generation of nitric oxide which can further harm the lining of the bowel. Sounds like alcohol consumption is trouble. Sounds like alcohol could lead to one very insidious disease.

So far, I have not differentiated between an occasional drink, and regular drinking. An occasional drink, perhaps okay. But regular drinking (which is actually alcoholism) and heavy drinking (which is actually alcoholism), not okay. In any event, drastically limit or avoid entirely the use of alcohol, say I. Regard alcohol as a destructive force (because it is a destructive force), say I.

Smoking cessation

In recent years, the most striking epidemiological finding in relation to ulcerative colitis is the recognition that it is predominately a disease of non-smokers and risk of its development in ex-smokers is between four and five times the expected risk in the general population. ~Zijlstra et al., 1994

This is a paradox (although I have a good idea what is going on): Astonishingly, smoking, as harmful as it is, reduces one's risk of contracting ulcerative colitis. This is quite surprising, is it not?

Smoking protects against ulcerative colitis in a couple of ways. **First**, it stimulates mucus secretion in the colon and rectum (Fries and Comunale, 2011; Bastida and Beltrán, 2011). **Second**, smoking—via nicotine—acts to modify the immune response. Nicotine binds a receptor (α7 nicotinic receptor) found in a variety of immune cells as well as in the intestinal epithelial cell and subsequently suppresses inflammation (Nielsen et al., 2009). We'll talk more about this later, but not over a drink.

So, now that you have ulcerative colitis, considering taking up smoking or, having previously quit, restarting the habit? I wouldn't. Ulcerative colitis patients who smoke have an increased risk of spin-off diseases such as ankylosing spondylitis (Apostolopoulos, 2006). And smoking may make ankylosing spondylitis symptoms worse and make for a more adverse outcome (Averns et al., 1996; Chen 2013). Some feel that a nicotine patch may do the trick. However, one team of investigators report that transdermal nicotine only offers a *"modest benefit"* as a therapy for ulcerative colitis (Molodecky and Kaplan, 2010).

Stress

The belief that stress may trigger IBD is popular among sufferers of CD and UC, but stress is more likely to modulate disease manifestations rather than being an initiating factor.

Stress also augments intestinal permeability, *and the entry of excessive amounts of luminal antigens could activate pre-sensitized mucosal T cells.* **~Danese et al., 2004, emphasis added**

Stress-related molecules dampen immune responses . . . bacteria can use these factors to enhance microbial pathogenesis during stress.

Collectively, increased sympathetic stimulation, presumably during periods of stress, may increase the susceptibility to the host to pathogenic infection by influencing virulence capacity related to adhesion and antimicrobial defenses. **~Radek, 2010, emphasis added**

Immune homeostasis does not arise passively from an absence of inflammatory stimuli; rather, ***maintenance of health requires specific mechanisms to restrain reactions to inflammatory stimuli that do not warrant a full response.*** *In this sense, the regulation of inflammation seems to be considered in terms of checkpoints. Among these mechanisms,* ***the nervous system is the main regulator of the immune system***. **~Peña et al., 2011, emphasis added**

*The vagus nerve prevents the release of TNF, HMGB1, IL-1 and other proinflammatory cytokines. As the activity of this pathway is controlled by neural signals, **it provides a way for the brain to regulate the cytokine response in a localized, controlled, and organ-specific manner**.* ~Tracey, 2005, emphasis added

*Parasympathetic impairment results in a **dominant sympathetic drive**, and it is known that this **enhances colonic inflammation**.* ~Ghia et al., 2007, emphasis added

Astonishingly (to me), some physicians and scientists question a role for stress in the pathogenesis of ulcerative colitis. If given the opportunity, I would simply ask the "non-believers" whether they have ever heard of the cholinergic anti-inflammatory pathway. From the looks of things, I doubt that many have. And if they have, they may not be paying attention to or making the connection between stress and the pathogenesis of ulcerative colitis. But since the cholinergic anti-inflammatory pathway is a relatively new discovery, I will cut them some slack. And, of course, you are clueless (as usual). Recent discoveries have shown that stress alters immune responses because ***the brain controls the immune response!*** (Peña et al., 2011) The brain communicates with the immune cells of the gut, wherein "stress" equals a more intense inflammatory response and "calm" actually calms the inflammatory response. Signals originating in the brain may even stop inflammation in its tracks! Later I will devote an entire chapter to the cholinergic anti-inflammatory pathway. You'll be blown away! I think we can exploit this pathway in the battle against ulcerative colitis.

Recently, a neural circuit has been identified that controls the inflammatory response in a reflex-like manner. This circuit involves the vagus nerve which is able to respond to it by releasing acetylcholine which, through an interaction with immune cells, dampens the inflammatory response. (Van Westderloo et al., 2010)

Let's get back to our discussion on stress and the pathogenesis of ulcerative colitis. It is clear, stress in the form of adverse life events is a factor in relapse and the severity of ulcerative colitis (Mawdsley and Rampton, 2005). But what may be missing in the conversation is this: Ulcerative colitis has small beginnings (Van Praet, et al., 2012). It can be unnoticeable at first, being isolated to a small area of involvement with the immune system acting to effectively deal with the issues at hand. The immune system just may succeed; an ulcerative-colitis-in-the-making may never take hold. "Tummy troubles" vanish, never to return. Remission may occur even before you have the disease! But add stressful events and all bets are off. Stress dysregulates everything! It can either depress or intensify the immune response (Mawdsley and Rampton, 2005), it can induce mucus barrier defects (Radek, 2010), and stress can increase the availability of iron for pathogen acquisition, increasing their virulence and ability to adhere to the intestinal epithelial cell and to penetrate (Radek, 2010). I could go on and on about the negative consequences of stress. (But that might be stressful.) Stress actually changes who you are, from an immunological standpoint. Therefore, we should not underestimate the negative impact of stress on the health and function of our mucosal barrier of defense. And we should probably not *monkey* around with stress, either. Tamarins are monkeys. Gibbons are monkeys.

> Cotton top tamarins are at increased risk of a colitis that closely resembles UC when subjected to the chronic stress of living in captivity, with remission being induced by return to natural living conditions. Similarly, Siamese gibbons can also develop a fatal colitis when held in captivity. (Mawdsley and Rampton, 2005)

NSAIDS

> NSAIDs have been implicated not only in exacerbations of IBD, but also as a potent precipitant of new cases, perhaps by blockade of protective

prostaglandins, by altering mucosal immune reactivity and by increasing intestinal permeability. **~Apostolopoulos, 2006**

NSAIDs can cause damage to the intestinal mucosa of the stomach, small bowel, and colon. NSAIDs can also <u>increase intestinal permeability</u> by inhibiting cyclooxygenase, which reduces prostaglandin production. **~Molodecky and Kaplan, 2010, emphasis added**

There is substantial evidence that exacerbation of IBD happens after treatment with NSAIDs, but the available data remain conflicting, and it is not clear whether selective COX-2 inhibitors are safer than traditional NSAIDs. However, there is some evidence that selective COX-2 inhibition and COX -1 inhibition (with low-dose aspirin) appear to be well-tolerated in the short term. Regarding the mechanisms of relapse, the reduction of prostaglandins appears to be the hallmark of the NSAIDs adverse effects. **~Kefalakes et al., 2009**

Well, things here are almost self-explanatory. So, I will need to comment only a little. NSAIDs can harm, so try to avoid them. But we as a society turn to this class of drugs all too frequently, and sometimes we pay a heavy price. The disease burden from NSAIDs is greater than one might expect, and the death penalty risk is quite astounding. Thousands of individuals die per year in the USA, traced to NSAID use! Yet many individuals take these medications like they are candy (sort of)—to control headache, everyday aches and pains, and to treat a disease process. We won't go into details here—discussing COX-1, COX-2, prostaglandins, and selective inhibition and the like. All of this is beyond the scope of this chapter and this book. I simply want to warn you of names like Aspirin, Advil, Motrin, Aleve, Bufferin, Excedrin, Ecotrin, Celebrex, and Naprosyn. Some of these are over-the-counter drugs. Some, only by prescription. All should be used with caution, and, with prolonged use, could lead to IBD. Here is some good advice:

If NSAIDs administration is necessary, there is a need for careful follow up of IBD patients, mainly those in remission, during the first few days of treatment, as disease aggravation of clinical relapse requires drug discontinuation. (Kefalakes et al., 2009)

Dietary disruption of barrier function

Diet is one of the major determinants for the persistence of a given bacterium in the gastrointestinal tract because the diet provides nutrients not only for the host but also for the bacterium. **~Blaut and Claver, 2007**

Emerging evidence has also identified dietary lipid intake as an important factor contributing to the etiology of IBD. At least one study, in a Danish population, found that excessive consumption of omega-6 PUFA [polyunsaturated fatty acid] increases ulcerative colitis risk by **30%**; *whereas consumption of docosahexaenoic acid [DHA], an omega-3 PFUA, reduced the burden by* **77%**. **~Brown et al., 2012, emphasis added**

Depletion of short-chain fatty acid-producing organisms possibly deprives already vulnerable intestinal epithelial cells, **leading to invasion of commensal or low-pathogenic bacteria with subsequent activation of immunocompetent cells.** *~Sasaki and Klapproth, 2012, emphasis added*

The capacity to acquire iron during intestinal inflammation is an important virulence trait for survival in the inflamed gut.

Pathogens which have adapted to this hostile environment have acquired a range of virulence factors that provide access to nutrients in the inflamed gut, including glycoproteins in the mucus layer and metal ions. **~Blaschitz and Raffatellu, 2010**

Why is diet such an important topic regarding the pathogenesis of ulcerative colitis? **First,** *"dietary factors alter the microbial community resulting in biological changes in the host."* (Brown et al., 2012) **Second,** *"the 'Western' diet, which is high in sugar and fat [and particularly rich in the omega-6 fatty acids], causes dysbiosis which affects both host GI tract metabolism and immune homeostasis."* (Brown et al., 2012) **Third,**

"Experimental studies indicate that commonly used food ingredients can alter the intestinal barrier, thereby causing intestinal inflammation." (Ruemmele, 2016) **Fourth** (and there are many more), a diet that consists of refined, processed foods is generally a low-fiber diet. A low-fiber diet adversely affects the epithelial cells of the rectum and colon (colonocytes), in as much as it is the breakdown of dietary fibers by gut bacteria that supplies short-chain fatty acids that fuel these cells so they can function properly. *"In fact, a major part of the energy used by the colonocytes is derived from short [chain] fatty acids (acetate and butyrate)."* (Johansson et al., 2011) So, the Western diet is basically a "starvation diet" for the intestinal epithelial cell, a cell that is also an immune cell, a cell that needs energy to adequately perform its many duties and to adequately protect.

> *Depletion of short-chain fatty acid-producing organisms possibly deprives already vulnerable intestinal epithelial cells, leading to invasion of commensal or low-pathogenic bacteria with subsequent activation of immunocompetent cells.* (Sasaki and Klapproth, 2012)

Low-fiber diets, like the lousy one you are probably on now, also increase the risk of colon cancer (and so does vitamin D deficiency). The risk of colon cancer is automatically elevated in patients with ulcerative colitis. The Western diet is a good reason why. You will learn more about this disaster (the Western diet) later.

Fortunately, there is a diet perfect for the ulcerative colitis patient. It is the vegetarian diet. Sorry, all you meat-lovers out there (including myself)!

> *Vegetarianism alters intestinal microbiota in humans because high amounts of fiber result in increased short chain fatty acid production by microbes which decreases the intestinal pH. This*

prevents the growth of potentially pathogenic bacteria such as E coli and other members of Enterobacteriaceae. (Brown et al., 2012)

But in order to "weaponize" the vegetarian diet, that is, make it more effective in the battle against ulcerative colitis, one should limit or eliminate a few food additives that are known to stir up trouble and actually damage the colon. The big three problem areas (in my opinion) are emulsifyers like carrageenan, foods preserved with sulfates, and iron-fortified foods.

With respect to carrageenan (a common sulphated food additive) and sulfate-preserved foods (and beer), *"the strongest evidence for a dietary factor is that sulphur and sulphate may be implicated in relapses of ulcerative colitis."* (Lukas et al., 2006)

With respect to iron fortification . . . where do I start? I'll keep this short. Iron fuels the virulence of pathogens, allowing them to become more adherent and more invasive. Iron creates and perpetuates dysbiosis. Iron irritates the intestinal mucosa, and particularly the inflamed intestinal mucosa. Yes, iron is pure evil! Yet, we need it for our very survival. Here is the point: Iron consumed in excess of our need— and in excess of our ability to sequester and escort it within protective molecules that we ourselves make (or eat)—travels downstream in the GI tract and complicates our lives in so many unpleasant ways. It promotes and perpetuates diseases like IBD. It also promotes the growth of certain cancers. Just so you know, as an ulcerative colitis patient you are at increased risk of contracting colorectal cancer. I will document all this later. Just believe (and prepare to do things differently).

We will spend more time on dietary and iron issues in upcoming chapters, of that you can be sure—so important! So very important! But before I leave this section, I need to share this:

Co-administration of ferrous salts [as per iron supplements] with vitamin C exacerbates oxidative stress in the gastrointestinal tract leading to ulceration in healthy individuals, exacerbation of chronic gastrointestinal inflammatory disease and can lead to cancer. (Fisher and Naughton, 2004)

Are you beginning to see how important appropriate dietary advice can be? It can be so important. It can change everything!

One more topic to discuss and we can move on to the next chapter.

Turning darkness into light

Advances in our understanding of the molecular machinery of the circadian clock, and the discovery of clock genes in the GI tract are opening up new avenues of research for a role of sleep in IBD. Altering circadian rhythm significantly worsens the development of colitis in animal models, and preliminary human studies have shown that patients with IBD are at increased risk for altered sleep patterns.

With prolonged sleep loss, there are elevations in monocytes and natural killer cells, which form the source for the secretion of inflammatory cytokines. Thus, disturbed sleep and chronic inflammation in IBD could form a self-perpetuating feedback loop with the chronic inflammation of IBD worsening sleep, and decreased sleep exacerbating the production of inflammatory cytokines and the inflammatory milieu. **~Swanson et al., 2011**

"Burning the candle at both ends" is an expression that often refers to doing too much at the expense of adequate sleep. This certainly occurs when one is writing a book on ulcerative colitis. Surprisingly, lack of adequate sleep is recognized as a risk factor for ulcerative colitis. (Boy, am I in trouble!) All of this revolves around the hormone melatonin, a hormone generated by darkness, and preferably at night when the human animal should be sleeping (in a cave). An individual's melatonin level takes a big hit when one does not sleep (in the dark) and does not sleep for an adequate amount of time. Beware Night-Shift Workers of America, you may be at greater risk for contracting ulcerative colitis! In fact, your risk of many diseases is significantly greater due to night shift work. So what is this melatonin?

Melatonin is a hormone produced by the pineal gland located somewhere at the base of that crazy brain of yours and regulates a myriad of physiological processes. It helps you regulate your immune system, even in the gut. It promotes repair. It makes you a better person. My advice: Study, diligently study, ways to promote adequate, restorative sleep. **Make it happen!** You are free to try melatonin supplements if you choose—some have found this helpful—but I believe generating melatonin the old-fashioned way is perhaps the best way. Do not underestimate the power of restorative sleep. (Okay, you can if you want to.)

Well, I think I have covered the most relevant risk factors for ulcerative colitis fairly well. Now we can move on.

The immune response in the gut

Want to be blown away? Watch the following the video. It will give you a sense of just how complicated the immune response is.

—Immunology in the Gut Mucosa
www.youtube.com/watch?v=gnZEge78_78

Thoughts on remission in ulcerative colitis

These are my thoughts, and perhaps the thoughts of many others: Remission in ulcerative colitis occurs when reasons for its expression are resolved. *"By lowering the inflammation in IBD patients, induction or maintenance of remission may be achieved."* (Sharifi et al., 2016) Drugs may do this, in that, by modifying the inflammatory response, things may reset, the mucus layer may once again become a formidable layer of protection, and life goes on . . . sometimes without the need of further medical attention. In my view, each of the risk factors needs to be addressed or this thing will just keep on coming at you. The resolution of inflammation is not always achieved by forceful suppression of the immune response. Success may be achieved by simply doing things that tip the scales in your favor, by doing things that allow healing to occur, and by not doing things that interfere with the healing process. I doubt, very seriously, if little attention is given to the various layers of defense, that success (remission without immunosuppression) will be achieved. There is so much that can be done to give you an edge in the battle against ulcerative colitis. And I know just where to begin. But we'll have to wait. We have a few other important things we need to discuss.

(More on) The genetics behind the disease

> *Genetics alone cannot determine risks of developing UC since the rate among identical twins is between **16–18.5%**.* ~**Awad and Jasion, 2015, emphasis added**

> *Genetic variants associated with ulcerative colitis, reduced expression of peroxisome proliferator-activated receptor γ (PPAR-γ) by colonocytes, mucus abnormalities, and abnormalities of regulatory T cells (Treg) may also contribute to selective autoimmune-mediated events in the pathogenesis of ulcerative colitis.* ~**Danses and Fiocchi, 2011**

We briefly discussed this issue in the previous gray box, but I sensed you wanted to learn more. Here is more:

Unfortunately, for you the ulcerative colitis patient, things have progressed too far. Now, the genetics you have make a difference and define how effectively (and less awkwardly) the battle will be waged and how quickly it will resolve. Genetic predisposition, while it may make it easier to contract ulcerative colitis, does not necessarily mean an individual will fall victim. It is stated that the various genetic abnormalities associated with ulcerative colitis exert only a *"small additive effect"* in the pathogenesis of ulcerative colitis (Danses and Fiocchi, 2011) with environmental factors of far greater significance in the pathogenesis of ulcerative colitis (Fries and Comunale, 2011). Furthermore, identical twins, whose genetics are identical, have only a **16%** chance that both will both develop the disease (Fries and Comunale, 2011), illustrating the power of other forces at work in the pathogenesis of ulcerative colitis. Genetic issues, however, will define the expression of the disease and act to make its resolution more difficult to achieve. Remarkably, there are at least two genetic abnormalities that increase the risk of contracting Crohn's disease that are *"protective for ulcerative colitis."* (Kaunitz and Nayyar, 2016)

There is little one can do about genetics, except for the fact that one can prevent genetics from becoming a factor. For you, this is too late. At one point in time, however, your genetics were not an issue. Back then (the good 'ol days, when the price of toilet paper really didn't matter), you did not have the disease . . . even though your genes were basically no different than they are now. But, as barriers were breached and defenses were impaired by predisposing factors, genetic issues came into play. Fortunately, there are no major genetic defects in MUC2 gene, the gene responsible for the production and the general character of mucus (Salim and Söderholm, 2011), but there are genetic defects found in the ulcerative colitis patient that make the battle so difficult to win. You can read about these in some other book or in some research paper. We just don't have the time to dwell on genetics in this presentation. I'm stressed enough as it is.

~References~

Aamodt G, Bukholm G, Jahnsen J, Moum B, Vatn MH, IBSEN Study Group. **The association between water supply and inflammatory bowel disease based on a 1990–1993 cohort study in southeastern Norway.** American journal of epidemiology. 2008 Sep 18;168(9):1065-72.

Attene-Ramos MS, Wagner ED, Gaskins HR, Plewa MJ. **Hydrogen sulfide induces direct radical-associated DNA damage.** Molecular cancer research. 2007 May 1;5(5):455-9.

Apostolopoulos P. **Environmental Factors in IBD.** Annals of Gastroenterology. 2006;19(2):152–154.

Averns HL, Oxtoby J, Taylor HG, Jones PW, Dziedzic K, Dawes PT. **Smoking and outcome in ankylosing spondylitis.** Scandinavian journal of rheumatology. 1996 Jan 1;25(3):138-42.

Awad A, Jasion VS. **Use of a nutritional therapy, serum-derived bovine immunoglobulin/protein isolate (SBI), to achieve improvement in two different cases of colitis.** J Gastrointest Dig Syst. 2015;5(2):274.

Bager P, Simonsen J, Nielsen NM, Frisch M. **Cesarean section and offspring's risk of inflammatory bowel disease: a national cohort study.** Inflammatory bowel diseases. 2012 May 1;18(5):857-62.

Bastida G, Beltrán B. **Ulcerative colitis in smokers, non-smokers and ex-smokers.** World journal of gastroenterology: WJG. 2011 Jun 14;17(22):2740.

Bevins CL, Salzman NH. **The potter's wheel: the host's role in sculpting its microbiota. Cellular and Molecular Life Sciences.** 2011 Nov 1;68(22):3675.

Blanck S, Aberra F. **Vitamin d deficiency is associated with ulcerative colitis disease activity.** Digestive diseases and sciences. 2013 Jun 1;58(6):1698-702.

Blaschitz C, Raffatellu M. **Th17 cytokines and the gut mucosal barrier. Journal of clinical immunology.** 2010 Mar 1;30(2):196-203.

Blaut M, Clavel T. **Metabolic diversity of the intestinal microbiota: implications for health and disease.** The Journal of nutrition. 2007 Mar 1;137(3):751S-5S.

Brady DM. **Molecular mimicry, the hygiene hypothesis, stealth infections and other examples of disconnect between medical research and the practice of clinical medicine in autoimmune disease.** Open Journal of Rheumatology and Autoimmune Diseases. 2013 Feb 18;3(01):33.

Brown K, DeCoffe D, Molcan E, Gibson DL. **Diet-induced dysbiosis of the intestinal microbiota and the effects on immunity and disease.** Nutrients. 2012 Aug;4(8):1095-119.

Cantorna MT, Zhu Y, Froicu M, Wittke A. **Vitamin D status, 1, 25-dihydroxyvitamin D3, and the immune system.** The American journal of clinical nutrition. 2004 Dec 1;80(6):1717S-20S.

Chen CH, Chen HA, Lu CL, Liao HT, Liu CH, Tsai CY, Chou CT. **Association of cigarette smoking with Chinese ankylosing spondylitis patients in Taiwan: a poor disease outcome in systemic inflammation, functional ability, and physical mobility.** Clinical rheumatology. 2013 May 1;32(5):659-63.

Chen SJ, Liu XW, Liu JP, Yang XY, Lu FG. **Ulcerative colitis as a polymicrobial infection characterized by sustained broken mucus barrier.** World Journal of Gastroenterology: WJG. 2014 Jul 28;20(28):9468.

Comito D, Romano C. **Dysbiosis in the pathogenesis of pediatric inflammatory bowel diseases.** International journal of inflammation. 2012;2012.

Danese S, Sans M, Fiocchi C. **Inflammatory bowel disease: the role of environmental factors.** Autoimmunity reviews. 2004 Jul 1;3(5):394-400.

Danese S, Fiocchi. **Ulcerative colitis.** N Engl J Med 2011; 365:1713-1725 DOI: 10.1056/NEJMra1102942.

de Groot PF, Frissen MN, de Clercq NC, Nieuwdorp M. **Fecal microbiota transplantation in metabolic syndrome: history, present and future.** Gut Microbes. 2017 May 4;8(3):253-67.

Detzel CJ, Horgan A, Henderson AL, Petschow BW, Warner CD, Maas KJ, Weaver EM. **Bovine immunoglobulin/protein isolate binds pro-inflammatory bacterial compounds and prevents immune activation in an intestinal co-culture model.** PloS One. 2015 Apr 1;10(4):e0120278.

Du J, Chen Y, Shi Y, Liu T, Cao Y, Tang Y, Ge X, Nie H, Zheng C, Li YC. 1, 25-**Dihydroxyvitamin D protects intestinal epithelial barrier by regulating the myosin light chain kinase signaling pathway.** Inflammatory bowel diseases. 2015 Aug 17;21(11):2495-506.

Feldmann M, Steinman L. **Design of effective immunotherapy for human autoimmunity.** Nature. 2005 Jun 1;435(7042):612.

Fisher AE, Naughton DP. **Iron supplements: the quick fix with long-term consequences.** Nutrition journal. 2004 Dec 1;3(1):2.

Fries W, Comunale S. **Ulcerative colitis: pathogenesis.** Current drug targets. 2011 Sep 1;12(10):1373-82.

Ghia JE, Blennerhassett P, Collins SM. **Vagus nerve integrity and experimental colitis. American Journal of Physiology-Gastrointestinal and Liver Physiology.** 2007 Sep;293(3):G560-7.

Gill N, Wlodarska M, Finlay BB. **Roadblocks in the gut: barriers to enteric infection.** Cellular microbiology. 2011 May;13(5):660-9.

Gubatan J, Mitsuhashi S, Longhi MS, Zenlea T, Rosenberg L, Robson S, Moss AC. **Higher serum vitamin D levels are associated with protective serum cytokine profiles in patients with ulcerative colitis.** Cytokine. 2018 Mar 31;103:38-45.

Johansson ME, Gustafsson JK, Sjöberg KE, Petersson J, Holm L, Sjövall H, Hansson GC. **Bacteria penetrate the inner mucus layer before inflammation in the dextran sulfate colitis model.** PloS one. 2010;5(8).

Johansson ME, Larsson JM, Hansson GC. **The two mucus layers of colon are organized by the MUC2 mucin, whereas the outer layer is a legislator of host–microbial interactions.** Proceedings of the national academy of sciences. 2011 Mar 15;108(Supplement 1):4659-65.

Johansson ME, Gustafsson JK, Holmén-Larsson J, Jabbar KS, Xia L, Xu H, Ghishan FK, Carvalho FA, Gewirtz AT, Sjövall H, Hansson GC. **Bacteria penetrate the normally impenetrable inner colon mucus layer in both murine colitis models and patients with ulcerative colitis.** Gut. 2014 Feb 1;63(2):281-91.

Jowett SL, Seal CJ, Pearce MS, Phillips E, Gregory W, Barton JR, Welfare MR. **Influence of dietary factors on the clinical course of ulcerative colitis: a prospective cohort study.** Gut. 2004 Oct 1;53(10):1479-84.

Kaunitz J, Nayyar P. **Bugs, genes, fatty acids, and serotonin: Unraveling inflammatory bowel disease?.** F1000Research. 2015;4.

Kaur N, Chen CC, Luther J, Kao JY. **Intestinal dysbiosis in inflammatory bowel disease.** Gut microbes. 2011 Jul 1;2(4):211-6.

Kefalakes H, Stylianides TJ, Amanakis G, Kolios G. **Exacerbation of inflammatory bowel diseases associated with the use of nonsteroidal anti-inflammatory drugs: myth or reality?.** European journal of clinical pharmacology. 2009 Oct 1;65(10):963-70.

Kortman GA, Raffatellu M, Swinkels DW, Tjalsma H. **Nutritional iron turned inside out: intestinal stress from a gut microbial perspective. FEMS microbiology reviews.** 2014 Nov 1;38(6):1202-34.

Li YC. **Investigating the role of vitamin D in IBD pathophysiology and treatment.** Gastroenterology & hepatology. 2008 Jan;4(1):20.

Looft T, Allen HK. **Collateral effects of antibiotics on mammalian gut microbiomes.** Gut microbes. 2012 Sep 20;3(5):463-7.

Lukas M, Bortlik M, Maratka Z. **What is the origin of ulcerative colitis? Still more questions than answers.** Postgraduate medical journal. 2006 Oct 1;82(972):620-5.

Mawdsley JE, Rampton DS. **Psychological stress in IBD: new insights into pathogenic and therapeutic implications.** Gut. 2005 Oct 1;54(10):1481-91.

McGuckin MA, Eri R, Simms LA, Florin TH, Radford-Smith G. **Intestinal barrier dysfunction in inflammatory bowel diseases.** Inflammatory bowel diseases. 2008 Jul 11;15(1):100-13.

McGuckin MA, Lindén SK, Sutton P, Florin TH. **Mucin dynamics and enteric pathogens.** Nature Reviews Microbiology. 2011 Apr;9(4):265.

Molodecky NA, Kaplan GG. **Environmental risk factors for inflammatory bowel disease.** Gastroenterology & hepatology. 2010 May;6(5):339.

Mutlu EA, Gillevet PM, Rangwala H, Sikaroodi M, Naqvi A, Engen PA, Kwasny M, Lau CK, Keshavarzian A. **Colonic microbiome is altered in alcoholism. American Journal of Physiology-Gastrointestinal and Liver Physiology.** 2012 Jan 12;302(9):G966-78.

Neurath MF, Travis SP. **Mucosal healing in inflammatory bowel diseases: a systematic review.** Gut. 2012 Jan 1:gutjnl-2012.

Nguyen GC **Bugs and Drugs: Insights into the Pathogenesis of Inflammatory Bowel Disease.** Am J Gastroenterol 2011;106:2143–2145.

Nielsen OH, Bjerrum JT, Csillag C, Nielsen FC, Olsen J. **Influence of smoking on colonic gene expression profile in Crohn's disease.** PloS One. 2009 Jul 15;4(7):e6210.

Ohkusa T, Yoshida T, Sato N, Watanabe S, Tajiri H, Okayasu I. **Commensal bacteria can enter colonic epithelial cells and induce proinflammatory cytokine secretion: a possible pathogenic mechanism of ulcerative colitis.** Journal of Medical Microbiology. 2009 May 1;58(5):535-45.

Peña G, Cai B, Ramos L, Vida G, Deitch EA, Ulloa L. **Cholinergic regulatory lymphocytes re-establish neuromodulation of innate immune responses in sepsis.** The Journal of Immunology. 2011 Jul 15;187(2):718-25.

Peyrin-Biroulet L, Oussalah A, Bigard MA. **Crohn's disease: the hot hypothesis.** Medical hypotheses. 2009 Jul 1;73(1):94-6.

Pravda J. **Radical induction theory of ulcerative colitis.** World journal of gastroenterology: WJG. 2005 Apr 28;11(16):2371.

Radek KA. **Antimicrobial anxiety: the impact of stress on antimicrobial immunity.** Journal of leukocyte biology. 2010 Aug;88(2):263-77.

Rehman A, Lepage P, Nolte A, Hellmig S, Schreiber S, Ott SJ. T**ranscriptional activity of the dominant gut mucosal microbiota in chronic inflammatory bowel disease patients.** Journal of medical microbiology. 2010 Sep 1;59(9):1114-22.

Roediger WE. **Nitric oxide from dysbiotic bacterial respiration of nitrate in the pathogenesis and as a target for therapy of ulcerative colitis.** Alimentary pharmacology & therapeutics. 2008 Apr;27(7):531-41.

Ruemmele FM. **Role of diet in inflammatory bowel disease.** Annals of Nutrition and Metabolism. 2016;68(Suppl. 1):32-41.

Purohit V, Bode JC, Bode C, Brenner DA, Choudhry MA, Hamilton F, Kang YJ, Keshavarzian A, Rao R, Sartor RB, Swanson C. **Alcohol, intestinal bacterial** growth, intestinal permeability to endotoxin, and medical consequences: summary of a symposium. Alcohol. 2008 Aug 1;42(5):349-61.

Salim SA, Söderholm JD. **Importance of disrupted intestinal barrier in inflammatory bowel diseases.** Inflammatory bowel diseases. 2011 Jan 1;17(1):362-81.

Sartor RB. **Probiotics for gastrointestinal diseases.** UpToDate. Graphic. 2013;50560.

Sasaki M, Klapproth JM. **The role of bacteria in the pathogenesis of ulcerative colitis.** Journal of signal transduction. 2012;2012.

Schneider H, Braun A, Füllekrug J, Stremmel W, Ehehalt R. **Lipid based therapy for ulcerative colitis—modulation of intestinal mucus membrane phospholipids as a tool to influence inflammation.** International journal of molecular sciences. 2010 Oct;11(10):4149-64.

Shaw SY, Blanchard JF, Bernstein CN. **Association between the use of antibiotics and new diagnoses of Crohn's disease and ulcerative colitis.** The American journal of gastroenterology. 2011 Dec;106(12):2133.

Sharifi A, Hosseinzadeh-Attar MJ, Vahedi H, Nedjat S. **A randomized controlled trial on the effect of vitamin D3 on inflammation and cathelicidin gene expression in ulcerative colitis patients.** Saudi journal of gastroenterology: official journal of the Saudi Gastroenterology Association. 2016 Jul;22(4):316.

Steidler L. **Microbiological and immunological strategies for treatment of inflammatory bowel disease.** Microbes and infection. 2001 Nov 1;3(13):1157-66.

Swanson GR, Burgess HJ, Keshavarzian A. **Sleep disturbances and inflammatory bowel disease: a potential trigger for disease flare?.** Expert review of clinical immunology. 2011 Jan 1;7(1):29-36.

Swidsinski A, Loening-Baucke V, Theissig F, Engelhardt H, Bengmark S, Koch S, Lochs H, Dörffel Y. **Comparative study of the intestinal mucus barrier in normal and inflamed colon.** Gut. 2007 Mar 1;56(3):343-50.

Swidsinski A, Loening-Baucke V, Bengmark S, Scholze J, Doerffel Y. **Bacterial biofilm suppression with antibiotics for ulcerative and indeterminate colitis: consequences of aggressive treatment.** Archives of medical research. 2008 Feb 1;39(2):198-204.

Tanaka M, Saito H, Kusumi T, Fukuda S, Shimoyama T, Sasaki Y, Suto K, Munakata A, Kudo H. **Spatial distribution and histogenesis of colorectal Paneth cell metaplasia in idiopathic inflammatory bowel disease.** Journal of gastroenterology and hepatology. 2001 Dec;16(12):1353-9.

Tracey KJ. **Fat meets the cholinergic antiinflammatory pathway. The Journal of experimental medicine.** 2005 Oct 17;202(8):1017-21.

Ubeda C, Pamer EG. **Antibiotics, microbiota, and immune defense. Trends in immunology.** 2012 Sep 1;33(9):459-66.

Van den Abbeele P, Verstraete W, El Aidy S, Geirnaert A, van de Wiele T. **Prebiotics, faecal transplants and microbial network units to stimulate biodiversity of the human gut microbiome.** Microbial biotechnology. 2013 Jul 1;6(4):335-40.

Van Praet L, Jacques P, Van den Bosch F, Elewaut D. **The transition of acute to chronic bowel inflammation in spondyloarthritis.** Nature Reviews Rheumatology. 2012 May;8(5):288.

Van Westerloo DJ. **The vagal immune reflex: a blessing from above.** Wiener Medizinische Wochenschrift. 2010 Mar 1;160(5-6):112-7.

Vrieze A, Holleman F, Zoetendal EG, De Vos WM, Hoekstra JB, Nieuwdorp M. **The environment within: how gut microbiota may influence metabolism and body composition.** Diabetologia. 2010 Apr 1;53(4):606-13.

Wang TT, Dabbas B, Laperriere D, Bitton AJ, Soualhine H, Tavera-Mendoza LE, Dionne S, Servant MJ, Bitton A, Seidman EG, Mader S. **Direct and indirect induction by 1, 25-dihydroxyvitamin D3 of the NOD2/CARD15-defensin β2 innate immune pathway defective in Crohn disease.** Journal of Biological Chemistry. 2010 Jan 22;285(4):2227-31.

Willing BP, Russell SL, Finlay BB. **Shifting the balance: antibiotic effects on host–microbiota mutualism.** Nature Reviews Microbiology. 2011 Apr;9(4):233.

Wu S, Yoon S, Zhang YG, Lu R, Xia Y, Wan J, Petrof EO, Claud EC, Chen D, Sun J. **Vitamin D receptor pathway is required for probiotic protection in colitis.** American Journal of Physiology-Gastrointestinal and Liver Physiology. 2015 Jul 9;309(5):G341-9.

Xu L, Lochhead P, Ko Y, Claggett B, Leong RW, Ananthakrishnan AN. **Systematic review with meta-analysis: breastfeeding and the risk of Crohn's disease and**

ulcerative colitis. Alimentary pharmacology & therapeutics. 2017 Nov 1;46(9):780-9.

Xu XR, Liu CQ, Feng BS, Liu ZJ. **Dysregulation of mucosal immune response in pathogenesis of inflammatory bowel disease.** World journal of gastroenterology: WJG. 2014 Mar 28;20(12):3255.

Zijlstra FJ, Srivastava ED, Rhodes M, van Dijk AP, Fogg F, Samson HJ, Copeman M, Russell MA, Feyerabend C, Williams GT. **Effect of nicotine on rectal mucus and mucosal eicosanoids.** Gut. 1994 Feb 1;35(2):247-51.

Chapter 4
Straight talk

I believe physicians have fallen into an incorrect pattern of using steroids without considering other therapeutic options. The toxicity associated with oral steroids occurs so frequently and is so severe that physicians should now take another look at administering these agents indiscriminately. **~Present, 2000**

T alk about a mine field! I will need to be careful what I say here! I'll do my best. But I will be bold! As we continue, please keep in mind I am in favor of the use of drug therapy in the battle against ulcerative colitis and I hold physicians in high regard. With that out of the way . . .

The physician is and should be trained in the skillful use of drugs, even the skillful use of dangerous drugs—the more skillful the better! And drug therapy is by far the easiest route to take. All it takes is a patient in need, an exceptional intellect, a terrific, intense education, a license, a current trend, and a pen and pad of paper. And, certainly, people are helped, oftentimes quite dramatically. But sometimes people do not respond as anticipated, and some are seriously harmed. And Medicine, even Medicine, longs for something else. There *is* something else, and it is right under its nose. "Something else" can be found in the research literature. It is called alternative and complementary therapies. But there are barriers raised when it comes to embracing the use of alternatives.

The pressures to rely primarily and almost exclusively on drugs, including the use of drugs to treat the symptoms created by the use of drugs, is very strong in our society. The public, even the physician, has been conditioned to expect this—saturated with incoming messages that a drug is the answer to all our medical needs. Too few individuals want to drastically change their lifestyle, alter their diet in a profound way, or forsake their negative habits in order to manage a disease. So, what then are physicians to do? By far, the easiest thing to do is to prescribe drugs and focus on drug therapy to address the problems that come to their attention. Are you getting the point? I certainly hope so.

My goal in writing this chapter, indeed writing the entire book, is to encourage individuals—patient and physician alike—to start doing other things. Experiment! You, the patient, are being experimented on anyway (and the physician is experimenting on everyone who walks through the office door). Have you heard "let's try this" enough times to make you sick? Admittedly, drug therapy is trial and error (Terry et al., 2009), as the right dosage, the right drug, and the right combination of drugs is frequently under review. But stick with the drug route and little else, say I, unless you are exceptionally motivated to do something different (and can get your physician to climb on board).

I do not want to seem too critical of a profession I highly respect and greatly admire, but I do need to point out a few problems that are, admittedly, associated with the drugs in current use—particularly those used to treat ulcerative colitis. I will let the chips fall where they may. Keep in mind, Medicine knows the truth of what I am saying.

Just where am I going with all this? I want this little chapter to be a pep talk, not only for you but also for the physician. Drug therapy has its advantages along with its pitfalls. In view of the pitfalls, there is a clear need to reduce our dependency on drugs, drugs that can help but can also harm. *"Carve out opportunities to do this,"* say I. In my mind, speaking of ways to limit the use of dangerous drugs is a *very* noble thing. Furthermore, questioning the drug-only approach to ulcerative colitis— particularly when there are so many complementary and alternative therapies available—is also a *very* noble thing.

So, what follows, is a little motivational talk, taken directly from the medical literature and placed here with the hopes that you will pay close attention to the various therapies and strategies we will discuss within the pages of this book. These are therapies and strategies that may allow an individual to limit or possibly avoid the use of immunosuppressants and biologics in his or her personal battle against ulcerative colitis. Listen to what the experts say about conventional therapy:

> *Current treatment [of IBD] relies heavily on corticosteroids and broad-spectrum immunosuppressives that have significant side effects. The situation is unsatisfactory for both the patient and the attending physician.* (Hunter and McKay, 2004, emphasis added)

> *The toxic side effects of steroids are marked and include cushingoid features, psychological effects (including euphoria, inability to sleep and steroid psychosis), ocular effects (including cataracts and glaucoma), peptic disease, hypertension, diabetes, dermatological problems (including acne and stria), myopathy, osteoporosis, aseptic necrosis of the hip of other joints, and increased susceptibility to infections and renal calculi, including others.* (Present, 2000)

There's more:

> *Modern-day therapeutics for IBD have limited efficacy and are not without their danger.* (Weinstock and Elliott, 2009, emphasis added)

> *Modern therapy, especially biological therapy, is both expensive and potentially dangerous, and yet only a subgroup of IBD patients gain significant clinical benefit.* (Colombel et al., 2008)

> *Because they suppress the immune system, all biologics carry an increased risk of infections, which in rare cases can be serious. Cimzia, Humira, and Remicade carry a boxed warning for increased risk of serious infections leading to hospitalization or death. If*

*someone taking a biologic develops a serious infection, the drug
should be discontinued. People with tuberculosis, heart failure, or
multiple sclerosis should not take biologics because they can bring
on these conditions or make them worse.*

*In rare cases, some people taking TNF inhibitors have
developed certain cancers such as lymphoma. Lymphoma is a
type of cancer that affects the lymph system, which is part of the
body's immune system.* (WebMD, 2013, emphasis added)

I think I've made my point here. And by now, no doubt you have a
sense as to why I have strong feelings regarding the reliance principally
upon drugs and little else in the treatment of disease, any disease! And
we're in luck! With respect to ulcerative colitis, there are many
alternative and complementary therapies available to battle this disease.
You will see.

An excellent guide

It is probably safe to assume that you are currently taking
medications to treat your ulcerative colitis. And things may be going
quite well in this respect. Congratulations! But there *are* things you
should know. The following is an excellent guide on IBD medications,
and the side affects you should be aware of. You can find this guide on
the web by searching for it by title. It is presented by the Crohn's &
Colitis Foundation of America, so we know it can be trusted. You really
should do this! Search for:

—Understanding IBD Medications and Side Effects
https://www.crohnscolitisfoundation.org/sites/default/files/legacy/
assets/pdfs/understanding-ibd-medications-brochure-final.pdf

~*References*~

Colombel JF, Watson AJ, Neurath MF. **The 10 remaining mysteries of inflammatory bowel disease.** Gut. 2008 Apr 1;57(4):429-33.

Hunter MM, McKay DM. **Helminths as therapeutic agents for inflammatory bowel disease. Alimentary pharmacology & therapeutics.** 2004 Jan;19(2):167-77.

Present DH. **How to do without steroids in inflammatory bowel disease. Inflammatory bowel diseases.** 2000 Feb 1;6(1):48-57.

Terry PD, Villinger F, Bubenik GA, Sitaraman SV. **Melatonin and ulcerative colitis: evidence, biological mechanisms, and future research. Inflammatory bowel diseases.** 2009 Jan 1;15(1):134-40.

*Web*MD **Taking a Biologic for Crohn's Disease: Risks and Benefits.** 2005-2013

Weinstock JV, Elliott DE. **Helminths and the IBD hygiene hypothesis. Inflammatory bowel diseases.** 2009 Jan 1;15(1):128-33.

Chapter 5
Good news! Healing is possible

The mucosal lesion in active colitis is characterized by intense inflammatory cell infiltrate, crypt abscesses, mucin depletion, and surface ulceration. <u>During the healing phase</u> epithelial continuity is restored, the infiltrate and abscesses begin to resolve, and epithelial mucin content improves. **~Riley et al., 1991, emphasis added**

Mucosal healing in IBD is therefore a tightly controlled process associated with suppression of inflammation and improvement of intestinal function. **~Neurath and Travis, 2012**

We are now nearing the therapy portion of the book—and we know healing can occur, we know how to read. After the last chapter, I thought we could use a more positive chapter, so I came up with this one.

As we enter our discussion of the alternative and complementary therapies, I want you to keep in mind (like, never forget) <u>the fundamental problem</u> in ulcerative colitis. **The fundamental problem in ulcerative colitis is a disruption of the mucus layer of protection, allowing bacteria to be where they should not be, leading to an ongoing inflammatory response (war)**. But there are other things I want you to keep in mind.

Although the battle you are experiencing may have begun out of necessity, its continuation is not at all as it should be. Initial efforts to achieve resolution have failed. And **over time, and in the absence of remission and presence of ongoing threat, ulcerative colitis is self-perpetuating, taking on a life of its own.** Non-resolving inflammation leads to more non-resolving inflammation, and the end of all the madness seems nowhere in sight.

Due to a variety of factors, your initial inflammatory response has evolved into an exaggerated, dysregulated catastrophe—aided by defective genetics, faulty living, and continual threat. And you are still dealing with the same problem you started out with—the absence or disruption of the mucus layer of protection in locations along the rectum and colon *and* bacteria living on or acting upon the surface of intestinal epithelial cells, invading or threatening invasion. Of course, it takes war to control all the madness.

But even so, healing is possible, even in difficult cases. Indeed, *"The mucosa of the colon is more likely to heal in patients with ulcerative colitis than in those with Crohn's disease."* (de Chambrun et al., 2010) And we're in luck! The *". . . current goal of IBD therapy has been set to 'mucosal healing', instead of improvement in clinical symptoms."* (Okamoto, 2011) Unfortunately, this goal was not always the goal medicine had in mind.

Before, say 2001, it was thought that symptom control in ulcerative colitis was good enough, and the control of symptoms became the therapeutic goal (Kane et al., 2009)—who can argue with the absence of symptoms and a life returned to normal? But given time, a change in thought has occurred. (We came to our senses.) It became clear, and is now well-established, that symptom control, while noble and essential, is no guarantee the disease process has stopped and the danger has passed. The disease can continue under the radar, silent yet unresolved. In the absence of microscopic healing, relapse is much more likely to occur. Also, in the absence of microscopic healing, colorectal cancer is more likely to complicate and possibly destroy a life (Bryant et al., 2014). So, merely controlling symptoms and taking a wait-and-see attitude (and keeping fingers crossed) is no longer acceptable. Thankfully, microscopic healing is now the goal, a goal most noble and clearly within reach. *This should be your goal!*

Fortunately, we have several drugs that have a good track record of achieving remission, even microscopic healing! (see Neurath and Travis, 2012) This *is* good news. And although this book will discuss alternatives to drug therapy, drug therapy is certainly an acceptable route to take, even in view of the side effects (my opinion). That being said, I believe a better route to take is to carefully combine the best drug therapy has to offer with the best alternative and complementary therapies have to offer—**with the goal of making drug therapy more effective, perhaps of shorter duration, or perhaps, under certain circumstances, completely unnecessary.** This viewpoint seems very reasonable, given the knowledge we currently have, and the existence of many successful alternative and complementary modalities found in the medical literature.

So, all things under consideration, let's begin our tour of the promising alternatives to the drugs-and-little-else approach to ulcerative colitis. We'll take a deep dive into the medical literature, and we'll come up with at least something I'm sure can help you in the battle against ulcerative colitis. And in all this, we'll do our best to deal with the fundamental problem in ulcerative colitis. And we'll be all into healing.

> *The structural basis of mucosal healing is an intact barrier function of the gut epithelium that prevents translocation of commensal bacteria into the mucosa and submucosa with subsequent immune cell activation.* (Neurath and Travis, 2012)

What to expect

In the management of ulcerative colitis, drug therapy does have a pretty impressive track record. Here, I will share the statistics of remission associated with the various drugs in current use in the battle against ulcerative colitis. Be aware, the statistics I share, although relatively recent, may not be the latest statistics available. Also, be aware I will not be mentioning the statistics on the degree of risk these medications pose, at least not here. So, here are the favorability statistics on current drug therapy:

—**5-aminosalicylates** (5-ASA; Asacol; Pentasa; sulfasalazine, and others) may allow as many as **78%** of patients achieve mucosal healing within 8 weeks. (Neurath and Travis, 2012)

—**Steroids** (prednisone; etc.)—high dose—may allow as many as **30%** of patients achieve remission. (Neurath and Travis, 2012)

—**Azathioprine** (AZA; Imuran; Azafalk; Azapress) use may achieve mucosal healing in **69%** of patients placed on this medication. (Neurath and Travis, 2012)

—**Calcineurin inhibitors** (cyclosporine; tacrolimus) may allow **44%** of patients receiving these drugs to achieve mucosal healing (Neurath and Travis, 2012).

—**Biologicals** (Infliximab; Remicade; Humira) may allow mucosal healing to occur in as many as **62%** of patients placed on Infliximab, and in **42%** of patients placed on Humara. (Neurath and Travis, 2012)

The intestinal epithelial cell during healing

The capacity for the epithelial cell to play a role in healing is truly amazing. Remission does not take place without the extraordinary efforts of this cell. When conditions are just right, these cells will change their shape, transforming from a stubby, "sausage-like" form into a more flattened, "pancake-like" shape. (I'm a little hungry at the moment.) Remarkably, *"epithelial cells surrounding the wound lose their columnar polarity, take on a flattened morphology, and rapidly migrate into the denuded area to restore barrier integrity."* (Iizuka and Konno, 2011) Then, the intestinal epithelial cells will multiply like crazy

(Iizuka and Konno, 2011). (More pancakes?) Finally, the cells transform themselves back into stubby little sausages, resuming the life of a normal intestinal epithelial cell (Iizuka and Konno, 2011).

So, you see, healing *is* possible. The intestinal epithelial cell will do it for you. It only needs to be given a chance. As for me, it's time for breakfast.

Once remission is achieved . . .

Confidence is high, if you're new to ulcerative colitis, with proper medical management you will go into remission—and hopefully soon! But relapse does occur . . . and all too often.

> *For the patient being treated with UC,* **70%** *with active disease are likely to relapse with another flair within the following year while* **30%** *in remission are likely to relapse within the following year.* (Good and Panas, 2015, emphasis added)

Once achieved, what can be done to maintain remission? Ongoing drug therapy may be required. Alternately, you may be able to succeed with one or more of the alternative and complementary approaches we will discuss in the chapters to follow. Before you act, however, get your physician's approval first. As you continue reading, you will be impressed with all that can be done that can give you an edge and help you achieve and maintain remission.

What does remission look like?

> *. . . in UC patients with active disease, bacteria were shown to be in contact with epithelial cells, while almost all patients in remission showed a thicker mucus barrier and bacterial penetration similar to that of healthy subjects.* (Ijssennagger et al., 2016)

~References~

Bryant RV, Winer SS, Travis SP, Riddell RH. **Systematic review: Histological remission in inflammatory bowel disease. Is 'complete' remission the new treatment paradigm? An IOIBD initiative.** Journal of Crohn's and Colitis. 2014 Dec 1;8(12):1582-97.

de Chambrun GP, Peyrin-Biroulet L, Lémann M, Colombel JF. **Clinical implications of mucosal healing for the management of IBD.** Nature reviews Gastroenterology & hepatology. 2010 Jan;7(1):15.

Good L, Panas R. **Case series investigating the clinical practice experience of serum-derived bovine immunoglobulin/protein isolate (SBI) in the clinical management of patients with inflammatory bowel disease.** J Gastrointest Dig Syst. 2015;5(2):268.

Iizuka M, Konno S. **Wound healing of intestinal epithelial cells.** World journal of gastroenterology: WJG. 2011 May 7;17(17):2161.

Ijssennagger N, van der Meer R, van Mil SW. **Sulfide as a mucus barrier-breaker in inflammatory bowel disease?.** Trends in molecular medicine. 2016 Mar 1;22(3):190-9.

Kane S, Lu F, Kornbluth A, Awais D, Higgins PD. **Controversies in mucosal healing in ulcerative colitis. Inflammatory bowel diseases.** 2009 Feb 11;15(5):796-800.

Neurath MF, Travis SP. **Mucosal healing in inflammatory bowel diseases: a systematic review.** Gut. 2012 Jan 1:gutjnl-2012.

Okamoto R. **Epithelial regeneration in inflammatory bowel diseases.** Inflammation and Regeneration. 2011;31(3):275-81.

Riley SA, Mani V, Goodman MJ, Dutt S, Herd ME. **Microscopic activity in ulcerative colitis: what does it mean?.** Gut. 1991 Feb 1;32(2):174-8.

Chapter 6

Serum-Derived Bovine Immunoglobulin Therapy (SBI)

An impaired intestinal barrier allows unprocessed luminal antigens to interact with the mucosal immune system, thereby leading to an abnormal immune response.

Proinflammatory cytokines can disassemble the tight junction proteins, resulting in a further increase of epithelial permeability, which triggers and perpetuates local inflammation in IBD.

The present study shows that **SBI inclusion reduces the mucosal expression of inflammatory cytokines and prevents the increase in crypt permeability associated to the colitis syndrome.** ~Pérez-Bosque et al., 2015, emphasis added

SBI is uniquely composed of immunoglobulins which remain biologically active throughout the GI tract and have affinity for common intestinal antigens associated with GI inflammation. ~Detzel et al., 2015

Immunoglobins are protein molecules that function as antibodies against many pathogenic as well as potential pathogenic microorganisms. ~Rountree, 2002

My initial thought was to place this chapter later in the book, but I decided to place it here because I could wait no longer to tell you about **Serum-Derived Bovine Immunoglobulin/Protein Isolate (SBI)**. There is so much promise here! And this therapy has a track record of rescuing people in whom drug therapy has failed. So, what is it, this thing called SBI?

SBI is a medicinal food product derived from bovine (cow) blood—sounds kinda gross, but if you eat meat, you are eating blood. So, relax. Besides, SBI is a purified product; and, as such, is probably a lot safer and healthier than that big fat juicy steak you ate the other day, and with no intention of sharing with me. (I notice these things.) This product is classified as a food, and has no known negative interaction with drug therapy. In fact, you can take SBI along with your usual ulcerative colitis medications without concern that it will interfere with their actions. And you may want to, should your current medication(s) be underperforming, the side effects are too much to bear, or you just cannot live with the thought of relapse.

So, what does SBI do?

The mode of action for this specially formulated bovine immunoglobin preparation is multifaceted. SBI binds microbial components, maintains GI immune balance, manages gut barrier function and improves nutrient utilization. (Shafran et al., 2015)

SBI is a high protein dietary supplement that is jam-packed with immunoglobulins, IgG, IgA, and IgM (Detzel et al., 2015). These are some of the same, beneficial ingredients found in breast milk—particularly concentrated in mother's first milk, known as **colostrum** (Hurley and Theil, 2011). So, perhaps taking clues from this form of therapy (yes, breast milk, colostrum included, is therapy for the newborn baby), a new treatment for IBD has emerged.

Immunoglobulins, by their innate action of 1) binding bacteria (Van Arsdall et al., 2016), 2) binding bacterial breakdown components (Beauerle et al., 2015), and 3) binding bacterial toxins (Arikapudi et al., 2017), form complexes too large to pass beyond the not-so-tight-because-of-disease junctions that exist between neighboring intestinal epithelial cells (Beauerle et al., 2015), and are eventually flushed away.

Immunoglobulins, by their presence and actions within the bowel, reduce the immune response required to deal with all the madness. Less immune system stimulation means less immune-cell activation and an increased opportunity for healing programs to be set in motion. Someone gets to life a normal life. Sound good? Let's review a few case reports.

Case report: Kayla

We'll call her Kayla. Kayla is 14 years old at the moment. She has plans for her life, plans that do not include 20 bloody, watery mucus-laden stools daily, and which is currently occupying so much of her time. Over the past 6 months she endured abdominal pain, decreased appetite, and incurred a 10-pound weight loss due to her illness. Surprise, surprise! After a comprehensive workup, Kayla received the diagnosis of ulcerative colitis. She also received excellent, standard medical care—an initial series of mesalamine enemas, sulfasalazine 4 times a day, and a short course of prednisone. Yet despite all this, a repeat colonoscopy performed 7 months after the initiation of therapy demonstrated persistent inflammation. This finding lead to more steroids and a switch from sulfasalazine to oral mesalamine.

Three months into Kayla's revised treatment regime, no real symptomatic improvement occurred. It was time to do something different. SBI is something different.

Kayla was started on a nightly course of SBI, a product called **EnteraGam®**, 5 grams of which was added to her treatment plan, taken nightly. Mesalamine was continued. And guess what? *"Crampy abdominal symptoms, blood in the stools, and diarrhea resolved within 2 months of SBI intake."* (Soriano and Ramos-Soriano, 2017) Furthermore, a follow-up colonoscopy revealed a normal looking colon. In addition, biopsy findings *"demonstrated a normal colonic mucosa showing no* *significant inflammatory activity."* (Soriano and Ramos-Soriano, 2017) I am impressed.

Read the entire story in an article entitled, *Clinical and Pathologic Remission of Pediatric Ulcerative Colitis with Serum-Derived Bovine Immunoglobin Added to the Standard Treatment Regime*, written by Soriano and Ramos-Soriano, 2017. Just type this title in the Google search box, and before you know it, the article will magically appear. As a bonus, this article shows before and after colonoscopy pictures on page 342—very impressive! Print out this article and share it with your physician. See what happens. Maybe it's time to be a little assertive. It's your colon, right?

Case report: Brenda

We'll give this individual the name Brenda. This is her story. She is 60 years old at this point in time, but this has not always been the case and is certain to change. (I'm seeing if you are paying attention.)

Brenda is lucky, compared to Kayla, as she is having only 8 watery, bloody stools per day to deal with. And I mean each and every day! Additionally, abdominal cramping also frequently occurs.

Prior to her present illness, Brenda had been treated for pan- (all over) colitis, and for the past couple of years she had achieved and maintained remission thanks to anti-TNF therapy (Humira). But things they would change, and not for the good.

Brenda developed a knee infection that required antibiotic therapy to address this issue. Due to this unfortunate turn of events, anti-TNF therapy was discontinued. She also underwent multiple surgeries to wash out the infection in her knee. If all that wasn't enough, during all this, Brenda twice developed an enteric (gut) bacterial infection caused by *C. difficile* (*C-diff*). This is an often-encountered occurrence associated with antibiotic therapy, and it can kill. Brenda's *C-diff* was successfully managed with vancomycin.

Following a successful management of her knee infection, Brenda began to experience what was likely to be a flare of ulcerative colitis symptoms. Steroids, given in response, were prescribed yet failed to reduce her symptoms. Two years prior, Brenda was kept in remission by anti-TNF therapy. So, in view of an apparent return of her ulcerative colitis (a test for *C-diff* was negative), restarting anti-TNF therapy was placed under serious consideration. But this time, she wanted none of this.

Apparently, Brenda credited anti-TNF therapy for a serious bout of septic arthritic knee and did not want to experience *this* ever again. In view of her previous experience with anti-TNF therapy, she was offered EnteraGam®—good call! In addition, she was also prescribed a higher dose of steroids, (despite the fact they were previously ineffective). Perhaps not surprisingly (to Kayla), before the start of EnteraGam®, Brenda began to experience *"10 to 15 watery stools per day, accompanied by frequent bleeding during the approximately 3-week period on the higher steroid dose."* (Beauerle et al., 2015) Her EnteraGam® dose was 5 grams 4 times a day for one week, then 5 grams daily. Good news was on the horizon.

"At the follow-up, four-weeks after initiating SBI (EnteraGam®), the patient reported 1–2 formed bowel movements per day. She denied rectal bleeding and abdominal cramps." (Beauerle et al., 2015) Three cheers for Brenda! And three cheers for her physician!

At two months (only two months, mind you) after initiating SBI therapy, a colonoscopy was performed. Brenda's colon looked completely normal, with no evidence of disease.

One year later, maintained only on SBI, 5 grams per day (no medication), Brenda remains symptom free. Remember hearing me say, "Healing is possible?" Now do you believe me?

This story is also available free on the internet. In the article reporting Brenda's story, there are the before and after images of her transformed colon. Search for this article in the same manner you searched for the article featuring Kayla's story, using the title *Successful Management of Refractory Ulcerative Colitis with Orally Administrated Serum-Derived Bovine Immunoglobulin Therapy.* It was written by Beauerle et al.

Case report: Aaron

After much thought (not really), I gave our next ulcerative colitis patient the name Aaron. Aaron was 24, at a time he had had it with loose/watery stools. "The madness needs to end! I have other things to do! Let someone else do all the suffering! *Why me?*" With thoughts like these, it was high time to get things under control.

In one respect, Aaron may have been one very fortunate individual, given the fact that he was caught early-on in the disease process and did not require aggressive drug therapy, such as steroids and anti-TNF biologicals, to salvage what is left of him. He was started on mesalamine suppositories in addition to SBI. Why wait to start SBI? Why wait for the more powerful drugs to be given the opportunity to fail? (And they do fail, quite frequently.) Apparently, SBI can be started at any point during the disease process. And in Aaron's case, the results of early intervention with SBI along with first-response therapy (mesalamine), was very, very satisfying.

> At the follow-up exam, no diarrhea (loose/water stools) or rectal blood was noted. The mesalamine suppositories were discontinued but the patient was continued on the SBI therapy at 5 g/day. At 3 months of SBI therapy, the patient remained asymptomatic. Because the patient was well managed, no follow up sigmoidoscopy was performed. The patient continues to be asymptomatic and has remained on SBI therapy at 5 g/day for approximately 9 months. (Good and Panas, 2015)

Aaron's story can be found in the paper entitled, *Case Series Investigating the Clinical Practice Experience of Serum-Derived Bovine*

Immunoglobulin/Protein Isolate (SBI) in the Clinical Management of Patients with Inflammatory Bowel Disease by Good and Panas, 2015. It is available free on the net. Search for it in the usual fashion.

I just glanced at the clock and it looks like we have time for one more SBI success story. I will tell you about the individual I have named Bill.

Case report: Bill

Bill was 26 years at the time he was diagnosed with moderately severe pan-ulcerative colitis. The symptoms he was experiencing prior to diagnosis is a tightly held secret, perhaps too ghastly to mention in the article featuring his story. Following diagnosis, he was placed on oral and rectal mesalamine and received repeated doses of steroids. This combination therapy was continued for a year. And each time the physician tried to wean the steroids, Bill would experience 5–10 loose, bloody stools per day. And like Aaron, Bill had other things to do. Even after adding adalimumab (Humira) to the mix, and tapering off steroids, he would still experience flares of cramping, loose stools, and rectal bleeding. Well, something else needed to be done. Bill was not responding to conventional therapy. "So, let's try more conventional therapy!"

In order to manage these repeated flares different therapeutic regimens consisting of oral and rectal mesalamines, antibiotics (ciprofloxin and metronidazole), probiotics and oral steroids were attempted for nearly 8 months. (Awad and Jasion, 2015)

"Okay, things aren't working out too well here! Now it's time to really get serious!" So, in the fullness of time, SBI was started—prescribed at a dose of 5g twice daily. After 8 weeks, Bill was delighted to report 1–2 formed stools per day, and without any symptom of ulcerative colitis. And the rest is history.

He [Bill] was completely removed from oral steroids at this time and SBI was decreased to 5 g QD [once daily]. The patient continued to do well and has remained on adalimumab, oral mesalamine and SBI 5g QD for the past year. He remains in a complete clinical and endoscopic remission. Colonoscopy was performed a year after starting SBI during which time quiescent colitis was observed with no active inflammation. Random biopsies confirmed chronic inactive colitis. (Awad and Jason, 2015).

This story, including both before and after colonoscopy photos as well as other case reports, can be found in: *Use of a Nutritional Therapy, Serum-Derived Bovine Immunoglobulin/Protein Isolate (SBI), to Achieve Improvement in Two Different Cases of Colitis*, written by Awad and Jason and published in 2015. Search, find, read, rejoice, share.

So, I may have piqued your interest in SBI. If you want to try this form of therapy, you'll need to discuss this with your physician. EnteraGam® is available only by prescription. You will probably need to arm yourself with knowledge, with papers, and with a printout or two from the company, **Entera Health, Incorporated**. Go to enteragam.com and explore the website. There are a number of videos to watch while on this website.

Besides EnteraGam®, there are two other SBI products available that I should mention. One is called **IgG Plus®**. This product is promoted by **Extreme Immunity** at www.extremeimmunity.com, and appears to be very similar to EnteraGam®. It is available in both powder and encapsulated form. The other SBI product, similar to EnteraGam®, is called **SBI Protect**, available from **Ortho Molecular Products** at https://www.orthomolecularproducts.com/. SBI Protect is available in both powder and encapsulated form. One advantage of IgG Plus® and SBI Protect is a prescription is not required for purchase. One disadvantage: With no prescription requirement, an individual is tempted to go out on his or her own and not first seek and obtain physician approval. My recommendation is that you work with a physician in all things in the treatment of ulcerative colitis. Mistakes can be made. Things can be overlooked. Feathers can be ruffled. Are we clear?

EnteraGam® TV

Although the EnteraGam® website (http://enteragam.com/) has all the videos on SBI you will ever need, YouTube is another source. I like the convenience of YouTube. I recommend:

—**EnteraGam® MOA animation** – General (2015)
https://www.youtube.com/watch?v=EQITOgLNpQ4

—**EnteraGam® MOA Tight Junction Proteins** – General (2016)
https://www.youtube.com/watch?v=Zf4C-Plk908

This may be of help

I mentioned **colostrum** earlier, near the beginning of this chapter. It, too, contains immunoglobulins, particularly IgG (Solomons, 2002). In addition, colostrum contains other components that are believed to be helpful in reducing inflammation and promoting healing in ulcerative colitis. These include growth factors and antimicrobial factors, such as lactoferrin, lysozyme and lactoperoxidase (Pakkanen and Aalto, 1997). And it's not like colostrum has not been previously considered in the battle against ulcerative colitis. It has.

There are several reports on YouTube and in the lay press that claim colostrum is useful in the treatment of ulcerative colitis. And one study in the medical literature takes colostrum to a whole other level. In this study, bovine colostrum was given as an enema. They report:

We have shown, in this initial study, using a double-blind, randomized protocol, that colostral enemas induced a rapid reduction in symptom scores and disease remission in a large proportion of patients with active left-sided colitis, when administered in combination with the 5-aminosalicylic acid mesalazine. In contrast, patients receiving mesalazine with placebo enema showed minimal improvement. (Khan et al., 2002)

Perhaps taking a colostrum supplement, per your physician's direction, along with EnteraGam® (or IgG Plus®), may synergistically help usher in remission. Seems logical. Perhaps after achieving remission with EnteraGam®, one could use colostrum to maintain remission. This course of action would be a cost-saving measure, as EnteraGam® is relatively expensive.

Colostrum is more fragile than EnteraGam®, more at risk for damage by stomach acidity. So, some proponents recommend enteric-coated colostrum. You can easily find enteric-coated colostrum online. Or you can enteric coat colostrum all by yourself. If you cannot find enteric coated colostrum, I have the solution. I'll share my enteric re-encapsulation method with you in the gray box at the end of the following chapter.

One colostrum-based product, **IgG Protect®**, appears promising as it is a highly concentrated formula of the good things found in colostrum, including IgG, lactoferrin (an iron-binding and anti-inflammatory molecule), proline-rich peptides (regulators and modulators of cytokines), and growth factors that aid in promoting repair and reducing intestinal permeability. It is available from **Ortho Molecular Products.** https://www.orthomolecularproducts.com/igg-protect/ . Physician approval first!

Oh! One last thing. If I were you, I wouldn't do the colostrum enema thing without first seeking physician approval and guidance. You need to work closely with a physician to make sure it is appropriate and is done correctly.

A place for lactoferrin

*Lf [lactoferrin], a natural compound of mammalian secretions, exerts a plethora of biological activities. Its protective effects range from direct **antimicrobial** activities against a variety of pathogens, including bacteria, viruses, fungi and parasites, to **anti-inflammatory** and anti-tumor activities. These multiple functions rely not only on the capacity of Lf to **bind iron** but also on its marked capacity to interact with molecular and cellular components of both host and pathogens.*

Lf can also favor the activation, differentiation, and proliferation of immune cells, and this promoting activity has been related to a direct effect of Lf on immune cells through the recognition of specific Lf binding sites.
~Puddu et al., 2009, emphasis added

It would appear, lactoferrin is underappreciated as a therapy for ulcerative colitis. The reason I suggest this, is I never see it promoted as an adjunct therapy for this disease. I think it should at least be investigated to see if it can come to the aid of the ulcerative colitis patient. Lactoferrin is a generally safe therapy, and doses as high as 7.2 grams/day has been used in the treatment of hepatitis C (Okada et al., 2002) and doses as high as 9 grams/day have been used in the treatment of cancer (Wolf et al., 2007). Lactoferrin binds iron, withholding it from pathogens (Puddu et al., 2009). Iron withholding is a valuable host defense against pathogens (Nairz et al., 2010). Lactoferrin can also bind and inactivate LPS, the wall component of Gram-negative bacteria, and in so doing reduce inflammatory responses generated by LPS exposure (Ono et al., 2010; Ho et al., 2013). Furthermore, lactoferrin can disturb biofilm formation, disrupting a mechanism bacteria can use to protect themselves from attack and to promote colonization (Singh et al., 2002).

Additionally, lactoferrin decreases intestinal epithelial barrier permeability and strengthens barrier function (Zhad et al., 2019)—just one of the many reasons to take a good hard look at lactoferrin.

As far as ulcerative colitis is concerned, lactoferrin seems to work in experimental models of this disease. In one study, using rats, one group of investigators were able to successfully use oral lactoferrin to treat experimental colitis and report: *"Oral administration of lactoferrin in TNBS-treated rats attenuated all of the inflammatory responses."* (Togawa et al., 2002)

Lactoferrin supplementation sounds like an ideal therapy for ulcerative colitis. However, as in all things, caution is warranted: *"In very high doses, skin rash, loss of appetite, fatigue, chills, and constipation have been reported."* (*Web*MD, 2005-2019) In the future, I hope to see studies and case reports relaying the efficacy of lactoferrin as a successful therapy for ulcerative colitis. Iron binding, and withholding it from pathogens, are reasons enough to conduct such investigations.

~References~

Arikapudi S, Rashid S, Al Almomani LA, Treece J, Baumrucker SJ. **Serum Bovine Immunoglobulin for Chemotherapy-Induced Gastrointestinal Mucositis.** American Journal of Hospice and Palliative Medicine®. 2017 Jan 1:1049909117735831.

Awad A, Jasion VS. **Use of a Nutritional Therapy, Serum-Derived Bovine Immunoglobulin/Protein isolate (SBI), to Achieve Improvement in Two Different Cases of Colitis.** J Gastrointest Dig Syst. 2015;5(2):274.

Beauerle B, Burnett B, Dryden G. **Successful management of refractory ulcerative colitis with orally administered serum-derived bovine immunoglobulin therapy.** Clin Case Rep Rev. 2015;1(4):90–92.

Detzel CJ, Horgan A, Henderson AL, Petschow BW, Warner CD, Maas KJ, Weaver EM. **Bovine immunoglobulin/protein isolate binds pro-inflammatory bacterial compounds and prevents immune activation in an intestinal co-culture model.** PloS One. 2015 Apr 1;10(4):e0120278.

EnteraGam website: http://enteragam.com/

EnteraGam prescription order form: https://www.foundcare.com/wp-content/uploads/2017/09/EnteraGamRxorder-FINAL.pdf

Good L, Panas R. **Case series investigating the clinical practice experience of serum-derived bovine immunoglobulin/protein isolate (SBI) in the clinical management of patients with inflammatory bowel disease.** J Gastrointest Dig Syst. 2015;5(2):268.

Ho S, Pothoulakis C, Wai Koon H. **Antimicrobial peptides and colitis.** Current pharmaceutical design. 2013 Jan 1;19(1):40-7.

Hurley WL, Theil PK. **Perspectives on immunoglobulins in colostrum and milk.** Nutrients. 2011 Apr 14;3(4):442-74.

Khan Z, Macdonald C, Wicks AC, Holt MP, Floyd D, Ghosh S, Wright NA, Playford RJ. **Use of the 'nutriceutical', bovine colostrum, for the treatment of distal colitis: results from an initial study.** Alimentary pharmacology & therapeutics. 2002 Nov 1;16(11):1917-22.

Nairz M, Schroll A, Sonnweber T, Weiss G. **The struggle for iron–a metal at the host–pathogen interface.** Cellular microbiology. 2010 Dec;12(12):1691-702.

Okada S, Tanaka K, Sato T, Ueno H, Saito S, Okusaka T, Sato K, Yamamoto S, Kakizoe T. **Dose-response trial of lactoferrin in patients with chronic hepatitis C.** Japanese Journal of Cancer Research. 2002 Sep;93(9):1063-9.

Ono T, Murakoshi M, Suzuki N, Iida N, Ohdera M, Iigo M, Yoshida T, Sugiyama K, Nishino H. **Potent anti-obesity effect of enteric-coated lactoferrin: decrease in visceral fat accumulation in Japanese men and women with abdominal obesity after 8-week administration of enteric-coated lactoferrin tablets.** British journal of nutrition. 2010 Dec;104(11):1688-95.

Pakkanen R, Aalto J. **Growth factors and antimicrobial factors of bovine colostrum.** International Dairy Journal. 1997 May 1;7(5):285-97.

Pérez-Bosque A, Miró L, Maijó M, Polo J, Campbell J, Russell L, Crenshaw J, Weaver E, Moretó M. **Dietary intervention with serum-derived bovine immunoglobulins protects barrier function in a mouse model of colitis.** American Journal of Physiology-Gastrointestinal and Liver Physiology. 2015 Apr 16;308(12):G1012-8.

Puddu P, Valenti P, Gessani S. **Immunomodulatory effects of lactoferrin on antigen presenting cells.** Biochimie. 2009 Jan 1;91(1):11-8.

Rountree R. **Proven therapeutic benefits of high quality probiotics.** Applied Nutritional Science Reports. 2002;4:1-6.

Shafran I, Burgunder P, Wei D, Young HE, Klein G, Burnett BP. **Management of inflammatory bowel disease with oral serum-derived bovine immunoglobulin.** Therapeutic advances in gastroenterology. 2015 Nov;8(6):331-9.

Singh PK, Parsek MR, Greenberg EP, Welsh MJ. **A component of innate immunity prevents bacterial biofilm development.** Nature. 2002 May;417(6888):552-5.

Solomons NW. **Modulation of the immune system and the response against pathogens with bovine colostrum concentrates.** European Journal of Clinical Nutrition. 2002 Jul 25;56(S3):S24.

Soriano RA, Ramos-Soriano AG. **Clinical and pathologic remission of pediatric ulcerative colitis with serum-derived bovine immunoglobulin added to the**

standard treatment regimen. Case reports in gastroenterology. 2017;11(2):335-43.

Togawa J-I, Nagase H, Tanaka K, Inamori M, Sato S, Saito T, Sekihara H 2002 **Lactoferrin Reduces Colitis in Rats via Modulation of the Immune System and Correction of Cytokine Imbalance.** J Gastroenterol Hepatol; December; 17(12):1291–1298.

Van Arsdall M, Haque I, Liu Y, Rhoads JM. **Is There a Role for the Enteral Administration of Serum-Derived Immunoglobulins in Human Gastrointestinal Disease and Pediatric Critical Care Nutrition?.** Advances in Nutrition. 2016 May 9;7(3):535-43.

Wolf JS, Li G, Varadhachary A, Petrak K, Schneyer M, Li D, Ongkasuwan J, Zhang X, Taylor RJ, Strome SE, O'Malley BW. **Oral lactoferrin results in T cell–dependent tumor inhibition of head and neck squamous cell carcinoma in vivo.** Clinical Cancer Research. 2007 Mar 1;13(5):1601-10.

Zhao X, Xu XX, Liu Y, Xi EZ, An JJ, Tabys D, Liu N. **The in vitro protective role of bovine lactoferrin on intestinal epithelial barrier.** Molecules. 2019 Jan;24(1):148.

Chapter 7
Probiotics

The onset and progress of the disease [UC] are <u>directly</u> influenced by the nature of the intestinal microflora, the intestinal barrier function, and the immunological responses of the host. ~**Sung and Park, 2013, emphasis added**

Gut dysbiosis can be defined as a stable, perturbed ecosystem that has reduced capacity for protection and is associated with disease. ~**McCarville et al., 2016**

Probiotics are live, nonpathogenic bacteria that confer health benefits beyond their nutritional value. ~**Dotan and Rachmilewitz, 2005**

*In addition to competing with pathogens for niches and nutrients, "competitively excluding" disease causing microbes from the host, **certain probiotic bacteria have also been shown to produce potent antimicrobial peptides (bacteriocins) which specifically target the invading pathogen.*** ~**Sleator, 2010, emphasis added**

T he concept is simple enough—send in a bunch of good bacteria to counteract the effects of a bunch of bad bacteria, and all the while creating a little magic. And there is some real science behind doing this. So, let's take a look at what probiotics are all about. Perhaps probiotics are just what you need in your battle against ulcerative colitis.

The promises

*Accumulating evidence demonstrates **that probiotics communicate with the host by modulating key signaling pathways,** such as **NFκB** and MAPK, to either enhance or suppress activation and influence downstream pathways.* **~Thomas and Versalovic, 2010, emphasis added**

The sticky outer mucus surface offers the opportunity for probiotic strains to grow and build protective interlaced layers, preventing bacterial accumulation and microcolony formation on the colorectal surface. **~Chen et al., 2014**

Probiotics are viable agents conferring benefits to the health of the human host. They can provide a beneficial effect on intestinal epithelial cells in numerous ways. ***Some strains can block pathogen entry into the epithelial cell*** *by providing a physical barrier or by creating a mucus barrier; other probiotics maintain intestinal permeability acting on tight junctions. Some probiotic strains produce antimicrobial factors, other strains modulate the immune response.* **~Scaldaferri et al., 2016, emphasis added**

Probiotics are typically bacteria, typically alive, regarded as beneficial, prepared for oral consumption, sent into the GI tract to therapeutically improve the microbiome of the host and to create special effects that benefit the host. I can give an example.

One probiotic strain, *Lactobacillus* GG, *"has shown beneficial effects on intestinal immunity, it increases the number of cells that secrete immunoglobulin G and other immunoglobulins in the intestinal mucosa, and it stimulates the local release of interferon."* (D'Souza et al., 2002) You might not remember *"interferon"* because I haven't mentioned it before, but you are sure to remember *"immunoglobulin G"*—we talked about it in *Chapter 6* (please review). My hunch? You could use some immunoglobin G right about now.

So, what are the promises offered by probiotics, promises that if kept, shall we say, hold promise in the battle against ulcerative colitis. Here is a list of the beneficial actions attributed to various probiotics:

- *"Suppression of pathogen growth through release of antimicrobial factors such as lactic and acetic acid, hydrogen peroxide, and bacteriocins."* (Fedorak and Madsen, 2004)

- Inhibition of pathogen adherence to intestinal epithelial cells (Dotan and Rachmilewitz, 2005)

- Reduction of intestinal inflammation by *"directly blocking the signaling pathways hijacked by pathogens."* (Thomas and Versalovic, 2010)

- Competition with receptors that identify pathogenic bacteria, thereby reducing a provoked inflammatory response (Fedorak and Madsen, 2004; Shanahan, 2010)

- Promotion of mucus production (Mach, 2006)

- Promotion of epithelial barrier integrity by positively influencing the junctions between epithelial cells (Thomas and Versalovic, 2010; Shanahan, 2010)

- Reduction of proinflammatory cytokine production, including inhibiting NF-κB activation (Shanahan, 2010; Thomas and Versalovic, 2010)

- Stimulation of anti-inflammatory pathways (Mach, 2006)

- Stimulation of anti-inflammatory cytokine production, including IL-10 and TGF-β (Fedorak and Madsen, 2004; Mach, 2006)

- Expansion of immune cells that act to suppress inflammation (e.g., Treg cells) (Van den Abbeele et al., 2013; Dwivedi et al., 2016

- Capacity to adhere to the intestinal epithelial cell (thereby blocking the adherence of other bacteria) (Kumari et al., 2015)

- Suppression of pathogen generated biofilms (biofilm, a tight-knit bacterial colony protectively enclosed in a protective film-like structure) (Chen et al., 2014)

- Colonization in *"protective interlaced layers, preventing bacterial accumulation and microcolony formation on the colorectal surface."* (Chen et al., 2014)

- Competitive exclusion of pathogens by competing for space and nutrients (Sleator, 2010)

The above list of probiotic actions is probably more than you need to know, but your physician may read this book and appreciate this review. For you, the layperson, the take-home message is simple: Probiotics have a lot of positive actions to offer the individual with ulcerative colitis. Now if we can only get them to work. Some experts hold the view that probiotics have little to offer in achieving remission in ulcerative colitis (Sang et al., 2010), believing that they are not very effective under the circumstances of a disease that is so aggressive and hell-bent on destruction (Bengmark, 2010). Besides, there are problems that one may encounter when taking probiotics, problems you should be aware of.

The downside

The combined results demonstrate conclusively that ingested strains [of probiotic bacteria] do not become established members of the normal *microbiota but **persist only during periods of dosing or for relative short periods thereafter.*** ~Corthésy et al., 2007, emphasis added

*Other probiotics **increase NF-κB activation** through enhanced translocation into nucleus.* ~Thomas and Versalovic, 2010, emphasis added

Probiotics have a long and impressive record of safety, but there is no such thing as zero risk. ~Shanahan, 2010

The above quotations should be sufficient to warn that probiotics do have drawbacks, making guidance by your physician most appropriate, and probably mandatory. I will list some of the problems associated with the use of probiotics, as follows:

- Not all probiotics produce the same effects, even when they belong to the same species (Almeghaiseeb, 2007)

- Some probiotics antagonize the effects of other probiotics (Shanahan, 2010)

- Not all probiotics come from reputable sources (Shanahan, 2010), and may not be as advertised or be effective. *"**The choice of a high-quality probiotic product is one of the most important factors that determine efficacy of the probiotic.**"* (Kelesidis and Pothoulakis, 2012, emphasis added)

- Probiotics may not be appropriate for those who are seriously ill, due to the risk of probiotic bacterial sepsis (bacteria in the blood) (Verna and Lucak, 2010)

The problem of sepsis, mentioned directly above, is serious business. There are several reports in the medical literature of sepsis caused by probiotic use by immunodeficient individuals, by immunosuppressed individuals (such as occurs while taking anti-TNF-α drugs like Infliximab or other immunosuppressant drugs), and by those who are critically ill

(Verna and Lucak, 2010; Gouriet et al., 2012; Vahabnezhad et al., 2013; Meini et al., 2015). And in so many of the reports, the name *Lactobacillus rhamnosus* GG comes up, the same species mentioned earlier in the chapter. So, be careful with this probiotic! Physician approval and monitoring, a must.

One case report in a patient with <u>severe</u>, <u>active</u> ulcerative colitis, identified *Lactobacillus rhamnosus* GG in his bloodstream, identifying the cause of the sepsis. The patient just so happened to be taking this probiotic species. (Meini et al., 2015) This experience lead to the following precaution: *"Pending conclusive evidence, use of probiotics should be considered with caution in case of active severe inflammatory bowel diseases with mucosal disruption."* (Meini et al., 2015)

Apart from the above precautions, one of the challenges we face, ulcerative colitis or not, is the fact that the bacterial communities we have assembled over the years simply do not want to fade away into the night. They cherish life. They will do all they can to survive. They love to reproduce (like, who doesn't). I suppose, their love of life and family will compel them to kill probiotic bacteria, too, just like they are compelled to kill resident bacteria at first opportunity (see Be'Er et al., 2009). That being said, probiotics, if done right, appear to be beneficial in the battle against ulcerative colitis. However,

> ***The reason why attempts to reduce inflammation with the use of probiotics sometimes failed in the past might be that the pro-inflammatory pressure is simply too high due to the underlying disease, but also due to the consumption of too much of pro-inflammatory foods and prescription drugs, all with inflammation-enhancing abilities.*** (Bengmark, 2010, emphasis added)

The above quotation strongly suggests that addressing inflammation on many fronts may be necessary before the promises of probiotics can be fulfilled.

Your best bet

Several studies have indicated that probiotic preparation, including VSL#3, Escherichia coli Nissle 1917 and Saccharomyces boulardii, can effectively treat active UC. We previously found that bifidobacterium-fermented milk (BFM) containing live Bifidobacterium (Bifidobacterium breve strain Yakult, BbY) is effective in maintaining remission in UC patients and in treating patients with active UC. ~**Ishikawa et al., 2011**

Keeping in mind the positive benefits offered by probiotics as outlined earlier in the chapter, let's get right to it. The following probiotics are the ones most studied with respect to ulcerative colitis. They are also the ones most likely to be ordered or approved by the gastroenterologist.

Nissle 1917

The most extensively studied probiotic in IBD is Escherichia coli Nissle 1917, a strain purportedly isolated from a German soldier in World War I who had withstood a severe outbreak of gastroenteritis that devastated his unit. ~**Korzenik and Podolsky, 2006**

Well, you can't win a battle or win a war while you are pooping your brains out, day in and day out! (Can you identify?) Fortunately for one German soldier, during an outbreak of gastroenteritis in his regiment, he remained healthy while his comrades were filling their pants and dropping like flies. Fortunately for all of humanity, a scientist, Prof. Nissle, in 1917, discovered the reason why. He isolated a unique bacterium from the soldier's stool that apparently protected him from the outbreak. The Professor propagated this *E. coli* strain, and perhaps developed the first probiotic supplement to hit the market. It was sold in 1917, and you can still buy it today in Germany, Italy, and perhaps a few other European countries, under the trade name **Mutaflor®** (Scaldaferri et al., 2016). I looked, and you can purchase it in the USA online. Of note, since this probiotic is a refrigerated product, it should be promptly placed in the refrigerator after the shipment has been received, or it will lose potency. Here are some of the benefits offered by this probiotic:

- Stimulation of beta-defensin 2, *"a molecule that has proven to be crucial in the protection of mucosal barrier against the adhesion and invasion of pathogenic bacterial species."* (Losurdo et al., 2015)

- *"Inhibitory effect towards other pathogenic E coli."* (Scaldaferri et al., 2016)

- Direct killing of other pathogens by producing bacteriocins (Scaldaferri et al., 2016)

- Colonizes quickly and lasts for months after administration (Scaldaferri et al., 2016)

- Ability to displace pathogenic E coli species from attachment sites (Korzenik and Podolsky, 2006).

- Stimulates anti-inflammatory cytokines (Scaldaferri et al., 2016)

- *"Strengthens junctions of intestinal epithelial cells . . . so it has an effect on the repair of the 'leaky gut.'"* (Scaldaferri et al., 2016)

As promising as Nissle 1917 sounds, from what I have read, the evidence is less than robust (weak) to support its effectiveness in achieving and maintaining remission in ulcerative colitis, over standard drug therapy. On the other hand, in some European countries, Nissle 1917 is embraced, and is considered an *"effective alternative to mesalazine in maintenance of remission in UC patients."* (Scaldaferri et al., 2016)

In one early report (Rembacken et al., 1999), which may have influenced the European decision to embrace Nissle 1917 in the battle against ulcerative colitis, this probiotic appeared to show effectiveness in maintaining remission; yet, this study also demonstrated relapse rates that were similar to 5-ASA administration (Langman and Allan, 1999). I'm a little impressed, but I want more.

What about rectal administration of Nissle 1917? No thanks! Okay, maybe. One study showed a shorter time to remission with an enema containing Nissle 1917 compared to placebo (Matthes et al., 2010; Losurdo et al., 2015).

I wish I had a more optimistic view of the effectiveness of Nissle 1917 in the treatment of ulcerative colitis, yet the purported actions are most impressive. It may be that this single strain of probiotic could be combined with other probiotics to achieve greater clinical success. And taking this probiotic could be all it takes to give someone an edge and help them achieve and maintain remission. So, it may be exactly what someone needs. I guess the jury is still out on Nissle 1917. Others may not agree, as there seems to be a strong following for the effectiveness of this probiotic. As for me, before jumping onboard I would like to see studies reporting a better response rate than the studies I have reviewed to date.

Let's move on the next probiotic. It may be a better bet than Nissle 1917 in the treatment of ulcerative colitis.

VSL#3

While Nissle 1917 is the most extensively studied probiotic, the best-known probiotic in clinical use is VSL#3 (Furrie et al., 2005). This probiotic is the "gold standard" for a condition called pouchitis (Losurdo et al., 2015). We'll talk about pouchitis a bit later. But for now, let's focus on VSL#3 as a therapy for ulcerative colitis.

The recognized advantages/actions offered by VSL#3 are:

- Increased expression of genes that promote mucus secretion (Sood et al., 2009)

- Reduction of signaling associated with elevated inflammatory responses (Chapman et al., 2006)

- Increased production of the anti-inflammatory cytokine Il-10 (Chapman et al., 2006; Sood et al., 2009)

- Inhibition of proinflammatory T-cell generation (Chapman et al., 2006)

- Decreased production of the proinflammatory cytokine TNF-α (Sood et al., 2009)

VSL#3 is a combination of eight different probiotic strains. They are alive yet held in suspended animation (freeze-dried). Good luck pronouncing their names. *L paracasei, L plantarum, L acidophilus,* and *L delbrueckii subspecies bulgaricus* are all *Lactobacilli. B longum, B breve,* and *B infantis* belong to the *Bifidobacteria* family. *Streptococcus thermophilus* completes the list of the eight members of the VSL#3 family of good bacteria just waiting to serve (Sood et al., 2009).

In several studies, VSL#3 administration resulted in *"superior"* outcomes, compared to both the use of a placebo and no probiotic treatment at all, in achieving and maintaining remission in various forms of IBD (see Pagnini et al., 2013). This probiotic combination is particularly suitable for children with ulcerative colitis (a patient population you have be careful with because of the dangers that accompany drug therapy) (Huynh et al., 2009), and for those with pouchitis (Losurdo et al., 2015). Based on the evidence, this probiotic appears to be a great option to consider in the treatment of ulcerative colitis.

Back to children for a few moments, one study reports: *"Treatment of pediatric patients diagnosed with mild to moderate UC with VSL#3* resulted in a remission rate of **65%** and a combined remission/response rate of **61%**." (Huynh et al., 2009, emphasis added)

In adults, one study reported treatment of patients with mild to moderate ulcerative colitis, who did not respond to conventional therapy with VSL#3, "resulted in a combined induction of remission/response rates of **77%** with no adverse events." (Bibiloni et al., 2005, emphasis added)

I think it is safe to say that VSL#3 clearly holds promise to those suffering from ulcerative colitis. But it will probably do you no good at all to just read about it. And it will probably be of no value to you if this form of therapy is not embraced by your physician and not offered to you.

Saccharomyces boulardii

> S boulardii has a unique action on inflammation by a specific alteration of the migratory behavior of T cells, which accumulate in mesenteric lymph nodes. Therefore, S boulardii treatment limits the infiltration of T-helper 1 cells in the inflamed colon and the amplification of inflammation induced by proinflammatory cytokines production. **~Dalmasso et al., 2006**

This probiotic is not a bacterium. It is a yeast. It is also something special. It offers the following beneficial actions:

- Neutralization of bacterial toxins (Kelesidis and Pothoulakis, 2012; Zanello et al., 2009)

- "S boulardii acts on the epithelial barrier in improving tight-junctions structure and in restoring membrane permeability disrupted by infectious pathogens." (Zanello et al., 2009)

- Ability to "trap T-cells" in the lymph nodes of the gut, limiting their interaction with other cells and restricting their ability to amplify inflammation (Guslandi, 2010)

- Inhibition or pathogen growth and translocation beyond the epithelial barrier (Kelesidis and Pothoulakis, 2012)

- Reduction in levels of pro-inflammatory cytokines while stimulating the production of IL-10, an anti-inflammatory cytokine (Kelesidis and Pothoulakis, 2012)

- Increase in short-chain fatty acids, the fuel most beneficial to the colonocyte (Zanello et al., 2009)

Similar to ulcerative colitis patients, Crohn's disease patients exhibit an increase in intestinal permeability. In one study, *"Those treated with S. boulardii were found to have a significant reduction in colonic permeability compared with those given placebo, thus reducing the risk of bacterial translocation in these patients."* (Kelesidis and Pothoulakis, 2012)

In another study, 17 out of 24 patients (**68%**) achieved clinical remission, confirmed with endoscopy, by the use of *S. boulardii* (Guslandi et al., 2010). And keep in mind, these were patients with a history of poor tolerance to steroid use. (They must have been the tougher cases.) In this study, the dose of *S. boulardii* was 250 mg, three times a day, for a period of four weeks. I'm impressed.

Others in the mix

Bifidobacteria-fermented milk decreased the relapse rate of UC from 90 to 27%. ~**Bibiloni et al., 2005**

There are other probiotics that we should consider putting to use in our battle against ulcerative colitis. Some have long, difficult-to-pronounce names. These are common bacteria that live in the gut and include the types of bacteria found in yogurt, kefir, and other fermented foods. The names to remember are *bifidobacteria* and *lactobacteria.*

These probiotics can be easily purchased at a supplement store or online. And these probiotics are true warriors:

> *Bifidobacteria and lactobacilli produce harmful substances for Gram-positive and Gram-negative bacteria, and they compete with pathogens (i.e., Clostridium, Bacteriodetes, Staphylococcus, and Enterobacter) for cell adhesion.* (Chen et al., 2014)

So, don't underestimate the commonplace probiotic. The two species mentioned directly above were included in the VSL#3 formula because of their effectiveness in dealing with a problem or two. *Bifidobacteria* and *lactobacilli*, not only produce harmful substances directed against pathogens, they also compete with pathogens for adhesion sites. Furthermore, these probiotics consume soluble fibers to produce butyrate, the energy source most preferred by the cells that line the colon. Butyrate not only fuels the colonocyte, it lowers colonic pH, stunning the growth of pathogenic bacteria. We'll cover all this in the next chapter.

To close this section out: There is a staggering array of probiotics on the market from which to choose, including probiotics composed of live bacteria found in soil. To be wise, discuss each probiotic choice with your physician. You can also ask your physician about the use of symbiotics.

Symbiotics

Consumption of synbiotic twice daily over four weeks significantly reduced mucosal inflammatory markers in active UC. This was concurrent with a reduction in colitis at the macroscopic and microscopic level.
~Furrie et al., 2005

You may have run across the term symbiotic and wondered what a symbiotic is. Simple! A symbiotic (also called synbiotic) is a probiotic combined with a prebiotic, in pill form (Damaskos and Kolios, 2008). So, what is a prebiotic, you ask?

A prebiotic is typically a dietary fiber that is capable of being fermented by bacteria, an action that produces byproducts that are beneficial to the host by creating conditions which suppress the growth of pathogenic bacteria. We'll cover prebiotics in greater detail in the next chapter. The supposed advantage of a probiotic, combined with a prebiotic to create a symbiotic, is to encourage the growth of the probiotic bacteria involved as well as the growth of the good bacteria already present in the gut (Flesch et al., 2014). And ostensibly, the combination will provide increased benefits to the consumer. There does appear to be an advantage of symbiotics over probiotics.

One small study, the first study to assess the effect of a symbiotic on ulcerative colitis patients, eight patients received a symbiotic supplement and eight patients received a fake pill (placebo) (Furrie et al., 2005). Of the eight patients who received the symbiotic, five experienced improvement. The use of a symbiotic, twice daily over four weeks, *"significantly reduced mucosal inflammatory markers in active UC. This was concurrent with a reduction in colitis at the macroscopic and microscopic level."* (Furrie et al., 2005) This initial study is a start, in testing the value of combining probiotics with prebiotics (symbiotics) in the treatment of ulcerative colitis.

A subsequent study of symbiotics, conducted in 2006, reported greater quality of life in the symbiotic test subjects compared with those who only received a probiotic and with those who only received a prebiotic (Fujimori et al., 2009). I guess I'm a little impressed, but not enough to personally consider the use of a symbiotic. Besides, I can make my own symbiotics, on site! To do this, all I would need to do is take a suitable probiotic and eat one of my favorite foods, potato salad. The starches in potato (therefore in potato salad), having been cooked then cooled, have been structurally transformed into what is called resistant starch. Resistant starch escapes digestion in the upper GI track and becomes available to good bacteria for fermentation, feeding them and creating prebiotic products like butyrate, problem solved.

The works!

As an extension of probiotic therapy, fecal bacteriotherapy comprises the entire normal human flora. **~Borody et al., 2004**

Sure, you can take a probiotic and receive benefit . . . maybe. Perhaps, you can take a prebiotic and receive benefit . . . hopefully! And, of course, you may benefit from a symbiotic . . . possibly. But why fool around? Why not take everything, all at once? And I'm talking *the works!* And you may only need to do so once. Some call it bacteriotherapy. I'll call it FMT.

FMT is short for <u>f</u>ecal <u>m</u>icrobial <u>t</u>ransplantation. Briefly, you take a complete microbiome from a healthy individual (an individual who has been tested and certified free of transmittable disease), and you "transplant" the microbiome into the gut of an individual suffering from ulcerative colitis. We're talking poop, here! Just keep in mind, FMT is the ultimate probiotic. It is also a symbiotic, as it contains dietary fibers and metabolic byproducts manufactured by bacteria, originally meant to benefit the donor. And FMT has an impressive track record. It has been remarkably successful for many, many individuals. I have one individual in mind. We'll call him Daniel.

Case report: Daniel

Daniel, age 61 in 2010, had what was described as extensive ulcerative colitis—verified by both endoscopic visualization and by analyzing collected tissue samples (Laszlo and Pascu, 2014). His ongoing therapy comprised steroids, 5-ASA (Asacol; Pentasa; sulfasalazine), and

Azathiorpim (Imuran), which gave him several periods of remission alternating with periods of relapse. This brings us up to 2012.

Due to a worsening of symptoms, Infliximab (Remicade) was started, and gave Daniel about a one year of remission . . . until it didn't. This unfortunate turn of events required an escalation of drug therapy, but to no avail. After a month or so of this (madness), it was time to get to the bottom of things. And I really mean *"get to the bottom of things!"* Someone said, "Let's see what FMT will do."

For FMT, a suitable donor is required. In Daniel's case, his son was tested and found to be free of transmissible disease. Now, with all the ducks in a row, the son of Daniel produced a stool specimen. The stool specimen was promptly placed in a blender, liquified, filtered, then infused into Daniel's colon by means of a colonoscope. (No one was smiling or chucking while any of this was going on. This is serious business.)

Well, Daniel, who received the ultimate in probiotics from his son, rapidly improved and was declared to be in complete clinical and endoscopic remission 5 months post-FMT. Immediately after the fecal transplant, Infliximab was discontinued. But just to make sure Daniel stays out of trouble, he is maintained on 5-ASA, 2 g/day.

This story is told in the paper entitled, *Full Clinical and Endoscopic Remission Following Fecal Microbiota Transplant with Moderate-Severe Treatment-Resistant Ulcerative Colitis*, by Laszlo and Pascu, 2014. Find it online and read it for yourself.

FMT case series

Others besides Daniel have experienced complete remission in ulcerative colitis by FMT. I have six individuals in mind.

A report released in 2003 details the experience of six patients who achieve complete remission from ulcerative colitis following <u>daily</u> fecal transplants for five consecutive days. Within a week, symptoms improved. Within a month all symptoms vanished. At various times, between 1 year to 13 years post-FMT, each patient's clinical remission was verified by endoscopy. *"To our knowledge, these 6 cases document for the first time the total disappearance of chronic UC without the need for maintenance treatment."* (Borody et al., 2003) Find the title of the Borody et al paper in the References section of this chapter, search for the paper online, and read the report for yourself. With FMT, you are playing with power (and poop). It is the ultimate probiotic. And this probiotic lasts.

A final comment here: Well, so much for the "loss-of-tolerance" theory! Those who believe that ulcerative colitis represents a loss of tolerance to normal bacteria may have a tough time explaining the success of a therapy that is nothing but normal bacteria (along with the molecules and metabolic byproducts bacteria produce). Because ulcerative colitis appears to be driven by dysbiosis, I'm sure the correction of dysbiosis by FMT is one of the answers the believers in the "loss-of-tolerance" therory will come up with. And they would be right. (Although there is so much more to the story.)

Later, I will dedicate an entire chapter to FMT. A most interesting chapter awaits.

A safe space for billions

Don't you just hate it? You pay good money for your probiotics—and do so with the full knowledge that every time you take them, stomach acid is going to kill many if not most of them, outright, and without hesitation and without mercy. This haunted me for years (actually, more like hours to days). All this killing—billions of friendly bacteria at a time—*must* come to an end. This sorry state of affairs finally got the best of me, so I devised a way around all the killing. I call it "enteric re-encapsulation." And it is so easy to do. Unless your probiotic is already enteric-coated (very few are), here are the steps to follow:

Step 1, shop around for the probiotic you wish to take, <u>making sure</u> to purchase one that comes in **capsule size 0 or smaller.** Later, you will place it inside a larger-sized capsule, size 00. (Note: Size 0 is smaller than 00, as is capsule size 1, 2, 3, and so forth—the larger the number, the smaller the capsule size.)

Step 2, place an order for empty **"enteric capsules, size 00"**—capsules specifically formulated to remain intact in the stomach, and only release its contents down-stream in the small intestine, far away from the stomach and all of its acid. Of course, the probiotic bacteria selected will need to survive the threat of bile acids, but many are more than capable of doing just that (Ruiz et al., 2013), so don't worry too much about this. If, however, you are worried too much about this and you want to reduce the bile-acid threat to your probiotic, you could do so by taking your enteric-encapsulated probiotic with a low-fat meal.

Once you have both probiotic and empty enteric capsules right in front of you, you are ready to advance to the next step.

Step 3, separate the empty enteric capsule, drop your probiotic within, unopened, capsule and all, then close the enteric capsule back up. Presto! You have enteric re-encapsulated your probiotic! How easy is this? Now, your probiotic, bacteria that number in the billions, are protected from stomach acid and more likely to survive the journey on the way to the colon. And while you are taking the time to place one probiotic into one enteric capsule, you might as well enteric re-encapsulate the entire bottle of probiotics, so you can stay ahead of the game.

Step 4, you may now take your probiotic, as directed.

Step 5, you get better, and do so to the astonishment of both you and your physician. Somewhere, a choir will be singing. I'll be smiling from ear to ear.

There is one company that that manufactures enteric capsules (identified below) and sells to the average Joe. Sure, you can search for and purchase empty enteric-coated capsules online if you want to (a little cheaper), but enteric capsules appear to be a better option—made entirely out of acid-resistant material, and purportedly more resistant to stomach acid than enteric-coated capsules. The company: **Capsuline**. The website: www.capsuline.com. When you go to their home page, you can find the product by clicking on "Speciality Capsules." This will take you to a page that lists the sizes of "Enteric Capsules." Click on "**Size 00**" and take it from there. A package of 1000 capsules, breaks down to a cost of about 4 cents each. I believe this nominal cost is well worth it, after all you are creating a safe space for billions. The same exact enteric capsule can also be purchased on Amazon. Warning: As there are many similar-looking products on the Capsuline website and on Amazon, be sure to choose the right product. The key words are "**Acid Resistant Enteric.**" If the product cost is less than $39.99, you are probably viewing the wrong product.

One thing I have noticed, Capsuline does not always have enteric capsules available. Not sure why. (I'll have to straighten them out.) So, I went looking for an alternative and found a company that sells (to the average Joe) size 00 enteric-coated capsules online. The company is **CapsuleSupplies.com**. Apparently, their name is their website address. 1,000 enteric-coated capsules will cost you $23.99. Shipping is free.

And this just in! I found another company that sells size 00 enteric-coated empty capsules, called **SuperDosing.com**. I ordered my first 1,000 off Amazon, at a cost of 2 cents each. Not bad!

Probiotics and pouchitis

You can get into a lot of trouble with ulcerative colitis. Unfortunately, the disease can progress to the point that the entire colon, often including the rectum, must be removed. Some physicians and experts call this a "cure" for ulcerative colitis. I think not. The disease is simply converted into a new set of problems.

Surgically (no fun here), the colon can be removed and one can live life with an ostomy . . . forever (no fun here). Alternatively, a surgical procedure can be performed to create what is called a "J-pouch." What is a J-pouch, you ask? Briefly, after the diseased colon is removed, the small intestine is connected directly to the rectum, if still present, or connected directly to the anal canal. First, however, the terminal portion of the small intestine is folded over to look like the letter "J," sliced to form longitudinal communications between the folded-over portions, then sewed together in a manner to form a large pouch— hence the name "J-pouch." The J-pouch serves as a reservoir, permitting stool to accumulate over time to allow the individual to pass stool periodically, just like in the good old days. And, overall, the ulcerative colitis patient can live a normal life. I guess, with all the pain, the bleeding, and all the other stuff gone, this is a "cure" after all.

Unfortunately, you can get into trouble with a J-pouch. It is called pouchitis.

> It [pouchitis] is characterized by urgency, faecal incontinence, rectal bleeding, abdominal cramping, diarrhea and fever. Pouchitis is most likely to occur during the first postsurgical year; however, at least 50% of patients experience one episode of pouchitis within 10 years of surgery. (Chapman et al., 2006, emphasis added)

Basically, pouchitis is inflammation of the ileal reservoir, the J-pouch, the cause of which is unknown (Fedorak and Madsen, 2004). "However, recent studies have demonstrated reduced counts of lactobacilli and bifidobacteria within the pouch. This suggests that this syndrome may be the result of altered luminal microflora." (Fedorak and Madsen, 2004)

Fortunately, antibiotics can "cure" pouchitis; but so can probiotics. In fact, VLS#3 can be very effective in this regard, and accordingly, is regarded as the "gold standard" in the treatment of pouchitis (Losurdo et al., 2015). Prebiotic fibers can also combat pouchitis. (see Gibson and Delzenne, 2008) And that's all I have to say about that.

J-pouch, information and perspectives

As previously mentioned, sometimes the disease in ulcerative colitis becomes too advanced, and the colon must go. A permanent ileostomy is one option, but not a great one. The J-pouch, or something similar, is usually the best option to pursue, under the circumstances. To become more informed, read the following:

From the perspective of the healthcare professional:

—**Pouch Living**, Cleveland Clinic
https://my.clevelandclinic.org/ccf/media/files/Digestive_Disease/HealthyPouch_Spring_2009.pdf

—**Ileal Pouch Owner's Manual**, University of Wisconsin Dept. of Surgery
https://www.uwhealth.org/files/uwhealth/docs/pdf6/ileal_pouch_reconstruction.pdf

From the perspective of the patient:

—**Finally Achieving a Normal Life**, by Ladonna Ashbrooks
https://my.clevelandclinic.org/ccf/media/files/Digestive_Disease/HealthyPouch_Spring_2009.pdf

—**What's Life Like with a J-Pouch? One Woman's Story.** By Brooke Bogdan
https://www.everydayhealth.com/columns/my-health-story/whats-life-like-with-j-pouch-one-womans-story/

—**Living with a J-Pouch**, by Edmund Murray
https://www.ibdrelief.com/learn/treatment/surgery/restorative-proctocolectomy-with-ileal-pouch-anal-anastomosis-ipaa/living-with-a-j-pouch

—**My J-Pouch Surgery**, by Alwine Jarvis
https://www.ibdrelief.com/learn/treatment/surgery/restorative-proctocolectomy-with-ileal-pouch-anal-anastomosis-ipaa/my-j- pouch-surgery-alwine-jarvis

(Note: You can find the above articles simply searching by title, but I provide the complicated URL just in case.)

~References~

Almeghaiseeb ES. **Probiotics: an overview and their role in inflammatory bowel disease.** Saudi Journal of Gastroenterology. 2007 Jul 1;13(3):150.

Be'Er A, Zhang HP, Florin EL, Payne SM, Ben-Jacob E, Swinney HL. **Deadly competition between sibling bacterial colonies.** Proceedings of the National Academy of Sciences. 2009 Jan 13;106(2):428-33.

Bengmark S. **Pre-, Pro-, Synbiotics and Human Health.** FOOD TECHNOL BIOTECH. 2010;48(4):464-475.

Bibiloni R, Fedorak RN, Tannock GW, Madsen KL, Gionchetti P, Campieri M, De Simone C, Sartor RB. **VSL# 3 probiotic-mixture induces remission in patients with active ulcerative colitis.** The American journal of gastroenterology. 2005 Jul;100(7):1539.

Borody TJ, Warren EF, Leis S, Surace R, Ashman O. **Treatment of ulcerative colitis using fecal bacteriotherapy.** Journal of clinical gastroenterology. 2003 Jul 1;37(1):42-7.

Borody TJ, Warren EF, Leis SM, Surace R, Ashman O, Siarakas S. **Bacteriotherapy using fecal flora: toying with human motions.** Journal of clinical gastroenterology. 2004 Jul 1;38(6):475-83.

Chapman TM, Plosker GL, Figgitt DP. **VSL# 3 Probiotic Mixture.** Drugs. 2006 Jul 1;66(10):1371-87.

Chen SJ, Liu XW, Liu JP, Yang XY, Lu FG. **Ulcerative colitis as a polymicrobial infection characterized by sustained broken mucus barrier.** World Journal of Gastroenterology: WJG. 2014 Jul 28;20(28):9468.

Corthésy B, Gaskins HR, Mercenier A. **Cross-talk between probiotic bacteria and the host immune system.** The Journal of nutrition. 2007 Mar 1;137(3):781S-90S.

Dalmasso G, Cottrez F, Imbert V, Lagadec P, Peyron JF, Rampal P, Czerucka D, Groux H. **Saccharomyces boulardii inhibits inflammatory bowel disease by** trapping T cells in mesenteric lymph nodes. Gastroenterology. 2006 Dec 1;131(6):1812-25.

Damaskos D, Kolios G. **Probiotics and prebiotics in inflammatory bowel disease: microflora 'on the scope'.** British journal of clinical pharmacology. 2008 Apr 1;65(4):453-67.

Dotan I, Rachmilewitz D. **Probiotics in inflammatory bowel disease: possible mechanisms of action.** Current opinion in gastroenterology. 2005 Jul 1;21(4):426-30.

D'Souza AL, Rajkumar C, Cooke J, Bulpitt CJ. **Probiotics in prevention of antibiotic associated diarrhoea: meta-analysis.** Bmj. 2002 Jun 8;324(7350):1361.

Dwivedi M, Kumar P, Laddha NC, Kemp EH. **Induction of regulatory T cells: a role for probiotics and prebiotics to suppress autoimmunity.** Autoimmunity reviews. 2016 Apr 1;15(4):379-92.

Fedorak RN, Madsen KL. **Probiotics and the management of inflammatory bowel disease. Inflammatory bowel diseases.** 2004 May 1;10(3):286-99.

Flesch AG, Poziomyck AK, Damin DD. **The therapeutic use of symbiotics.** ABCD. Arquivos Brasileiros de Cirurgia Digestiva (São Paulo). 2014 Sep;27(3):206-9.

Fujimori S, Gudis K, Mitsui K, Seo T, Yonezawa M, Tanaka S, Tatsuguchi A, Sakamoto C. **A randomized controlled trial on the efficacy of symbotic versus probiotic or prebiotic treatment to improve the quality of life in patients with ulcerative colitis.** Nutrition. 2009 May 1;25(5):520-5.

Furrie E, Macfarlane S, Kennedy A, Cummings JH, Walsh SV, O'neil DA, Macfarlane GT. **Synbiotic therapy (Bifidobacterium longum/Synergy 1) initiates resolution of inflammation in patients with active ulcerative colitis: a randomized controlled pilot trial.** Gut. 2005 Feb 1;54(2):242-9.

Gibson GR, Delzenne N. **Inulin and oligofructose: New scientific developments.** Nutrition Today. 2008 Mar 1;43(2):54-9.

Gouriet F, Million M, Henri M, Fournier PE, Raoult D. **Lactobacillus rhamnosus bacteremia: an emerging clinical entity.** European journal of clinical microbiology & infectious diseases. 2012 Sep 1;31(9):2469-80.

Guslandi M. **Saccharomyces boulardii plus rifaximin in mesalamine-intolerant ulcerative colitis.** Journal of clinical gastroenterology. 2010 May 1;44(5):385.

Huynh HQ, debruyn J, Guan L, Diaz H, Li M, Girgis S, Turner J, Fedorak R, Madsen K. **Probiotic preparation VSL# 3 induces remission in children with mild to moderate acute ulcerative colitis: a pilot study.** Inflammatory bowel diseases. 2009 May 1;15(5):760-8.

Ishikawa H, Matsumoto S, Ohashi Y, Imaoka A, Setoyama H, Umesaki Y, Tanaka R, Otani T. **Beneficial effects of probiotic bifidobacterium and galacto-oligosaccharide in patients with ulcerative colitis: a randomized controlled study.** Digestion. 2011;84(2):128-33.

Kelesidis T, Pothoulakis C. **Efficacy and safety of the probiotic Saccharomyces boulardii for the prevention and therapy of gastrointestinal disorders.** Therapeutic advances in gastroenterology. 2012 Mar;5(2):111-25.

Korzenik JR, Podolsky DK. **Evolving knowledge and therapy of inflammatory bowel disease.** Nature reviews Drug discovery. 2006 Mar;5(3):197.

Kumari R, Verma N, Verma AK, Ahuja V, Paul J. **Diversity and abundance of lactobacilli during ulcerative colitis in North Indian patients: a case control study.** Of. 2015;10:7-10.

Langman MS, Allan RN. **Escherichia coli for ulcerative colitis.** The Lancet. 1999 Dec 4;354(9194):2000-1.

Laszlo M, Pascu O. **Full Clinical and Endoscopic Remission Following Fecal Microbiota Transplant with Moderate-Severe Treatment-Resistant Ulcerative Colitis.** J Gastroint Dig Syst. 2014;4(183):2.

Losurdo G, Iannone A, Contaldo A, Ierardi E, Di Leo A, Principi M. **Escherichia coli nissle 1917 in ulcerative colitis treatment: systematic review and meta-analysis.** J Gastrointestin Liver Dis. 2015 Dec 1;24(4):499-505.

Losurdo G, Iannone A, Contaldo A, Ierardi E, Di Leo A, Principi M. **Escherichia coli nissle 1917 in ulcerative colitis treatment: systematic review and meta-analysis.** J Gastrointestin Liver Dis. 2015 Dec 1;24(4):499-505.

Mach T. **Clinical usefulness of probiotics.** J. Physiol. Pharmacol. 2006;57(2333):89.

Matthes H, Krummenerl T, Giensch M, Wolff C, Schulze J. **Clinical trial: probiotic treatment of acute distal ulcerative colitis with rectally administered Escherichia coli Nissle 1917 (EcN).** BMC complementary and Alternative medicine. 2010 Dec;10(1):13.

McCarville JL, Caminero A, Verdu EF. **Novel perspectives on therapeutic modulation of the gut microbiota.** Therapeutic advances in gastroenterology. 2016 Jul;9(4):580-93.

Meini S, Laureano R, Fani L, Tascini C, Galano A, Antonelli A, Rossolini GM. **Breakthrough Lactobacillus rhamnosus GG bacteremia associated with probiotic use in an adult patient with severe active ulcerative colitis: case report and review of the literature.** Infection. 2015 Dec 1;43(6):777-81.

Pagnini C, Delle Fave G, Bamias G. **Probiotics in inflammatory bowel disease: Pathophysiological background and clinical applications.** World Journal of Immunology. 2013 Nov 27;3(3):31-43.

Rembacken BJ, Snelling AM, Hawkey PM, Chalmers DM, Axon AT. **Non-pathogenic Escherichia coli versus mesalazine for the treatment of ulcerative colitis: a randomized trial.** The Lancet. 1999 Aug 21;354(9179):635-9.

Ruiz L, Margolles A, Sánchez B. **Bile resistance mechanisms in Lactobacillus and Bifidobacterium.** Frontiers in microbiology. 2013 Dec 24;4:396.

Sang LX, Chang B, Zhang WL, Wu XM, Li XH, Jiang M. **Remission induction and maintenance effect of probiotics on ulcerative colitis: a meta-analysis.** World journal of gastroenterology: WJG. 2010 Apr 21;16(15):1908.

Scaldaferri F, Gerardi V, Mangiola F, Lopetuso LR, Pizzoferrato M, Petito V, Papa A, Stojanovic J, Poscia A, Cammarota G, Gasbarrini A. **Role and mechanisms of action of Escherichia coli Nissle 1917 in the maintenance of remission in ulcerative colitis patients: an update.** World journal of gastroenterology. 2016 Jun 28;22(24):5505.

Shanahan F. **Probiotics in perspective.** Gastroenterology. 2010 Dec 1;139(6):1808-12.

Sleator RD. **Probiotic therapy-recruiting old friends to fight new foes. Gut pathogens.** 2010 Dec;2(1):5.

Sood A, Midha V, Makharia GK, Ahuja V, Singal D, Goswami P, Tandon RK. **The probiotic preparation, VSL# 3 induces remission in patients with mild-to-**

moderately active ulcerative colitis. Clinical Gastroenterology and Hepatology. 2009 Nov 1;7(11):1202-9.

Sung MK, Park MY. **Nutritional modulators of ulcerative colitis: clinical efficacies and mechanistic view.** World Journal of Gastroenterology: WJG. 2013 Feb 21;19(7):994.

Thomas CM, Versalovic J. **Probiotics-host communication: Modulation of signaling pathways in the intestine.** Gut microbes. 2010 May 1;1(3):148-63.

Vahabnezhad E, Mochon AB, Wozniak LJ, Ziring DA. **Lactobacillus bacteremia associated with probiotic use in a pediatric patient with ulcerative colitis.** Journal of clinical gastroenterology. 2013 May 1;47(5):437-9.

Van den Abbeele P, Verstraete W, El Aidy S, Geirnaert A, Van de Wiele T. **Prebiotics, faecal transplants and microbial network units to stimulate biodiversity of the human gut microbiome.** Microbial biotechnology. 2013 Jul 1;6(4):335-40.

Verna EC, Lucak S. **Use of probiotics in gastrointestinal disorders: what to recommend?.** Therapeutic advances in gastroenterology. 2010 Sep;3(5):307-19.

Zanello G, Meurens F, Berri M, Salmon H. **Saccharomyces boulardii effects on gastrointestinal diseases. Current issues in molecular biology.** 2009 Jan 1;11(1):47.

Chapter 8
Prebiotics

Prebiotic was defined more than a decade ago as a "non-digestible food ingredient that beneficially affects the host by selectively stimulating the growth and/or activity of 1 or a limited number of bacteria in the colon, and thus improves host health." **~Gibson and Delzenne, 2008**

Although a probiotic can increase the numbers of the particular bacteria, it is unlikely to alter concentrations of other bacteria present in the gut. ***A prebiotic might have a more profound influence on the intestinal environment,*** *increasing certain bacteria for which the prebiotic is a growth factor, usually Bifidobacteria, while changing the colonic pH, making it less hospitable for other bacteria.* **~Korzenik and Podolsky, 2006, emphasis added**

Feeding prebiotics changes the composition of the intestinal microflora toward more protective intestinal bacteria and alters systemic and mucosal responses of the host. **~Looijer–Van Langen et al., 2009**

The concept is simple enough—send in a bunch of fibers to increase the concentrations of good bacteria with the goal of limiting the numbers of bad bacteria, and all the while creating a little magic. As to be expected, there is real science behind doing this. The promise of prebiotics is, in one sense, the promise of probiotics—more good bacteria in the colon and available to benefit the likes of you and the likes of me. And, *"similar to probiotics,* ***only a continuous intake of prebiotics will maintain their beneficial effects."*** (Looijer–Van Langen et al., 2009, emphasis added)

Based on the lead quotations of this chapter, perhaps prebiotics are just what you need in your personal battle against ulcerative colitis. In the form of a question, the answer is "Yes!" However, under certain circumstances the answer may be "No," at least for the time being. Perhaps unexpectedly, there are a few contraindications and other things to consider before embarking on prebiotic supplementation in the context of ulcerative colitis—and particularly so when the disease has progressed beyond the initial or mild stages of the disease. We'll sort all this out in this most important chapter.

What are they? What do they do?

> An important role in the maintenance of colonic homeostasis has been attributed to SCFA [short chain fatty acids], mainly acetate, propionate and butyrate. They are produced in the large bowel by the anaerobic bacterial fermentation of undigested dietary carbohydrates and fiber poly-saccharides, with <u>butyrate being considered the major fuel source for colonocytes</u>. ~**Rodríguez-Cabezas et al., 2002, emphasis added**

> Butyrate has a <u>pivotal</u> role in the context of 'gut/body health'. Its production is dependent on diet and intestinal microflora, but it is also able to modulate intestinal microflora through regulation of luminal pH and to exert many beneficial extraintestinal effects . . .. ~**Canani et al., 2012, emphasis added**

Basically, this is what it takes to be a prebiotic: **1)** You need to be a dietary fiber (or other food component) that resists both digestion and absorption in the upper GI tract, **2)** you need to be able to be *"selectively fermented by one or a limited number of potentially beneficial bacteria"* present in the colon, and **3)** you *"must be able to alter the colonic microflora toward a healthier composition."* (Kolida et al., 2002). Just so you know, you would make a lousy prebiotic—too low in fiber and too high in protein and fat—so I'll scratch you off the list. You should be safe.

By the action of bacterial fermentation, a prebiotic will customarily be transformed into a beneficial compound like the short-chain fatty acid (SCFA) butyrate, a compound that feeds the intestinal epithelial cell, plays a *"critical"* role in maintaining the barrier integrity, and participates in a wide range of other beneficial actions (Rodríguez-Cabezas et al., 2002, Sasaki and Klapproth, 2012).

Furthermore, prebiotic use is, in effect, a method of creating probiotics out of the bacteria already present in the bowel. A prebiotic stimulates the replication of more bacteria, particularly good bacteria. And doing so is easy to accomplish. It does this simply by feeding them. And feeding them turns them into more of them.

Prebiotics can be taken as a dietary supplement or can be obtained by eating your vegetables (and fruits). If the lifeform you are eating is a plant, you are probably eating a prebiotic. Even an insoluble fiber like those found in whole grain wheat and whole grain corn can act as a prebiotic (Slavin, 2013); however, the beneficial effects most desired are perhaps best achieved with <u>soluble</u> fiber, such as we find in fruits and vegetables, in as much as *"Fruits and vegetables have, on a calorie per calorie basis, **two to eight times** more fiber than do whole grains."* (Carrera-Bastos, et al., 2011, emphasis added)

With a prebiotic, particularly a soluble fiber, you can expand the concentrations of the good bacteria you already have in the colon, and at the same time create environmental conditions unfavorable for pathogenic bacteria (by reducing colonic pH and by other mechanisms) (Looijer–Van Langen and Dieleman, 2009). Furthermore, **butyrate *"is <u>critical</u> for many aspects of barrier function including permeability, mucin and antimicrobial peptide production . . .."*** (McCarville et al., 2016, emphasis added). So soluble fiber consumption, so butyrate production, is not optional for the health of the colon, it is mandatory. Please take notice.

Now, let's get up to speed on the beneficial effects attributed to various prebiotics, beneficial effects the ulcerative colitis patient is likely in great need of. They include:

- Expansion in numbers of beneficial intestinal bacteria (Looijer–Van Langen et al., 2009)

- Modulation of genes that favor overall colon health (Jacobs et al., 2009)

- Increased production of the antimicrobial protein cathelicidin by colonocytes (Canani et al., 2012)

- Promotion of anti-inflammatory effects, including the suppression of the master regulator of inflammation, NF-κB (Hamer et al., 2008; Canani et al., 2012) and the activation of other anti-inflammatory pathways such as PPAR-γ (Hamer et al., 2008). (I'll tell you about PPAR-γ in a forthcoming chapter.)

- Expansion of anti-inflammatory Treg immune cell numbers (McCarville et al., 2016)

- *"Acidification [pH reduction] of the colonic environment, which is detrimental to some pathogenic strains of bacteria . . .."* (Lomax and Calder, 2008)

- *"Acidification of the colon favoring mucin production."* (Lomax and Calder, 2008)

- Prevention of attachment by harmful bacteria to intestinal epithelial cells (Sartor, 2004)

- Inhibition of the ability of harmful bacteria to secrete substances meant to kill their competitors, substances used by harmful bacteria to survive and thrive (Sartor, 2004)

- Reduction of several bacterial enzyme activities that can be harmful to the intestinal epithelium (Looijer–Van Langen and Dieleman, 2009)

- Enhancement of gut immune responsiveness against enteric (gut) pathogens (Gibson and Delzenne, 2008)

- Enhancement of antioxidant defenses in the colon (Hamer et al., 2009)

- Limitation of the chemical signaling that attracts pro-inflammatory immune cells, thereby limiting aggressive immune responses (Rodríguez-Cabezas et al., 2002)

- Promotion of normal cell turnover, cell migration, and regeneration capacity of the intestinal epithelial layer (Gibson and Delzenne, 2008; Hamer et al., 2008)

- Reduction in intestinal permeability (Hamer et al., 2008)

- Prevention of bacterial translocation beyond the intestinal epithelial barrier (Carrera-Bastos et al., 2011)

- Suppression of protein fermentation in the colon, subsequently limiting the production of toxic byproducts (Vanhoutvin et al., 2009; Mohan et al., 2017)

- Restraining uncontrolled growth in colonic epithelial cells, favoring a reduction in colon cancer risk in the ulcerative colitis patient (Scheppach et al., 2001)

Quite a list! (I could have added more.)

At this point in our conversation, you should be aware that many, if not most of the beneficial actions listed above, are attributed to the SCFA called butyrate. Although not the most abundant SCFA produced in the colon by bacterial fermentation (Holscher, 2017), butyrate is the big one!

Perhaps the one perhaps most necessary. This compound plays *"a pivotal role in the context of 'gut/body health.'"* (Canani et al., 2012) Fortunately, butyrate is easily produced by gut bacteria acting on soluble fibers. The good bacteria create it. You need it. The colonocytes love it! Soluble fibers should be in adequate supply. But for many, many individuals (millions upon millions), they are not. So, who can we turn to in our hour of need?

What are their names? What makes them so special?

*Examples of fermentable dietary and chemically modified fibers that are associated with a higher production of SCFAs . . . are **oligofructose**, **inulin**, **psyllium**, **germinated barley foodstuff**, **hydrolysed guar gum**, **oat bran**, corn starch, **isomalt**, **gluconic acid** and **butyrylated starch**.*

Although the beneficial effects of these fibers are often attributed to the increased butyrate production, these soluble fibers can also affect other intestinal characteristics influencing intestinal health, such as increased fecal bulk, shortened colonic transit time, changes in the composition of the gut microbiota, lowered intraluminal pH and changed bile acid profiles.
~Hamer et al., 2008, emphasis added

There are a wide variety of prebiotic fibers as well as other dietary components that are collectively referred to as soluble fibers (e.g., inulin and oligofructose) that ferment in the colon and, hence, provide a wide range of beneficial effects such as previously described. And, even if a particular prebiotic under discussion is not a true fiber, if it acts like a fiber, I will refer to it as a fiber. Other authors do this, too.

But before we get too far along in our conversation, let's take a moment to discuss real food and the beneficial fibers they possess. Real food is probably the best option when it comes to prebiotics, in as much as *"diets enriched in plant foods (e.g., semi-vegetarian diets) will increase the proportion of a range of different types of DF [dietary fibers] in the diet."* (Wong et al., 2016) A variety of different fibers are reported to be more effective than a limited variety of fibers in the effort to elicit beneficial effects and to correct dysbiosis.

Vegetables and fruit need fiber, shall we say, in order to be vegetables and fruits. The fibers in vegetables and fruit give them structure so that floppiness does not set in. And when you eat a vegetable or a fruit, you are saying, in effect, "I want what you've got." After you eat a vegetable or a fruit, including the fibers it contains, then you reap the rewards. This is the normal way to get your fiber. But the normal way may not be sufficient to modify a disease process as tenacious (and as dastardly) as ulcerative colitis, or to overcome a fiber deficiency due to the insane dietary practices followed in our society and probably followed by you. Enter prebiotic supplementation.

A prebiotic supplement is typically derived from vegetables and fruits, but let's just say "plants." Unfortunately, in our Western-diet society, our consumption of fibers from vegetables and fruit (plants) on average are about **50%** of what they should be (Bengmark, 2010; Slavin, 2013). A fiber deficiency could be a problem. A fiber supplement may be the answer.

There are distinct advantages to be a gained by prebiotic supplementation. With supplemental prebiotics you can consume greater amounts of dietary fiber (and other prebiotics) than you otherwise would or that is practical to accomplish by diet alone. Plus, by taking a particular type of prebiotic, you may be able to achieve a beneficial, targeted effect. Because many prebiotics are fermented and depleted in the proximal or beginning portion of the colon, and do not reach the lower or distal portions of the colon where they are clearly needed, one reason to supplement with a prebiotic is to target the distal colon. This can be done by supplementing with a prebiotic known to reach the distal colon, <u>sufficiently intact</u>, for fermentation in this region of the bowel (Cherbut et al., 2003). But there are other reasons to target the colon with prebiotics.

One example of a beneficial, targeted effect achieved by prebiotics, perhaps one of considerable importance, is the prevention of what is called proteolytic fermentation.

> As micro-organisms preferably ferment carbohydrates, most saccharolytic [carbohydrate] fermentation occurs in the proximal colon. Depletion of carbohydrate sources in the <u>distal</u> colon **leads to a switch from saccharolytic to proteolytic [protein] fermentation, which is less favorable due to the formation of potentially toxic products.** Both these toxic products and the lower availability of SCFAs in the distal colon are hypothesized to be involved in the pathogenesis of gastro-intestinal disorders such as ulcerative colitis (UC) and cancer. (Vanhoutvin et al., 2009, emphasis added)

Given the negative effect of proteolytic (protein) fermentation on colon health, certainly one goal in prebiotic supplementation should be to target the distal colon in a manner that reduces the generation of toxic byproducts generated by protein fermentation, for they are toxic. Toxic means danger. Toxic means stay away. Toxic means increased disease activity. Toxic means unhappiness. You want no part of toxic, and likely you want no part of unhappiness. *"Therefore, it is desirable to sustain prebiotic oligosaccharides as the dominate substrate in the colon for minimization of proteolytic [protein digesting] activity."* (Mohan et al., 2017) Just to drive the message home: *". . . **undigested protein metabolized to end products such as phenols, indoles, and ammonia may have detrimental effects on colon health."*** (Muir et al., 1995, emphasis added) Sounds dreadful! (It is.)

Fortunately for us, for therapeutic purposes, a wide variety of supplemental fibers are commercially available and offered to counteract the diseases and medical situations associated with, or impacted by, low fiber consumption. Not surprisingly, one such disease is ulcerative colitis. And in as much as some fibers may not be as effective as other fibers in the treatment of ulcerative colitis, making a wise choice here may be pivotal to achieving success (Slavin, 2013; Wong et al., 2016).

Here are the prebiotics you are likely to run across in your study of these issues and as you continue in your search to find ways to achieve or maintain remission in the battle against ulcerative colitis:

Inulin

> Currently, food components that seem to exert the best prebiotic effects are inulin-type frucans. ~**Roberfroid, 2001**

> Its slower fermentation rate and higher prebiotic potency makes inulin a more interesting compound than oligofructose to beneficially influence the microbial community from both the proximal and distal colon region. ~**van de Wiele et al., 2007**

Inulin (not to be confused with insulin)—which may be strategically combined with another prebiotic, oligofructose—is readily fermented by two major families of beneficial bacteria, *lactobacilli* and *bifidobacteria*, to produce lactic, acetic, propionic, and butyric acids (Gibson and Delzenne, 2008; Duncan et al., 2004). The immediate effect of all this acid production is a more acidic colonic environment, which stuns the growth of potentially pathogenic bacteria (Gibson and Delzenne, 2008; Looijer–Van Langen et al., 2009). And in the acidic environment so created, other beneficial effects can occur and occur with greater ease.

Inulin may indeed be very promising in the battle against ulcerative colitis. And if it is chicory-derived inulin, its peak fermentation time is 8 hours post consumption, giving it plenty of time to arrive in the distal colon, a place where it is most likely needed (Holscher, 2017). One more thing before we move on.

If ulcerative colitis progresses to the point of necessitating a total colectomy and the formation of an ileal pouch, inulin supplementation may be a good therapeutic option, should pouchitis occur. One study of 24 patients with pouchitis demonstrated decreased endoscopic and histological inflammation following 24 grams daily of supplemental inulin (Looijer–Van Langen and Dieleman, 2009).

Oligofructose

> *Nourishing beneficial bacteria, such as Bifidobacteria, with inulin or oligofructose allows them to "outcompete" potential detrimental organisms and thereby potentially contribute to the health of the host.* **~Niness, 1999**

> *A higher production of propionate and butyrate was noted during supplementation of both oligofructose and inulin.* **~van de Wiele et al., 2007**

Inulin can be combined with the related, inulin-degradation product, oligofructose—but perhaps not without potential adverse effects (Looijer–Van Langen and Dieleman, 2009). We will discuss this a bit later. Nevertheless, combined with inulin, or all by itself, oligofructose can be acted upon to produce a ton of butyrate. This could come in handy. *"Among the LDCs [low-digestible carbohydrates], fructo-oligosaccharides occupy a key position by **their ability to change <u>significantly</u> the composition of the colonic microflora**."* (Scheppach et al., 2001, emphasis added)

One reason for adding oligofructose to inulin is to achieve broader prebiotic coverage in the bowel. The easier and quicker-to-ferment oligofructose acting in the proximal, beginning portion of the colon and inulin, taking longer to ferment, acting in the more distal regions of the colon (van de Wiele et al., 2007; Holscher, 2017).

Germinated barley foodstuff (GBF)

> *Germinated barley foodstuff appears to be a safe and effective maintenance therapy to prolong remission in patients with UC.* **~Haskey and Gibson, 2017**

One advantage of GFB is the complete lack of side effects or toxicity.
~Mitsuyama et al., 1998

We observed a remarkable trend in the reduction of clinical signs in patients with UC after GBF consumption. **~Faghfoori et al., 2011**

Germinated barley foodstuff, an oddly named by-product of beer-brewing, is an insoluble fiber that is nothing but special—possessing a particularly delightful ingredient called glutamine (Wong et al., 2016). Germinated barley foodstuff has success written all over it.

Four-week administration of 20–30 g of germinated barley extracts to patients with mild to moderate ulcerative colitis decreased clinical and endoscopic evidence of inflammation in both a pilot and a small placebo-controlled trial. (Sartor, 2004)

Germinated barley foodstuff not only stimulates the growth of beneficial bacteria, it stimulates the production of butyrate and other short-chain fatty acids, as well as provides glutamine in therapeutically relevant amounts (Bengmark, 2010). Think of glutamine as a bowel healer. Think of glutamine as medicine. *"Glutamine is known to enhance the growth and repair of the gut mucosa."* (Wong et al., 2016) Indeed, glutamine may the reason why this prebiotic is so promising and shown to be particularly effective.

It can well be observed the observed effect was more due to increased supply of glutamine and other antioxidants such as B vitamins than to the fiber per se as these compounds are known to be rich in by-products from breweries. (Bengmark, 2010)

In one study, in active ulcerative colitis patients, germinated barley foodstuffs *"showed clinical and endoscopic improvements following intervention for four weeks. Furthermore, stool butyrate concentrations had increased in these patients."* (Wong et al., 2016) In another study,

"Germinated barley foodstuff prolonged remission in inactive UC patients." (Hamer et al., 2008) Foodstuffs for thought.

Glutamine, an amino acid and a *"major nutrient"* for the intestinal epithelial cell (Mitsuyama et al., 1998), is further credited with inhibiting intestinal permeability (Rapin and Wiernsperger, 2010). Reducing intestinal permeability is, of course, a win-win in the battle against ulcerative colitis.

Psyllium

> *Psyllium is a non-fermentable fiber but has unique therapeutic effects, based on its high solubility and viscosity.* ~**Holscher, 2017**

Psyllium may be characterized as a non-soluble fiber, but this appears not to be the case. It actually *"consists of a mixture of insoluble and soluble fibres, which may have different effects."* (Wong et al., 2016) Furthermore, this fiber is mainly composed of **hemicellulose**, which *"is not digested in the small intestine, but instead it is broken down in the colon where it acts as a food source for the intestinal flora."* (Dharmarajan, 2005) And add one more thing that psyllium definitely has going for it; that would be its reputation.

> *Psyllium, long used by clinicians to maintain stool consistency in both constipation and diarrhea, is a form of prebiotic by virtue of its ability to serve as a metabolic substrate for bacteria. Administration of psyllium was superior to placebo in decreasing symptoms of patients with inactive ulcerative colitis, with a consistent increase in fecal Bifidobacterium concentrations, and decreased free water in the stool.* (Sartor, 2004)

Whether by direct fermentation or by some other effect, psyllium increases butyrate in the stools of ulcerative colitis patients (Pituch-Zdanowska et al., 2015). If butyrate is in the stool, it is probably available in relevant amounts to directly benefit the cells that line the colon.

Oat bran

Oat is rich in soluble fibers, β-glycans, and is known for its antiseptic properties. ~**Bengmark, 2010**

The fibers in oats, referred to collectively as oat bran, appear to have much to offer the ulcerative patient.

Two other studies in UC patients in remission, evaluating the supplementation of psyllium and oat bran, showed that the supplementation was safe, increased faecal butyrate concentrations and were found to be effective in the maintenance of remission. (Hamer et al., 2008)

*A controlled intervention study adding 60 grams/day of oat bran (equivalent to 20 grams oat fiber/day) to the diet of subjects with quiescent UC reported no signs or symptoms of colitis relapse after 12 weeks. A subgroup of subjects noted a decrease in abdominal pain, reflux and diarrhea. The greatest impact of the oat bran intervention was seen on the fecal short chain fatty acid (SCFA) concentrations found in the stool. Fifteen subjects demonstrated a **36%** increase in fecal butyrate concentrations within four weeks of intervention which was maintained throughout the 12-week intervention. This finding is important as increasing evidence suggests SCFAs play an essential role in maintaining the health of colonic mucosa as butyrate is the main energy substrate for colonocytes. Butyrate also plays an important role in the prevention and treatment of distal UC.* (Haskey and Gibson, 2017, emphasis added)

I could go on and on about oat bran, but since I promised to be brief, we'll move on to the next prebiotic.

Pectin

> *Pectin is also an interesting fibre [British spelling], extensively used by the pharmaceutical and food industry. It has a unique ability to form gels and is commonly used as a carrier of pharmacological active substances and in baby foods. An important finding is that pectin is a very strong antioxidant . . ..* **~Bengmark, 2010**

Pectin ferments more proximally in the colon and therefore may not make it to the lower colon to produce all the region-specific special effects we are hoping to achieve (Holscher, 2017). *"This has been demonstrated to occur with a soluble pectin preparation that was degraded almost fully and mostly in the proximal colon."* (Wong et al., 2016) But just add a scoop of pectin to a helping of psyllium or inulin, and you have a rather promising prebiotic combo on your hands, one capable of feeding the good bacteria stationed in multiple areas of the colon. I mentioned previously that some fibers are better fibers than others. This assertion certainly seems to be a warranted, in that it has been reported that the fermentation of apple pectin resulted in greater SCFA production than oat fiber or corn bran (Shinohara et al., 2010).

Pectin supplementation may come in handy in one unique ulcerative colitis-related situation. One team of investigators found that apple pectin supplementation delayed the deterioration of bacterial diversity following fecal transplant (Wei et al., 2016). In other words, apple pectin was able to maintain bacterial diversity in this study population. If it can help maintain bacterial diversity post-FMT, likely pectin could help maintain bacterial diversity in other study populations as well, including a study of one—that would be you.

One of the properties of pectin, mentioned by Bengmark above, is its ability to serve as an antioxidant, acting to limit the damage to the lining of the colon caused by free radicals (Bengmark, 2010). We will discuss the issues surrounding free radicals and antioxidants in ulcerative colitis, momentarily.

Resistant starch (RS)

RS-enriched food may be a way to elevate glucose and butyrate levels in the colon in a more physiological, consistent, cost-effective, and less stressful way.

From these results, it is to be concluded that colonic epithelial cells have better regenerative properties when supplied with RS. ~**Jacobasch et al., 1999)**

Any discussion of prebiotics should unquestionably include a discussion on resistant starch. Resistant starch is regarded as *"an excellent substrate for production of SCFA butyrate"* (Muir et al., 1995), and can be taken as a supplement or obtained by doing something as simple as devouring a serving of potato salad. Oddly, once a starchy food is cooked, like the potatoes used to make potato salad, then allowed to cool, the starches undergo a molecular transformation that makes them difficult for humans to digest (Jacobash et al.,1999). This, of course, is good news for all the potato salad-loving bacteria in your colon (and there are many). They can dine on it and create a sizeable amount of butyrate just for you, making resistant starch one great little prebiotic, unless . . .

It has been discovered that if an individual is missing one species of bacteria, *Ruminococcus bromii*, the ability to ferment resistant starch is reduced by 70% to 80%; whereas, individuals with this species of bacteria in the gut ferment 100% of the resistant starch consumed (Holscher, 2017). If resistant starch doesn't seem to be working, perhaps this is the reason. But for everyone else (those of us with plenty *Ruminococcus bromii* on active duty), resistant starch may be readily fermented to produce pleasing results. And you can easily combine resistant starch prebiotics with supplemental prebiotics.

Because carbohydrates are the main substrate for microflora (bacteria), imbalances may be prevented by a sufficient dietary supply of about 15 g/day of nondigestible saccharides such as resistant starch (RS), inulin, and their derivatives, fructo-pligosaccharides. (Jacobasch et al., 1999)

One more thing about the benefits of resistant starch that bears mentioning: Resistant starch fermentation has been shown to produce relevant amounts of hydrogen, a byproduct known to exhibit anti-inflammatory and antioxidant effects (Muir et al., 1995). We'll discuss hydrogen and its benefits shortly, so stay tuned.

Finally, the use of resistant starch as a prebiotic is not at all straightforward, being best accomplished by dietary measures. So, to help you out in this regard, may I recommend a little reading assignment? If you want to learn more about resistant starch (and you should want to learn more about resistant starch), go online, find by title, print out, and read the following articles:

–**Who Can Resist Resistant Starch**, by Rosane Oliveira, DVM, PhD

–**The Healthiest Resistant Starch for Your Gut**, by Carla Hernandez, NTP

–**The Definitive Guide to Resistant Starch**, by Mark Sisson

–**9 Foods That Are High in Resistant Starch**, by Rudy Mawer, MSc

–**High-Amylose Foods**, by Jessica Bruso, Nutritionist

Hydrolyzed guar gum (PHGG)

PHGG results in greater amounts of butyrate and other SCFAs than do other types of fiber. **~De La Torre and Silleras, 2003**

This prebiotic fiber is typically made from a plant cultivated in India or Pakistan and is processed (partially hydrolyzed) to make one dandy little probiotic. You can buy this prebiotic online, and it is relatively inexpensive. PHGG is regarded as a great butyrate-producing prebiotic and offers clear benefits to the individual battling either irritable bowel syndrome or ulcerative colitis. However, there appears to be a problem with guar gum. The creation of gas and bloating may be more likely to occur than with psyllium, by way of example (Dharmarajan, 2005). This may limit the desirability of this prebiotic. Perhaps a lower dose may lessen the problem and make its use more acceptable.

With respect to ulcerative colitis, one team of investigators report that in addition to supporting the growth of key bacterial species, *Bifidobacterium* and *Lactobacillus*, PHGG stimulates the growth of a family of bacteria reported to be suppressed in ulcerative colitis, namely *Parabacteroides* (Carlson et al., 2016). This would suggest that this prebiotic has much to offer the ulcerative patient.

And then there is Lactulose

The balance between oxidant and antioxidant systems is <u>extremely important</u> in the pathogenesis of ulcerative colitis and in the progress of tissue injury. ~**Cetinykaya et al., 2006. Emphasis added**

*. . . lactulose is bacterially fermented in the colon to short chain fatty acids and gasses. The main content of the gasses is H_2 [hydrogen]. Therefore, **lactulose which <u>dramatically</u> increases endogenous H_2 production, may act as an ideal indirect antioxidant, safe and effective in IBD treatment**.* ~**Yuedong et al., 2013, emphasis added**

Lactulose is a prebiotic that has the ability to promote the growth of Lactobacillus, Bifidobacterium and Gram-positive bacteria but has an inhibitory effect on Gram-negative bacteria, thus attenuating gut-derived endotoxemia (bacterial components in the bloodstream). **~Abu-Shanab and Quigley, 2010**

I'm going to throw this prebiotic, lactulose, in the mix because I believe that this indigestible, synthetic sugar has much to offer the ulcerative colitis patient. However, just like anything else you can throw at ulcerative colitis, there could be a problem or two associated with its use—placing lactulose on the list of therapies you need to first clear with your physician. Besides, unless you live in Canada, for example, you'll need a prescription for it anyway. Not a lot of people are talk'n lactulose these days as a therapy for ulcerative colitis, but perhaps they should. Here I will share with you some of the reported benefits.

First, lactulose increases beneficial bacteria in the gut, especially *bifido-bacterial* but also *lactobacilli* (Bouhnik et al., 2004; Tuohy et al., 2002). And we all know what this means:

> *Lactobacillus and Bifidobacteria produce harmful substances for Gram-positive and Gram-negative bacteria, and they compete with pathogens (i.e., Bacteriodetes, Clostridium, Staphylococcus, and Enterobacter) for cell adhesion.* (Scaldaferri et al., 2013)

In as much as lactulose is a laxative, prescribed for constipation, diarrhea would be an obvious side effect. However, in two small studies lactulose seemed to be well-tolerated in both the healthy individual and the ulcerative colitis patient (Szilagyi et al., 2000; Hafer et al., 2007). To be anticipated, if the dose is inappropriately high, problems may occur. (Diarrhea is a problem. The cost of toilet paper is a problem.) However, low-dose, prebiotic-dose, lactulose seems to be well-tolerated, even by the diarrhea-prone ulcerative colitis patient (Hafer et al., 2007). In the Hafer study, a dose of 10 g/day seemed to do the trick. Beneficial effects have also been reported with doses as low as 5 g/day, and were *"well tolerated"* (Bouhnik et al., 2004). Of note, a dose that may be considered "high-dose" is in the range of 20–60 g/day, *"which could lead to intolerance symptoms such as abdominal pain and diarrhea."* (Bouhnik et al., 2004)

Second, as with other prebiotics, lactulose increases the SCFA production, which decreases the pH in the colonic environment (Liao, 1994; Chen et al., 2012). Of course, this is most desirable and is exactly what you would expect from a top-notch prebiotic.

Third, lactulose has one clearly defined property that may come in handy in the battle against ulcerative colitis. When bacteria ferment this prebiotic, substantial amounts of free hydrogen (H_2) are released (Scheppach et al., 2001). Hydrogen, with little else to do, then effortlessly diffuses into the intestinal epithelium where it acts locally as a powerful, indeed *"remarkable,"* antioxidant (Chen et al., 2012). It even penetrates cell membranes and targets the cellular structures like the mitochondria and the nucleus (Zhang et al., 2013). Let's briefly review what this free radical business is all about. First, consider this:

> *Inflamed tissues generate hydroxyl radicals, the most cytotoxic reactive oxygen species (ROS), which up-regulate TNF-α expression through [the] NF-κB signaling pathway . . ..* (Chen et al., 2011)

Due to all the inflammatory activity occurring in ulcerative colitis, excessive amounts of free radicals are generated (Vanhoutvin et al., 2009; Chen et al., 2013). Free radicals, in various forms, are collective called reactive oxygen species (ROS). Excessive generation of ROS, or inadequate antioxidant defenses, not only intensifies the inflammatory response but also damages tissues and individual cells—even DNA—and may lead to colon cancer (Chen et al., 2013). Unfortunately, colon cancer is a constant threat facing the ulcerative colitis patient; 2% of which will experience this within 10 years, 8% within 20 years, and 18% within 30 years (Chen et al., 2013). Cancer risk alone is reason enough to aggressively address excessive ROS in ulcerative colitis.

And we do address the battle against ROS, at least to a relevant degree, with standard drug therapy (Cetinkaya et al., 2006). 5-ASA, for example, is *"a very effective"* antioxidant (López-Alarcón et al., 2005). But is 5-ASA enough? Could 5-ASA need a little help? And what about individuals who simply cannot tolerate 5-ASA? Given the role of ROS in ulcerative colitis, there must be a pressing need to identify antioxidants suitable for use with this disease—in as much as numerous studies have been conducted to evaluate a variety of substances for their antioxidant potential in the treatment of ulcerative colitis (see Moura et al., 2015) And it looks like, in lactulose, we have found one dandy antioxidant. *"Lactulose mediates hydrogen production and is an **ideal** endogenous hydrogen inducer."* (Chen et al., 2012, emphasis added) It is ideal because it can be transformed into "dramatic" amounts of H_2 within the colon and for the colon. And so we read:

> Lactulose, when orally administered, can be fermented in the colon and induce <u>dramatic</u> amounts of H_2 production. (Chen et al., 2012, emphasis added)

Finally, another action that is certain to benefit the ulcerative colitis patient is the ability of lactulose to inhibit the degradation of proteins and blood (from blood loss) within the colon. When uninhibited, the degradation of intracolonic protein, including blood protein, leads to the formation of toxic byproducts (Mortensen et al., 1990).

Importantly, the four major benefits of lactulose supplementation outlined in this section can be accomplished by lactulose without noticeable side effects (think low dosage).

A small study found that oral lactulose administration was well tolerated in stable ulcerative colitis patients (Szilagyi et al., 2000). In another study, a dose of 10 g/d did not substantially increase the rate of defecation (did not produce diarrhea) in the ulcerative colitis patient, and reported *"Overall, the administration of lactulose was well tolerated, with no serious effects observed."* (Hafer et al., 2007) Furthermore, *"significant improvements of quality of life was observed in the UC patients receiving lactulose compared to the control group (those not receiving lactulose)."* (Hafer et al., 2007) Could you use a little improvement in your quality of life? Of course you could.

Lactulose is available as a powder, as a liquid, and can be administered by retention enema. Lactulose use is considered *"safe,"* and *"can be taken daily for decades"* without adverse effects, except for individuals who are *"galactose-intolerant."* (Chen et al., 2012) Given the reported beneficial effects of lactulose and its safety profile, perhaps you should discuss lactulose with your physician the next chance you get.

What <u>ever</u> could go wrong?

Prebiotics have an excellent safety profile. However, they have been associated with symptoms of dose-dependent abdominal pain, flatulence, bloating, and diarrhea. **~Looijer–Van Langen and Dieleman, 2009**

It is apparent that certain types of DF [dietary fiber] in certain patients, at certain times, can increase the severity of some adverse effects such as elevated incidence of flatulence and "gut rumbling" and/or further exacerbate other disease symptoms . . .. **~Wong et al., 2016**

Excellent safety profile or not, with prebiotic supplementation prepare to pass a lot of gas. Warn all those around you. And warn repeatedly. Friendships are a risk. Relationships can be saved.

Flatulence, the act of passing gas and sharing it with others, is, perhaps, a surrogate marker that there is enough dietary fiber on board to get down to business. However, as promising as prebiotic supplementation is, and regarded as a safe practice even for ulcerative colitis, a problem or two may appear from out of nowhere. Let's take a look.

Potential translocation of bacteria

Perhaps an uncommon event in humans (but perhaps more likely in the ulcerative colitis patient), the translocation of bacteria from intestinal lumen to regional tissues and beyond, is certainly a potential complication of fiber supplementation. In a rat, sure it can happen.

One team of investigators reported that **inulin and oligofructose** enhanced the translocation of Salmonella from the gut of a rat into regions beyond, prompting this comment: *"the effects of prebiotics on bacterial translocation are still unclear and further research is necessary."* (Looijer–Van Langen and Dieleman, 2009)

If you feel seriously ill sometime after beginning a fiber supplementation regimen, the possibility exists that bacterial translocation is occurring. Time to call the doctor. Do not delay

Not enough to do the trick

Although a little prebiotic is probably better than no prebiotic, it is recognized that prebiotic supplementation will be largely ineffective if not taken in sufficient amounts.

> *Maintenance of a healthy gut microbiota and hemostasis can be promoted by the consumption of indigestible carbohydrates or dietary fibers.* ***However, a sufficient fiber intake is <u>required</u> for a higher effect.*** (Vigsnæs et al., 2011, emphasis added)

Insufficient hang time

We addressed this issue before in our discussions on inulin, oligofructose, and others. If the prebiotic is rapidly fermented in the proximal colon, there may not be enough prebiotic "fire-power" to reach regions with greater need, like the distal portions of the bowel—and may lead to the following problem:

> *As microorganisms preferably ferment carbohydrates, most saccharolytic [carbohydrate] fermentation occurs in the proximal colon.* **Depletion of carbohydrate sources in the distal colon leads to a switch from saccharolytic to proteolytic [protein] fermentation, which is less favorable due to the formation of potentially toxic products.** (Vanhoutvin et al., 2009, emphasis added)

Sounds bad, this proteolytic fermentation. So, let's talk about it.

Excessive protein fermentation

So, you're trying to boost butyrate levels in your battle against ulcerative colitis. Great! And you are using supplemental fibers to pull this off. Good call! However, you unwittingly selected the wrong prebiotic, one that quickly vanishes in the proximal colon, leaving nothing left for the distal colon. You notice no results (although you are flatusing a lot). You are disappointed (and socially isolated). But wouldn't you know, depending on the diet you are following, you are likely doing the "proteolytic-fermentation" thing—producing toxic byproducts and thereby continually harming yourself. There are two ways to address this problem: **1)** supplement with prebiotics that ferment in the distal colon, like chicory-derived inulin or lactulose, and **2)** eat less protein, particularly red meat. You should probably be limiting red meat, anyway—strongly recommended by many authorities. You'll find out why in the next chapter. Proteolytic fermentation is nothing to fool around with. **The toxic products produced by proteolytic fermentation** *"lower availability of SCFAs in the distal colon* are hypothesized to be involved in the pathogenesis of gastro-intestinal disorders such as ulcerative colitis (UC) and cancer."* (Vangoutvin et al., 2009, emphasis added)

Army of one not enough

Pectin, oat bran, and gar gum readily ferment in the upper or proximal colon (Morita et al., 1999). This could be a problem should you want prebiotic actions to address problems occurring in the lower or distal colon. So, why not add psyllium to the mix?

> . . . PS [psyllium] may delay the fermentation rate of HAS [high amylose cornstarch] in the cecum and shift the fermentation site of HAS toward the distal colon, leading to the higher butyrate concentration in the distal colon and feces.
> For these reasons, highly fermentable dietary fibers such as pectin, guar gum and oat bran are fully fermented in the cecum and proximal colon and do not contribute n-butyrate to the distal colon." (Morita et al., 1999)

But what about resistant starch? *"This also might be the case for resistant starches (RS) such as high-amylose cornstarch (HAS) which has a fermentation rate that is relatively rapid."* (Morita et al., 1999)

All this suggests that multiple fibers, not just one fiber (monotherapy), should be used in a strategy aimed at reducing the impact ulcerative colitis has on a life. It also suggests that resistant starch is not the best prebiotic to deal with the problem of proteolytic (protein) fermentation.

Pushing the limit

And I quote:

> If the fiber of interest is highly fermentable, e.g., inulin-type fibers, this dosage is near the top of the tolerable limit for human consumption, and consumption at this level is likely to result in

unpleasant side effects such as gas, bloating, and diarrhea.
(Holscher, 2017)

Maybe your prebiotic is on some kind of blacklist

Some dietary fibers ferment too quickly to be handled without symptoms. A category of foods called FODMAPs contain readily fermentable, poorly absorbed carbohydrates which can cause problems in both IBS and IBD patients (Knight-Sepulveda et al., 2015). For example, foods high in inulin, such as artichoke and beetroot, can be found on this list. So here is the problem with FODMAPs:

> *Poorly digested complex carbohydrates (even those with defined pre-biotic properties) may lead to bacterial overgrowth and bowel injury with increased intestinal permeability. The waste products of fermentation of undigested carbohydrates including methane, carbon dioxide, lactic and acetic acid, which are all gastrointestinal irritants.* (Olendzki et al., 2014)

So, you were impressed with what you have learned thus far in this chapter, you began eating more prebiotic foods, and you ran into problems. It could be that you are eating too many FODMAPs.

Sure, you can return to your wayward, Western-diet ways (low in fiber and high in evil) and receive none of the benefits a higher fiber diet offers. Or you can start all over, following the advice presented in the following paper:

—**Diet and Inflammatory Bowel Disease**, by Knight-Sepulveda et al., 2015

This paper is free online. Print it out so you can easily refer to it, as needed. Pay close attention to Table 3 on page 514 and Figure 2 on page 516. They will guide you in making wise dietary choices as you begin again, carefully, the process of introducing prebiotics into your diet. For the ulcerative colitis patient, the lesson of this paper is: **Go low and go slow with foods high in fiber.** This principle probably applies to prebiotic supplements, as well, particularly in the setting of IBD. **Start with low dose prebiotic supplementation and increase slowly, as tolerated.** Of course, doing all this with your physician's approval and supervision.

Another thing to be aware of: Dietary fiber restriction, particularly as extreme as the Low FODMAP Diet, should only be of short-term duration.

> *A critical evaluation of the studies purporting to support a low-FODMAP diet, however, shows that the endpoints have largely involved short-term measures of discomfort such as gas and bloating, rather than considering longer term effects on intestinal dysbiosis or inflammatory measures. For these reasons, we would caution against the acceptance of such a regime. (Wong et al., 2016)*

> *The fibre-restricted diet should always be used only on a temporary basis, and it is indicated in a few cases, which are acute relapse (with diarrhea, cramping), intestinal stenosis, and small intestinal bacterial overgrowth and after some types of surgery.* (Pituch-Zdanowska et al., 2015, emphasis added)

Clearly, for some individuals, some prebiotics can offend. So beware and work closely with your physician if you are having trouble with your prebiotics. We've read this before:

> *Poorly digested complex carbohydrates (even those with defined pre-biotic properties) may lead to bacterial overgrowth and bowel injury with increased intestinal permeability. The waste products of fermentation of undigested carbohydrates including methane, carbon dioxide, lactic and acetic acid, which are all gastrointestinal irritants. (Olendzki et al., 2014)*

Perforation (worst-case scenario)

> *Certain types of NSPs [non-starch polysaccharides, such as found in germinated barley, oat bran, pectin, and guar gum] in certain patients, at certain times may even exacerbate IBD, such as when increased fermented gas further accelerates the perforation of severe UC cases.*
> ~Nie at al., 2017

A perforated (torn open) bowel is a medical emergency. Success in this situation means someone does not die. Surgery is required. Prayers are offered. Just be aware that this is a rare complication—much more likely to occur in severe ulcerative colitis, but it still is a possibility.

Possible increased bacterial virulence

There may be another concern with prebiotics to place under consideration: One prebiotic sweetener, trehalose, rarely used, may enhance the virulence of a certain pathogen named *Clostridium difficile* (*C. diff*) (Collins et al., 2018). Ulcerative colitis patents are particularly susceptible to *C. diff* (Zhang et al., 2017), so this rather uncommon prebiotic should probably be placed on the list of probiotics to use with caution or to not use at all.

Butyrate in excess

Another important consideration: High concentrations of butyrate may increase intestinal permeability, at least experimentally (Hamer et al., 2008). This may be a potential problem associated with excessive use of butyrate tablets or from excessive butyrate "uptake" from butyrate enemas—both administration methods available for the treatment of ulcerative colitis.

Sadly, you are a non-responder

Remember our discussion on resistant starch? Regarding some individuals who did not respond to resistant starch because of a missing bacterium, *Ruminococcus bromii*? This brings up the concept of a non-responder. Someone, apparently, has a lot to say on the subject:

> These phenotypic responses are related to a combination of host genetics, adequate dosages of the dietary polysaccharide of interest, and the unique microbiota composition of the individual. Thus, "responders" and "non-responders" to dietary modulation of the microbiota via specific fibers may be linked to inadequate dosages and/or lack of bacteria that can ferment the supplemented fiber(s). For example, consumption of 2.5 grams/day of short-chain FOS or galactooligosaccharide (GOS) did not increase bifidobacteria, but doses of 10 grams/day were adequate to induce a bloom in bifidobacteria in the gastrointestinal microbiota. Furthermore, **individuals without detectable levels of bifidobacteria failed to respond** to consumption of up to 7.5 grams/day agave inulin. Responses are also dependent on fiber intake in the context of the entire diet; for example, dietary fiber per kilocalorie has been shown to be positively related to both Bifidobacterium spp. Abundances and fecal butyrate concentrations. (Holscher, 2017, emphasis added)

Perhaps with the right probiotic, one supplying the missing bacterial species, an improved response to prebiotics can be achieved. Sounds reasonable.

Returning to the dark side

There is one sure-fire method of undoing all the good provided by living the prebiotic-enhanced life. It is a return to the Western diet. Listen up!

Pronounced shifts in bacterial diversity and production of microbial derived fecal fermentative end products have been demonstrated in as little as 24 hours in humans switching between an agrarian diet rich in fiber (> 30 grams/day) to a meat-based diet that was essentially devoid of fiber.

Dietary fiber intake is notably different across industrialized and unindustrialized parts of the world—Westernized diets are characterized by their high content of animal protein, fat, sugar, and starch, and low fiber content while the diets of inhabitants of unindustrialized rural communities in African countries, such as Burkina Faso and Tanzania, provide up to seven times more fiber due to increased intake of fibrous plants. (Holscher, 2017)

A few final thoughts

There is almost an endless variety of prebiotics and prebiotic foods from which to choose, and many, if not most, hold promise in the battle against the greatest evil you have ever known. However, you may not need to go all crazy here, buying a variety of exotic prebiotics and giving each one a try. (Although I would be tempted to do this.) It may be that one or perhaps a combination of two of the prebiotics we have previously discussed, plus eating a healthy, fiber-rich diet—all under physician approval and direction—is all that is needed to tip the scales in your favor. And keep in mind, some individuals are very happy indeed, having achieved and maintained a remission that lasts with the use of prebiotics. As far as prebiotic side effects go, generally they are dose related.

Prebiotics . . . may induce gaseousness and bloating. Abdominal pain and diarrhea only occur with large doses. (Marteau and Seksik, 2004)

Before we move on, I want to put in another plug for **lactulose**. With daily use of this prebiotic, in a tolerable dose, you and your physician may not have to worry (as much) should there be a lack of sufficient prebiotic fibers in the diet you follow. Plus, you get the added benefit of increased antioxidant production.

Look who else can be a prebiotic

Acarbose, a drug used in the treatment of diabetes, delays the release of glucose from complex carbohydrates—allowing glucose to escape digestion in the small intestine and enter the colon where friendly bacteria are eagerly waiting, knife and fork in hand (Chen et al., 2012; Zhang et al., 2013). As a result, a *"considerable amount of hydrogen"* is produced (Chen et al., 2012; Zhang et al., 2013). Hydrogen, as we have learned, is a remarkable, powerful antioxidant. Should Acarbose, with its ability to promote hydrogen production, be considered for use in the battle against ulcerative colitis? These guys seem to think so:

> Zhang DQ, Zhu JH, Chen WC. **Acarbose: a new option in the treatment of ulcerative colitis by increasing hydrogen production.** African Journal of Traditional, Complementary and Alternative Medicines. 2013;10(1):166-9.

Turmeric, the bioactive ingredient in curry, is another prebiotic that can be acted on by colonic bacteria to produce substantial amounts of hydrogen, which *"plays an important role in inactivating oxidative stresses."* (Shimouchi et al., 2009) Curcumin, a popular derivative of turmeric, also promotes the production of colonic hydrogen, allowing it to be, in effect, a powerful antioxidant (Chen et al., 2012). Therefore, both turmeric and curcumin are true prebiotics, and have a few other tricks up their sleeves as well. We'll look into this later.

Sugar alcohols, their names ending in -ol, like **sorbitol** and **xylitol**, are also prebiotics—fermented by friendly bacteria to produce butyrate, and, wouldn't you know, produce hydrogen in relevant amounts (Knight-Sepulveda et al., 2015; Sato et al., 2017; Lugani and Sooch, 2017). In fact, experimentally, xylitol produces more butyrate than does oligofructose (Sato et al., 2017). But beware, these sweeteners are on the FODMAP list, and may cause GI distress in those who's ulcerative colitis is acting a lot like IBS (Knight-Sepulveda et al., 2015).

What's up, Doc?

To modify a disease process occurring in the rectum and distal colon, a butyrate enema can be prescribed to be used at home. Butyrate enemas offer many of the benefits associated with prebiotics, allowing butyrate to be applied directly to the surface of the rectum and distal colon. Perhaps many (at least some) individuals have found butyrate enemas to be very helpful in their personal battle against ulcerative colitis. Here's a little something on this, taken from the medical literature:

> Butyrate was administered by rectal enemas, because this is a safe and reliable way to deliver a specific amount of substrate to the distal colon. Other techniques, such as oral intake of dietary fibers or encapsulated butyrate, do not allow to accurately target the distal colon in vivo. The distal colon was chosen as [a] target area for the butyrate intervention since the concentration of butyrate is lowest in this part of the colon due to rapid fermentation of commonly ingested dietary fibers in the proximal colon and the incidence of carcinomas and diseases in particularly the distal part of the colon is rising. (Vanhoutvin et al., 2009)

If interested in "going" this route, you'll need a prescription before you can purchase butyrate enema solutions. A local compounding pharmacy can prepare them for you. **Woodland Hills Pharmacy** will be happy to do this for you. After that, you are on your own.

https://www.woodlandhillspharmacy.com/compounds/gastro
enterology/short-chain-fatty-acid-enema/

Or you can make a butyrate enema yourself. An actual ulcerative colitis patient, **Terry Chattsworth**, will show you how. Physician approval first! Pay Terry a visit online by following this link:

https://gettinghealthiernow.wordpress.com/2014/07/17/sodium-butyrate-enemas-uc/

Honey, I shrunk the pathogens!

This is just for fun—but there may be something here!

Honey, due to its prebiotic effects, and particularly its *"powerful"* antioxidant properties (Medhi et al., 2008), may have some value in the treatment of ulcerative colitis (Bilsel et al., 2002; Medhi et al., 2008). As far as its prebiotic potential, *"Honey contains oligosaccharides that can be utilized by saccharolytic fermenters to yield beneficial metabolites that promote the prebiotic effect."* (Mohan et al., 2017) In keeping with other prebiotics, and their role in suppressing the growth of pathogens, with honey consumption you may be able to "shrink" the number of pathogens in your life.

Besides being both a prebiotic *and* a powerful antioxidant, honey contains a multitude of beneficial ingredients. Honey contains important nutrients, such as trace elements (minerals), vitamins such as vitamin C, amino acids, and proteins (Erejuwa et al., 2012) But that's not all . . .

Honey contains an array of chemicals endowed with antiradical/anti-inflammatory activity . . . which can play an important role, alone or in combination, in their antitumor, anti-inflammatory effects. (Alvarez-Suarez et al., 2010)

So, it should be of no surprise to read: *"Honey might also be of value in ulcerative colitis."* (Erejuwa et al., 2012) (Okay, you can be surprised.)

But just so you know, not all honeys are created equal. Some are exceptional. **Manuka honey** *"has greatly attracted [the] attention of researchers for its biological properties, especially its antimicrobial and antioxidant capacities."* (Alvarex-Suarez et al., 2014) Another exceptional honey, **buckwheat honey**, has *"the highest antioxidant activity of honeys from 14 different floral sources tested."* (Gheldof et al., 2003) Exceptional honeys may be worth the extra costs involved. Manuka is produced in New Zealand and eastern Australia, whereas buckwheat honey is produced in the USA and Canada. Both honeys can be purchased online.

But be aware, honey is on the list of foods high in FODMAPs (Knight-Sepulveda et al., 2015). Tummy trouble (aside from what you already have) is a possibility.

The fiber content of (almost) everything

The following web address leads to a comprensive guide entitled *The Fiber Content of Foods*, and lists the content of both insoluble and soluble fibers in many of the foods we eat, both natural foods and prepared foods. If something is not listed in the guide, it is probably low in fiber.

https://www.prebiotin.com/prebiotin-academy/fiber-content-of-foods/

~References~

Abu-Shanab A, Quigley EM. **The role of the gut microbiota in nonalcoholic fatty liver disease.** Nature reviews Gastroenterology & hepatology. 2010 Dec;7(12):691.

Alvarez-Suarez JM, Tulipani S, Romandini S, Bertoli E, Battino M. **Contribution of honey in nutrition and human health: a review.** Mediterranean Journal of Nutrition and Metabolism. 2010 Apr 1;3(1):15-23.

Alvarez-Suarez JM, Gasparrini M, Forbes-Hernández TY, Mazzoni L, Giampieri F. **The composition and biological activity of honey: a focus on Manuka honey.** Foods. 2014 Jul 21;3(3):420-32.

Bengmark S. **Pre-, Pro-, Synbiotics and Human Health.** FOOD TECHNOL BIOTECH. 2010;48(4):464-75.

Bilsel Y, Bugra D, Yamaner S, Bulut T, Cevikbas U, Turkoglu U. **Could honey have a place in colitis therapy? Effects of honey, prednisolone, and disulfiram on inflammation, nitric oxide, and free radical formation.** Digestive Surgery. 2002;19(4):306-12.

Bouhnik Y, Attar A, Joly FA, Riottot M, Dyard F, Flourie B. **Lactulose ingestion increases faecal bifidobacterial counts: a randomised double-blind study in healthy humans.** European journal of clinical nutrition. 2004 Mar;58(3):462-6.

Canani RB, Ci Costanzo M, Leone L 2012 **The Epigenetic Effects of Butyrate: Potential Therapeutic Implications for Clinical Practice.** Clinical Epigenetics 4(1):4.

Carlson J, Gould T, Slavin J. **In vitro analysis of partially hydrolyzed guar gum fermentation on identified gut microbiota.** Anaerobe. 2016 Dec 1;42:60-6.

Carrera-Bastos P, Fontes-Villalba M, O'Keefe JH, Lindeberg S, Cordain L. **The western diet and lifestyle and diseases of civilization.** Research Reports in Clinical Cardiology. 2011 Mar 9;2:15-35.

Cetinkaya A, Bulbuloglu E, Kantarceken B, Ciralik H, Kurutas EB, Buyukbese MA, Gumusalan Y. **Effects of L-carnitine on oxidant/antioxidant status in acetic acid-induced colitis.** Digestive diseases and sciences. 2006 Mar 1;51(3):488-94.

Chen X, Zuo Q, Hai Y, Sun XJ. **Lactulose: an indirect antioxidant ameliorating inflammatory bowel disease by increasing hydrogen production.** Medical hypotheses. 2011 Mar 1;76(3):325-7.

Chen X, Zhai X, Kang Z, Sun X. **Lactulose: an effective preventive and therapeutic option for ischemic stroke by production of hydrogen.** Medical gas research. 2012 Dec;2(1):3.

Chen X, Zhai X, Shi J, Liu WW, Tao H, Sun X, Kang Z. **Lactulose mediates suppression of dextran sodium sulfate-induced colon inflammation by increasing hydrogen production.** Digestive diseases and sciences. 2013 Jun 1;58(6):1560-8.

Cherbut C, Michel C, Lecannu G. **The prebiotic characteristics of fructooligosaccharides are necessary for reduction of TNBS-induced colitis in rats.** The Journal of nutrition. 2003 Jan 1;133(1):21-7.

Collins J, Robinson C, Danhof H, Knetsch CW, van Leeuwen HC, Lawley TD, Auchtung JM, Britton RA. **Dietary trehalose enhances virulence of epidemic Clostridium difficile.** Nature. 2018 Jan 3.

De La Torre AM. Silleras BD. **The use of partially hydrolyzed guar gum (PHGG)-containing formulas in the treatment of Inflammatory Bowel Disease (IBD).** Rivista Italiana di Nutrizione Parenterale ed Enterale/Anno. 2003;21(3):105-11.

Dharmarajan TS. **Psyllium versus guar gum: facts and comparisons.** Practical Gastroenterology. 2005 Feb:72.

Duncan SH, Louis P, Flint HJ. **Lactate-utilizing bacteria, isolated from human feces, that produce butyrate as a major fermentation product.** Applied and environmental microbiology. 2004 Oct 1;70(10):5810-7.

Erejuwa OO, Sulaiman SA, Ab Wahab MS. **Honey: a novel antioxidant. Molecules.** 2012 Apr 12;17(4):4400-23.

Faber F, Bäumler AJ. **The impact of intestinal inflammation on the nutritional environment of the gut microbiota.** Immunology letters. 2014 Dec 1;162(2):48-53.

Faghfoori Z, Navai L, Shakerhosseini R, Somi MH, Nikniaz Z, Norouzi MF. **Effects of an oral supplementation of germinated barley foodstuff on serum tumour necrosis factor-α, interleukin-6 and-8 in patients with ulcerative colitis.** Annals of clinical biochemistry. 2011 May;48(3):233-7.

Gheldof N, Wang XH, Engeseth NJ. **Buckwheat honey increases serum antioxidant capacity in humans.** Journal of agricultural and food chemistry. 2003 Feb 26;51(5):1500-5.

Gibson GR, Delzenne N. **Inulin and oligofructose: New scientific developments.** Nutrition Today. 2008 Mar 1;43(2):54-9.

Hafer A, Krämer S, Duncker S, Krüger M, Manns MP, Bischoff SC. **Effect of oral lactulose on clinical and immunohistochemical parameters in patients with inflammatory bowel disease: a pilot study.** BMC gastroenterology. 2007 Dec;7(1):36.

Hamer HM, Jonkers DM, Venema K, Vanhoutvin SA, Troost FJ, Brummer RJ. **The role of butyrate on colonic function.** Alimentary pharmacology & therapeutics. 2008 Jan 1;27(2):104-19.

Hamer HM, Jonkers DM, Bast A, Vanhoutvin SA, Fischer MA, Kodde A, Troost FJ, Venema K, Brummer RJ. **Butyrate modulates oxidative stress in the colonic mucosa of healthy humans.** Clinical Nutrition. 2009 Feb 1;28(1):88-93.

Haskey N, Gibson DL. **An examination of diet for the maintenance of remission in inflammatory bowel disease.** Nutrients. 2017 Mar 10;9(3):259.

Holscher HD. **Dietary fiber and prebiotics and the gastrointestinal microbiota.** Gut Microbes. 2017 Mar 4;8(2):172-84.

Jacobasch G, Schmiedl D, Kruschewski M, Schmehl K. **Dietary resistant starch and chronic inflammatory bowel diseases.** International journal of colorectal disease. 1999 Dec 1;14(4-5):201-11.

Jacobs DM, Gaudier E, Duynhoven JV, Vaughan EE. **Non-digestible food ingredients, colonic microbiota and the impact on gut health and immunity: a role for metabolomics.** Current drug metabolism. 2009 Jan 1;10(1):41-54.

Knight-Sepulveda K, Kais S, Santaolalla R, Abreu MT. **Diet and inflammatory bowel disease.** Gastroenterology & hepatology. 2015 Aug;11(8):511.

Kolida S, Tuohy K, Gibson GR. **Prebiotic effects of inulin and oligofructose.** British Journal of Nutrition. 2002 May;87(S2):S193-7.

Korzenik JR, Podolsky DK. **Evolving knowledge and therapy of inflammatory bowel disease.** Nature reviews Drug discovery. 2006 Mar;5(3):197.

Liao W. **Lactulose—a potential drug for the treatment of inflammatory bowel disease.** Medical hypotheses. 1994 Oct 1;43(4):234-8.

Lomax AR, Calder PC. **Prebiotics, immune function, infection and inflammation: a review of the evidence.** British Journal of Nutrition. 2008 Sep;101(5):633-58.

Looijer–Van Langen MA, Dieleman LA. **Prebiotics in chronic intestinal inflammation.** Inflammatory bowel diseases. 2009 Mar 1;15(3):454-62.

López-Alarcón C, Rocco C, Lissi E, Carrasco C, Squella JA, Nuñez-Vergara L, Speisky H. **Reaction of 5-aminosalicylic acid with peroxyl radicals: protection and recovery by ascorbic acid and amino acids.** Pharmaceutical research. 2005 Oct 1;22(10):1642-8.

Lugani Y, Sooch S. **Xylitol, an emerging prebiotic: a review.** Int J Appl Pharm Biol Res. 2017;2:67-73.

Marteau P, Seksik P. **Tolerance of probiotics and prebiotics. Journal of clinical gastroenterology.** 2004 Jul 1;38:S67-9.

McCarville JL, Caminero A, Verdu EF. **Novel perspectives on therapeutic modulation of the gut microbiota.** Therapeutic advances in gastroenterology. 2016 Jul;9(4):580-93.

Medhi B, Prakash A, Avti PK, Saikia UN, Pandhi P, Khanduja KL. **Effect of Manuka honey and sulfasalazine in combination to promote antioxidant defense system in experimentally induced ulcerative colitis model in rats.** Indian Journal of Experimental Biology. 2008 Aug 46:583–90.

Mitsuyama K, Saiki T, Kanauchi O, Iwanaga T, Tomiyasu N, Nishiyama T, Tateishi H, Shirachi A, Ide M, Suzuki A, Noguchi K. **Treatment of ulcerative colitis with germinated barley foodstuff feeding: a pilot study.** Alimentary pharmacology & therapeutics. 1998 Dec;12(12):1225-30.

Mohan A, Quek SY, Gutierrez-Maddox N, Gao Y, Shu Q. **Effect of honey in improving the gut microbial balance.** Food Quality and Safety. 2017 May 1;1(2):107-15.

Morita T, Kasaoka S, Hase K, Kiriyama S. **Psyllium shifts the fermentation site of high-amylose cornstarch toward the distal colon and increases fecal butyrate concentration in rats.** The Journal of nutrition. 1999 Nov 1;129(11):2081-7.

Moura FA, de Andrade KQ, dos Santos JC, Araújo OR, Goulart MO. **Antioxidant therapy for treatment of inflammatory bowel disease: Does it work?.** Redox biology. 2015 Dec 1;6:617-39.

Mortensen PB, Holtug K, Bonnén H, Clausen MR. **The degradation of amino acids, proteins, and blood to short-chain fatty acids in colon is prevented by lactulose.** Gastroenterology. 1990 Feb 1;98(2):353-60.

Muir JG, Lu ZX, Young GP, Cameron-Smith D, Collier GR, O'Dea K. **Resistant starch in the diet increases breath hydrogen and serum acetate in human subjects.** The American journal of clinical nutrition. 1995 Apr 1;61(4):792-9.

Nie Y, Lin Q, Luo F. **Effects of Non-Starch Polysaccharides on Inflammatory Bowel Disease.** International journal of molecular sciences. 2017 Jun 27;18(7):1372.

Niness KR. **Inulin and oligofructose: what are they?.** The Journal of nutrition. 1999 Jul 1;129(7):1402S-6s.

Olendzki BC, Silverstein TD, Persuitte GM, Ma Y, Baldwin KR, Cave D. **An anti-inflammatory diet as treatment for inflammatory bowel disease: a case series report.** Nutrition journal. 2014 Dec;13(1):5.

Oliveira RP, Florence AC, Perego P, De Oliveira MN, Converti A. **Use of lactulose as prebiotic and its influence on the growth, acidification profile and viable counts of different probiotics in fermented skim milk.** International journal of food microbiology. 2011 Jan 31;145(1):22-7.

Pituch-Zdanowska A, Banaszkiewicz A, Albrecht P. **The role of dietary fibre in inflammatory bowel disease.** Przeglad gastroenterologiczny. 2015;10(3):135.

Rapin JR, Wiernsperger N. **Possible links between intestinal permeablity and food processing: a potential therapeutic niche for glutamine.** Clinics. 2010;65(6):635-43.

Roberfroid MB. **Prebiotics: preferential substrates for specific germs?.** The American journal of clinical nutrition. 2001 Feb 1;73(2):406s-9s.

Rodríguez-Cabezas ME, Galvez J, Lorente MD, Concha A, Camuesco D, Azzouz S, Osuna A, Redondo L, Zarzuelo A. **Dietary fiber down-regulates colonic tumor necrosis factor α and nitric oxide production in trinitrobenzenesulfonic acid-induced colitic rats.** The Journal of nutrition. 2002 Nov 1;132(11):3263-71.

Sartor RB. **Therapeutic manipulation of the enteric microflora in inflammatory bowel diseases: antibiotics, probiotics, and prebiotics.** Gastroenterology. 2004 May 1;126(6):1620-33.

Sasaki M, Klapproth JM. **The role of bacteria in the pathogenesis of ulcerative colitis.** Journal of signal transduction. 2012;2012.

Sato T, Kusuhara S, Yokoi W, Ito M, Miyazaki K. **Prebiotic potential of L-sorbose and xylitol in promoting the growth and metabolic activity of specific butyrate-producing bacteria in human fecal culture.** FEMS microbiology ecology. 2017 Jan 1;93(1).

Scaldaferri F, Gerardi V, Lopetuso LR, Del Zompo F, Mangiola F, Boškoski I, Bruno G, Petito V, Laterza L, Cammarota G, Gaetani E. **Gut microbial flora, prebiotics, and probiotics in IBD: their current usage and utility.** BioMed research international. 2013;2013.

Scheppach W, Luehrs H, Menzel T. **Beneficial health effects of low-digestible carbohydrate consumption.** British Journal of Nutrition. 2001 Mar;85(S1):S23-30.

Shimouchi A, Nose K, Takaoka M, Hayashi H, Kondo T. **Effect of dietary turmeric on breath hydrogen.** Digestive diseases and sciences. 2009 Aug 1;54(8):1725-9.

Shinohara K, Ohashi Y, Kawasumi K, Terada A, Fujisawa T. **Effect of apple intake on fecal microbiota and metabolites in humans.** Anaerobe. 2010 Oct 1;16(5):510-5.

Slavin J. **Fiber and prebiotics: mechanisms and health benefits.** Nutrients. 2013 Apr 22;5(4):1417-35.

Szilagyi A, Rivard J, Bitton A, Cohen A, Mishkin S, Shrier I, Wild G. **Short term effects of lactulose in patients with stable IBD: Coladapt study.** Gastroenterology. 2000 Apr 1;118(4):A1372.

Tuohy KM, Ziemer CJ, Klinder A, Knöbel Y, Pool-Zobel BL, Gibson GR. **A human volunteer study to determine the prebiotic effects of lactulose powder on human colonic microbiota.** Microbial Ecology in Health and Disease. 2002 Jan 1;14(3):165-73.

van de Wiele T, Boon N, Possemiers S, Jacobs H, Verstraete W. **Inulin-type fructans of longer degree of polymerization exert more pronounced in vitro prebiotic effects.** Journal of Applied Microbiology. 2007 Feb 1;102(2):452-60.

Vanhoutvin SA, Troost FJ, Hamer HM, Lindsey PJ, Koek GH, Jonkers DM, Kodde A, Venema K, Brummer RJ. **Butyrate-induced transcriptional changes in human colonic mucosa.** PloS one. 2009 Aug 25;4(8):e6759.

Vigsnæs LK, Holck J, Meyer AS, Licht TR. **In vitro fermentation of sugar beet arabino-oligosaccharides by fecal microbiota obtained from patients with ulcerative colitis to selectively stimulate the growth of Bifidobacterium spp. and Lactobacillus spp.** Applied and environmental microbiology. 2011 Dec 1;77(23):8336-44.

Wei Y, Gong J, Zhu W, Tian H, Ding C, Gu L, Li N, Li J. **Pectin enhances the effect of fecal microbiota transplantation in ulcerative colitis by delaying the loss of diversity of gut flora.** BMC microbiology. 2016 Dec;16(1):255.

Wong C, Harris PJ, Ferguson LR. **Potential benefits of dietary fibre intervention in inflammatory bowel disease.** International journal of molecular sciences. 2016 Jun 14;17(6):919.

Yuedong HA, Yu HO, Qi WA, Xudong LI, Dexi LI. **Lactulose mediates suppression of dextran sulfate sodium-induced colon inflammation.** Journal of Medical Colleges of PLA. 2013 Apr 1;28(2):65-79.

Zhang DQ, Zhu JH, Chen WC. **Acarbose: a new option in the treatment of ulcerative colitis by increasing hydrogen production.** African Journal of Traditional, Complementary and Alternative Medicines. 2013;10(1):166-9.

Zhang SL, Wang SN, Miao CY. **Influence of Microbiota on intestinal immune System in Ulcerative Colitis and its intervention.** Frontiers in immunology. 2017;8.

Chapter 9

Why bother

Experimental studies indicate that commonly used food ingredients can alter the intestinal barrier, thereby causing intestinal inflammation.

It is intriguing to learn that some frequently used food components impact on the quality of the intestinal barrier, as well as on the composition of the intestinal microbiome. **~Ruemmele, 2016**

Y ou're serious about getting well. You're making all the right moves—meds faithfully taken, avoiding foods that seem to annoy, and consuming your pre- and probiotics and whatever else that suits your fancy. But why bother, say I, when you continually harm yourself in many, many ways, and do so day in and day out. Some of what follows I have mentioned before, but important enough to discuss at greater length in this most important chapter.

There are dangers built into our society that you need to become aware of, dangers that not only predispose to ulcerative colitis but also promote its persistence. You, the ulcerative colitis patient, should probably avoid danger, at least as much as is reasonably possible. Exposing these dangers is what this chapter is all about. You may know some of this. But you don't know all of this. You may want to pay close attention to what follows. I believe this chapter is particularly relevant to those who are struggling in their battle against ulcerative colitis.

We have a lot of dangers to consider in this chapter, and it is anyone's guess which danger poses the greatest threat. But since we must start somewhere, I decided to begin with **emulsifiers,** substances also known as **surfactants**. Note: Since this as a long chapter, I'll break things up into small, bite-sized pieces (sections) just to make things easy on you, even though entire chapters, long arduous chapters, should be written on each item we will discuss. I don't know if I can scare you enough with small little sections, but I'll try. We'll cover a lot of ground here, so buckle up and we'll be on our way.

Emulsifiers (AKA Surfactants)

*Emulsifiers are detergents, and in view of the evidence that **they can increase bacterial translocation,** processed foods with a high emulsifier content may be better avoided by patients with IBD unless human challenge studies can be performed to establish safety.* **~Richman and Rhodes, 2013, emphasis added**

*These **emulsifiers act <u>directly</u> on the mucosal barrier** by decreasing the viscosity of the mucus, thereby **facilitating bacterial translocation** and potentially driving inflammation.* **~Ruemmele, 2016, emphasis added**

Imagine eating danger at every meal. You probably do so, without ever knowing. And there are consequences.

The emulsifiers of which I speak are food additives found in a wide variety of manufactured foods such as **dairy products**, including my favorite, **ice cream**—and also found in **bakery goods**, **chocolates**, **sausages**, such diverse items as **ketchup**, **mayonnaise**, **salad dressings**, **toothpaste**, **chewing gum**, even **baby formula** (Swidsinski et al., 2009; Csáki, 2011; Lerner and Matthias, 2015).

Emulsifiers are added for noble reasons—to make the product look and taste better, or perform better, as in not separating or by exhibiting a creamier texture. But there is a dark side. Sure, you can consume emulsifiers and not be adversely affected, at least not on the surface . . . like forever, but not everyone is so lucky. Emulsifiers seem to seek out the vulnerable in our society, setting them up and doing all they can to lead them down the path of disease and destruction. (Do I look like I'm kidding?)

And if you are an ulcerative colitis patient, or genetically predisposed, you are at particular risk from the negative effects of emulsifiers. Did you notice the words "bacterial translocation" in the quotations at the beginning of this section? Bacterial translocation, referring to bacteria and bacterial products that are not restrained by the mucus barrier but are allowed to establish contact with the intestinal epithelial lining, is the cause of much of the inflammatory and autoimmune disease burden in our society (Lerner and Matthias, 2015). Unfortunately for you, bacterial translocation is a way of life, in as much as in ulcerative colitis bacteria reside in physical contact with the intestinal epithelium and do so on an ongoing basis (Schneider et al., 2010). They also threaten to advance beyond the epithelial layer, and actually do (Kell and Pretorius, 2015). But even if bacteria never advance beyond the epithelial barrier, their offending molecules will, as will other small molecules that likewise amplify the inflammatory activity occurring in ulcerative colitis (Schulzke et al., 2009; Csáki, 2011; Michielan and D'Incà, 2015).

Avoiding emulsifiers, that is, avoiding the foods that they contain, limits the harm they cause. It's that simple. And you certainly don't need any more trouble than you already have. Although you can't escape all of them, you can escape a lot of them.

Emulsifiers not only damage the mucus layer but can also harm the intestinal epithelial cell, too—**by damaging both the cell membrane and its intracellular components** (Csáki, 2011). Such damage can *"enhance the permeability of the GI track"* through the intestinal epithelial cell itself (called the "transcellular pathway") and by increased permeability of the tight junctions adjoining the intestinal epithelial cell with its neighboring cell, a condition we commonly call "leaky gut" (Csáki, 2011; Lerner and Matthias, 2015).

"So why does all this matter?" (You're asking the right question.)

*The bacterial concentrations in the large intestine can reach extremely high concentrations of 10^{11} [hundred billion] bacteria/ml, but the <u>mucus barrier efficiently separates colonic bacteria from the colonic wall</u> **making any response unnecessary**.*

Viscous <u>mucus</u> covers the intestinal wall, <u>disables bacterial movements, and protects epithelial cells from contact with bacteria</u>. Leukocytes (white blood cells) migrate into and patrol within the mucus layer executing surveillance function without any collateral damage. The sticky outer mucus surface offers the opportunity for probiotic strains to grow and build protective interlaced layers, making it even more difficult for pathogenic strains to reach the mucosa.

The inflammation takes place <u>only</u> after the mucus barrier is broken and the defense is overwhelmed. *Since the beginning of the 20th century, there has been a steady increase in reported cases of both Crohn's disease and <u>ulcerative colitis</u> and the peak has obviously not been reached.* (Swidsinski et al., 2009, emphasis added)

You can't just keep on attacking your mucus layer without consequences. Dietary emulsifiers pose such a threat because an intact mucus barrier is so fundamentally important. It is trouble with this layer that has likely initiated your ulcerative colitis in the first place. It is trouble with this layer that is likely responsible for its persistence. Indeed,

As long as the mucus barrier is impaired, the inflammatory process cannot successfully clear bacteria from the mucosal surface and <u>immunosuppressive therapy remains the main therapeutic option</u>. (Swidsinski et al., 2009, emphasis added)

The emulsifiers in our Western diet are not present in tiny, inconsequential amounts. They are extensively used, and used in greater concentrations than the concentrations known to produce inflammatory bowel disease in laboratory animals—and particularly so with respect to one common emulsifier, **carrageenan** (Bhattacharyya et al., 2008). We will discuss carrageenan shortly.

It should be mentioned, there are natural surfactants in fat-containing foods, and you can get too much for your own good, but these surfactants are tame compared to the synthetic emulsifiers (surfactants) added to our manufactured foods (Csáki, 2011). And when it comes to emulsifiers, more is not better. *"As a given surfactant can increase the [intestinal] permeability in several ways simultaneously and, as surfactants are often applied in mixtures, we can expect a combined effect."* (Csáki, 2011, commas added for clarity) Say it with me: "We are so screwed!"

Let's examine some of the common emulsifiers that are added to our foods, after we carefully consider this:

> *Synthetic surfactant food additives are intensively applied even in the most frequently consumed foods such as bakery products. <u>Parallel with the excessive use of food surfactant additives, there has been an increase in the incidence of diseases related to intestinal hyperpermeability</u>.*

> *. . . the main trouble with food surfactants is not their own toxicity but the fact that they are consumed together with everyday foods, so <u>they increase intestinal permeability</u> for a short time – but <u>exactly and repeatedly when there are harmful antigens and pathogens in the [gut] lumen</u>. **Lasting damage occurs when chemicals, allergens, colloid particles or <u>microorganisms</u>, which enter the hyper-permeable mucosa, cause inflammation.** (Csáki, 2011, emphasis added)*

Mono- and diglycerides

It all started with these bad boys. In the 1930s, mono- and diglycerides were introduced to Western society, added to margarine (Csáki, 2011). Margarine was and is still a bad idea, a very bad idea—typically made from pro-inflammatory omega-6 seed oils (more on the omega-6s later). Margarine is not a healthy food, it is solidified vegetable oil, made to look like butter. (But I'm not fooled.) The added surfactants make things worse. Aside from fake butter, surfactants make other things worse, too.

Mono- and diglycerides are the most widely used synthetic surfactants in the food industry (Csáki, 2011). The biggest application is in **bakery products**, but are also found in **margarines, ice cream**, and **chewing gum** (Csáki, 2011). About 50% of all surfactants wind up in bakery products (Csáki, 2011), which may be one reason why people with various health problems often do better when they cut-out bread and related products, often credited to reduced gluten consumption. Rather, it could be due to less emulsifier consumption (or both). Surprisingly, **gluten** is itself an emulsifier (Swidsinski et al., 2009).

Mono- and diglycerides are generally regarded as safe, but their emulsifying behavior suggest otherwise. Even if, in isolation, mono- and diglycerides do not appear to be particularly harmful, their consumption will add to the emulsifier load to which an individual is exposed, and in this way may be particularly harmful (see Csáki, 2011).

All things considered, I personally feel it is wise to limit the consumption of mono- and diglycerides. To this end, I read labels. Since I can't completely avoid mono- and diglycerides, I do my best to avoid as many as I can, doing so by making wise food choices. For example: I would never purchase peanut butter containing mono- and diglycerides when it is so easy to find a **peanut butter** that does not contain these additives. I never use margarine (knowingly). I also limit bread and other commercial bakery products as a rule, but when I do throw caution to the wind and take the risk, I choose the bakery goods with the least amount of food additives. And I certainly go out of my way to limit the following:

Carrageenan

> *Carrageenan is a very common food additive in Western diets, but **predictably** causes inflammation in thousands of cell-based animal experiments.*

> *Carrageenan intake contributed to earlier relapse in patients with ulcerative colitis.* **~Bhattacharyya et al., 2017, emphasis added**

Carrageenan is often billed as a thickener and stabilizer, but it is also an emulsifier (Martino et al., 2017). It is also known to produce harm and destroy the lives of many (laboratory animals).

Carrageenan in animal studies **1)** alters the microbiome, **2)** disrupts the epithelial barrier, **3)** inhibits proteins that protect against pathogens, and **4)** stimulates the production of pro-inflammatory cytokines (Martino et al., 2017). None of this is good news. And get this: *". . . recent studies of human epithelial cells and the human microbiome support the findings from animal studies."* (Martino et al., 2017, emphasis added)

Carrageenan, given experimentally to rats, mice, monkeys, and guinea pigs, predictably creates colon ulcerations that resemble what we see in ulcerative colitis (Tobacman, 2001). In fact, as far back as 1969, oral carrageenan consumption was used to predictably create an animal model of ulcerative colitis, a strategy subsequently and repeatedly used to test different therapies to treat ulcerative colitis (Tobacman, 2001). All things considered, could carrageenan consumption lead to ulcerative colitis in humans? Many people believe that it does, or at least complicates the disease process and places remission further out of reach. Reflecting this sentiment: *"The signs/symptoms in UC patients may be attributable to some extent to ongoing exposure to carrageenan, as well as other pro-inflammatory exposures."* (Bhattacharyya et al., 2017)

Because it is not ethical to poison the bowel of people to the extent necessary to elucidate the harmful effects of carrageenan in humans, we study cultured human colon cells in the laboratory setting. Studies have shown that carrageenan activates pro-inflammatory pathways which lead to the production of pro-inflammatory cytokines, although not in high amounts. However, "... *the inflammation generated through these pathways <u>when a pathogen is additionally present</u> is high, supporting the hypothesis that an interaction is present in which carrageenan serves as a pro-inflammatory agent to **<u>amplify</u> <u>existing intestinal inflammation</u>.*" (Martino et al., 2017, emphasis added) It's a good thing we only consume a small amount of carrageenan per day—Oh, wait! Carrageenan is <u>generously</u> supplied in the Western diet; meaning, we eat a lot of it (whether we know it or not, whether we want to or not).

> *Carrageenan is routinely consumed in the typical Western diet, with average intake estimated to be about 250 mg/day. Intake by* ***some individuals may be as high as 2–4 grams/day*** . . ..
> (Bhattacharyya et al., 2017, emphasis added)

Let's see if we can find out where they put all that carrageenan. Look for it in

> . . . *a variety of manufactured food products, including **ice cream**, **yogurt**, **chocolate milk**, **ricotta cheese**, **soymilk**, **nutritional supplements**, **dietetic powders**, **condensed milk**, **infant formula**, and **low-fat sandwich meats**.* (Bhattacharyya et al., 2008, emphasis added)

The following is a more extensive list of foods to avoid in a personal quest to limit carrageenan exposure:

List of foods to avoid in the no-carrageenan diet

Almond milk
Bakery products with glazes, frostings
Beer
Candy; chocolate candies
Canned fish, meats
Chocolate and flavored milk mixes/powders, condensed milk, evaporated milk powders
Cottage cheese
Dietetic beverages
Deli meat
Flax milk
Frosting base mix, canned frostings
Gelled fruit snacks
Ice cream, frozen custard, frozen yogurt, sherbets, etc.
Infant formulas
Liquid coffee whitener
Maple Syrups
Meal Replacements
Nutritional drinks
Pie filling
Processed meats, fish or cheese
Pudding
Ricotta cheese
Soy Milks
Whipped cream (canned)
Yogurt

(Bhattacharyya et al., 2017)

Let me add this: Those who wish to reduce their fat intake often turn to low-fat prepared foods, but they may want to reconsider. Some manufacturers use carrageenan in their low-fat foods as a substitute for fat (Bhattacharyya et al., 2008). Along these lines, processed fatty foods typically contain emulsifiers, which, as we have learned, *"are detergents that alter the behaviors of the intestinal lining."* (Richman and Rhodes, 2013) These two authors, Richman and Rhodes, also recommend that all plates, bowls, and kitchen utensils be carefully rinsed after washing to avoid exposure to the detergents (emulsifiers) found in dishwashing soaps.

I almost forgot to mention this: Carrageenan increases the production of hydrogen sulphide in the gut (Gibson et al., 1991). Oh, oh! Hydrogen sulphide just happens to interfere with the utilization of butyrate by the colonocyte, and the cell thus affected is placed on a starvation diet and lives a life of dysregulation and quiet despair (Hamer et al., 2008).

There is a great source on all things carrageenan. It is called **The Cornucopia Institute**. The web address is https://www.cornucopia.org/. On the home page there is a **Reports** tab on the upper right-hand corner. Hover over the Reports tab, then click **Carrageenan Report**. About a quarter-way down the acquired page, look for: *Protect yourself and your family with Cornucopia's carrageenan buying guide.* Click on **buying guide**. This will lead you to a list of foods that do or do not contain carrageenan. Print out the list. Put it to use. And while you're at it, look near the bottom of the page for an article entitled: *Carrageenan: How a "Natural" Food Additive is Making Us Sick.* This article will reinforce the things I am saying about this insidious health threat.

I suppose you are wondering why carrageenan as well as other emulsifiers are added to our food when they pose such a threat. It might have something to do with scientists and thought leaders who just can't seem to get past well-entrenched opinions. It might have something to do with governing agencies having trouble recognizing that current regulations, regulations they have instituted in the past, are unsound. And, it might have something to do with food industry lobbying efforts, as this industry has much to lose if carrageenan were to be banned or severely limited. If I say any more, I'll probably get into trouble. So, I'll let these guys stir up a little trouble instead:

The last half-century has witnessed a steady increase in consumption of food additives, many of which have not been carefully tested as they were given GRAS [generally regarded as safe] status at the time government entities charged with regulating food safety were created and/or expanded. Moreover, the testing of food additives that has been performed has generally utilized animal models designed to detect acute toxicity and/or promotion of cancer. Our data herein suggests that such testing may be inadequate—a notion supported by the recent observation that artificial sweeteners [more later] induce dysglycemia [abnormal glucose regulation] in humans. (Chassaing et al., 2015)

Let's leave carrageenan for now and move on to the next emulsifier. It looks like there is another troublemaker in our midst, one we need to deal with and do so without delay.

Carboxymethylcellulose (CMC)

The commonly used food additives, carrageenan and carboxy-methylcellulose (CMC), are used to develop intestinal inflammation in animal models. **~Martino et al., 2017**

Carboxymethylcellulose (CMC) is a common food additive. In animal studies, CMC **1)** alters the microbiome, **2)** disrupts the epithelial barrier, **3)** inhibits proteins that protect against pathogens, and **4)** stimulates the production of pro-inflammatory cytokines (Martino et al., 2017). All this should sound familiar—*this is exactly what carrageenan does!* And for more bad news: Not only is CMC extensively used in the food industry, *"The annual amount of CMC utilized by the food industry is constantly increasing"* with *"no quantitative restrictions on its use"* (Swidsinski et al., 2009). And they don't even tell you about it, as there is apparently no requirement to list CMC as a food additive (Swidsinski et al., 2009).

*The substance is added to food to stabilize emulsions, for instance in **ice cream**, to dissolve ingredients such as **cacao** in order* *to make perfect **chocolate and sugar icing**, to boost the flavor of the natural aroma and to keep bread fresh and soft. It can be found in **toothpaste, chewing gum**, a variety of **baked goods, candies, sausages, ketchup** and other sources. It is a filling and stabilizing component of most **pills** and it is a main substitute for gluten in manufactured **gluten free products**.* (Swidsinski et al., 2009, emphasis added)

I'm trembling. Are you? Imagine, a food additive that predictably creates IBD in laboratory animals (Swidsinski et al., 2009), yet is unapologetically given to humans! And in unrestricted amounts! Just imagine! Just imagine adding polysorbate-80 to the mix.

Polysorbate-80

A primary means by which the intestine is protected from its microbiota is via multi-layered mucus structures that cover the intestinal surface, thereby allowing the vast majority of gut bacteria to be kept a safe distance from epithelial cells that line the intestine.

More specifically, our data suggest that one ubiquitous [abundantly present] class of food additives, namely emulsifiers, can disturb the host-microbiota relationship resulting in a microbiota with enhanced mucolytic [mucus destroying] and proinflammatory activity that promotes intestinal inflammation. ~**Chassaing et al., 2015**

Polysorbate-80 has been shown to integrate within cell membranes resulting in a change of membrane microviscosity. It is possible that alterations in the membrane fluidity could alter bacterial adhesion and translocation through epithelial cells. ~**Roberts et al., 2010**

It looks like I won't have to comment a lot on polysorbate-80, as the above quotations adequately tell the story—the same story that can be told about the other emulsifiers previously discussed. But I will say a few words before we move on.

Polysorbate-80, and its close cousin, polysorbate-60, are common food additives that have a dark little secret. They find a home in intestinal cell membranes and negatively alter membrane behavior, as in altering membrane fluidity (Roberts et al., 2010). And with respect to polysorbate-80, altered membrane fluidity may lead to *"bacterial adhesion and translocation through epithelial cells"* (Roberts et al., 2010).

Trouble seems to run in the polysorbate family. Polysorbate-20 also belongs to this family of troublemakers.

Other emulsifiers of concern

I can't go on forever about emulsifiers, time will not allow. So, to spare you and move things along, I'll wrap things up. Just be aware, if the additive has a name like diacetyltartaric acid esters of mono- diglycerides (DATEM), sodium stearoyl-2-lactylate (SSL), calcium stearoyl-2-lactylate (CSL), sucrose esters of fatty acids, polyglycerol esters of fatty acids (PGE), and sorbitan esters of fatty acids, it is an emulsifier that cannot be trusted, and probably should be avoided. (see Csáki, 2011).

Let's move on. More trouble ahead.

Maltodextrin (MDX)

Food additives are common in the Western diet, and animal and ex-vivo studies have suggested a detrimental effect of certain food additives, including polysorbate-80, carboxymethylcellulose, maltodextrin, carrageenan, and microparticles.

Moreover, artificial sweeteners and dietary emulsifiers adversely affect the gut microbiota and promote inflammatory responses. **~Yang et al., 2016**

The results of these experiments demonstrated that the modified starch, maltodextrin (MDX), markedly enhanced E. coli biofilm formation and epithelial cell adhesion. **~Nickerson and McDonald, 2012**

Maltodextrin (MDX) is a food additive that serves as a **thickener**, and shares some of the same negative effects we see with the emulsifiers (Ruemmele, 2016). MDX can be found in **snack foods, breakfast cereals, salad dressing, dietary fiber supplements,** and is added to **Equal®** and **Splenda®** as a bulking agent (Nickerson and McDonald, 2012).

The dangers of MDX seem to be related to its ability to impair the anti-bacterial responses by intestinal epithelial cells and the killer cell called the macrophage (Ruemmele, 2016). Furthermore, MDX enhances the ability of certain bacteria to adhere to the intestinal epithelial cell as well as form protective biofilms (Nickerson and McDonald, 2012).

How bad is all this? I'm not sure. But it sounds kinda bad to kinda very bad. So, it may be worthwhile limiting foods that contain MDX, particularly if an individual has a tattered mucus membrane (allowing bacterial translocation) and has a disease that requires a robust defense against pathogens—oh, that would be you.

There is a low MDX diet, of sorts. It is called **The Specific Carbohydrate Diet** (Nickerson et al., 2015). The dietary restrictions in the diet eliminate MDX, as well as carrageenan and many other questionable additives, and it does so by excluding pre-packaged and processed foods (Nickerson et al., 2015). Another diet, the **IBD-AID** diet, basically does the same thing, and is a promising dietary option for the treatment of IBD, ulcerative colitis included (Nickerson et al., 2015). I'll discuss these two diets later in the book, and at greater length.

There is a MDX-related food additive, xanthan gum, that seems to share some of the same negative effects of MDX, such as an impaired antimicrobial response to bacteria (Ruemmele, 2016). It might be appropriate to place xanthan gum on the list of things to limit or avoid. My oh my, the list is getting long!

Artificial sweeteners

Artificial sweeteners sound like a good idea, unfortunately they are a bad idea. Extensive use of artificial sweeteners in our society (composed of mostly fat people) has failed to make a dent in the battle of the bulge. In fact, they likely have added fuel to the fire (Fowler et al., 2008). One reason artificial sweeteners lead to obesity is due to the fact that they contribute to dysbiosis (Suez et al., 2014; Chia et al., 2016; Rodriguez-Palacious et al., 2018). Oh! You have trouble with dysbiosis, remember? Did you know dysbiosis negatively effects the intestinal mucosa? It does.

> *The secretion of mucus droplets by goblet cells is regulated by the microbiota, thus **dysbiosis plays a key role in disruption of the mucus layer.*** (Chan et al., 2013, emphasis added)

With dysbiosis in ulcerative colitis, there can be a preponderance of mucus-foraging bacteria that degrade (eat) the mucus layer of the bowel (Tailford et al., 2015). The actions of such bacteria weaken this essential layer of protection, which may stand directly in the way of healing in ulcerative colitis.

One investigator, nearly 20 years ago, began to suspect that there was something dreadfully wrong with artificial sweeteners, and wrote:

> *A decade ago, a series of accidental findings made me suspect that the impaired inactivation of digestive proteases due to the inhibition of gut bacteria by dietary chemicals, such as saccharin, play a causative role in IBD as a result of the accelerated degradation of the mucus layer and underlying endothelium.* (Qin, 2011)

The investigator in question initially focused on saccharin, then sucralose (Splenda®) became suspect, and a warning was issued:

As I suggested a decade ago, regarding the possible risk of saccharin on IBD, sucralose may have a similar but stronger impact on gut bacteria, digestive protease inactivation and gut barrier function. This may provide a possible explanation for the more pronounced high incidence of IBD observed in Canada. The use of sucralose is soaring, and is now being used in thousands of food products. Therefore, it would be worthwhile to investigate whether possible links between sucralose intake and IBD exist, before it is too late. (Qin, 2011)

And so it came to pass, others became involved and began to relate artificial sweeteners to IBD, with one report stating: *"Epidemiological studies indicate that the use of **artificial sweeteners double the risk** of Crohn's disease."* (Rodriguez-Palacious et al., 2018, emphasis added) And there is a reason for such findings. Artificial sweeteners create a disturbed microbiota (Suez et al., 2014; Rodriguez-Palacious et al., 2018). Furthermore, Rodriguez-Palacious et al report that Splenda® (the oh so popular Splenda®) promotes *"bacterial penetration of the intestinal epithelial and an increased predominance of E. coli."* (Rodriguez-Palacious et al., 2018) So, is it any wonder that some authorities strongly discourage the use of artificial sweeteners?

Another problem associated with artificial sweeteners is the inclusion of maltodextrin in some formulations (Nickerson and McDonald, 2012; Rodriguez-Palacious et al., 2018). We just discussed this a couple of pages back, but you probably forgot. I'll work on your memory later, unless I forget.

At this point in the conversation, you are undoubtedly wondering about high-fructose corn syrup (HFCS). Is it healthy? No. It is not particularly healthy. HFCS, too, contributes to dysbiosis as well as to obesity (Payne et al., 2012). Consider it an artificial sweetener, or at least a somewhat unnatural one.

Fructose as a naturally occurring monosaccharide present in many fruits and vegetables provides only modest amounts of free fructose to the host. Conversely, the soring use of HFCS as sweetener in soft drinks, baked goods and condiments is imparting a new challenge upon the intestinal environment in managing free fructose overloads. (Payne et al., 2012, emphasis added)

With HFCS, there is no compensatory insulin secretion; therefore, the brain does not get a strong signal (by the gut hormone leptin) that enough is enough, and then we get the munchies (Payne et al., 2012). In other words, HFCS fails to stimulate satiety, and overeating is often the result (Payne et al., 2012). And when you overeat, you are most likely eating far too many of the following:

Microparticles

Ultrafine and fine particles . . . cause inflammation in susceptible individuals.

In isolation such microparticles are biologically inert, but during transit through the intestinal track they absorb luminal constituents, such as calcium ions and bacterial lipopolysaccharide [a bacterial cell wall component]. **~Lomer et al., 2001**

Powell et al have proposed that billions of microparticles, mostly titanium, aluminum, and silicon oxides, are ingested principally from food additives.

*While not leading to inflammation in themselves, they are proposed to act as adjuncts, <u>permitting the absorption of other antigens</u> [molecules that trigger an immune response] and <u>preventing their appropriate disposition</u> by the immune system, **altering the normal intestinal immune tolerance, and stimulating an immune response.** ~Korzenik, 2005,* **emphasis added**

We are continually exposed to microparticles. They are in the air we breathe. They are in the water we drink. They are in the food we eat. And with respect to the food we eat:

> Significant quantities of titanium dioxide [TiO2] and silicate are swallowed, both as natural contaminants of food and as additives. In fact, **more than 10^{12} [1 Trillion] particles _per day_ are ingested.** (Schneider, 2007, emphasis added)

That's a lot of microparticles for our gut to deal with—*1 trillion per day!* And unfortunately for us, the gut seems to be having a little trouble dealing with all the madness.

What is gradually being recognized is that the microparticles added to our foods can adversely affect the gut—being both pro-inflammatory in some respects, and at the same time, being capable of depressing certain components of the immune system (Kish et al., 2013; Bettini et al., 2017). And they are added in large amounts, in the form of titanium dioxide (TiO2), iron oxide, silicon dioxide, zinc oxide, and the silver added to food packaging and applied as coatings on toothbrushes (Gatti, 2004)—potentially adding to our microparticle intake of approximately **20–80 micrograms per day** (McClements and Xiao, 2017).

Of the above mentioned microparticles, TiO2 is the most common microparticle added to our food (Becker et al., 2014). We like things that are gleaming white. Toothpaste is gleaming white. Sugary toppings are gleaming white. Mayonnaise is gleaming white. TiO2 makes things white. That's its job. Obviously, manufacturers *love* this additive.

Turning our attention to the negative effects microparticles have on the gut, the small intestine seems to be more of a target than the colon; but the colon does not get off Scott-free as it, too, can be adversely affected (Nogueira et al., 2012). In laboratory animals, studies have shown that TiO_2 microparticles favor the development of low-grade inflammation in the colon and are particularly pro-inflammatory at a time ***"when the gut is already faced with pathogenic challenges, such as a*** *preexisting colitis."* (Bettini et al., 2017, emphasis added) Historically, in the 1950s, disease resembling Crohn's was created simply by feeding dogs finely divided sand (Evans et al., 2002). Did we take notice? Answer: Apparently not.

Microparticles, in this discussion, certainly include the engineered, super small particles called **nanoparticles**. Nanoparticles are way too small to be seen by the naked eye. To put things in perspective, a large nanoparticle is about 800 times smaller than the width of a human hair, with a medium-sized nanoparticle being about 1,600 times smaller than the width of a human hair and about half the size of the virus that causes the flu (Yokel and MacPhail, 2011). Get the picture? Nanoparticles are, indeed, very, very small. With respect to TiO_2, *"Previous investigators of TiO_2 particles found that* ***TiO_2 as nano-sized particles is more toxic than similarly composed, but larger sized particles."*** (Nogueira et al., 2012, emphasis added) Indeed, *"Exposure to NPs [nanoparticles] was reported to induce greater inflammation than exposure to larger particles with identical chemical composition and mass concentration."* (Zhang et al., 2012) Furthermore, the smaller the particle, the *"greater its intracellular bioavailability."* (Achtschin and Sipahi, 2017)

Leave it to scientists and engineers to push the envelope and create particles so small they are heinous in character. In fact, their smallness makes them particularly dangerous, as their surface-to-weight ratio gives them more absorbing capacity (Powell, 1996; Richman and Rhodes, 2013; McClements and Xiao, 2017). **And what are they absorbing?** Among other things, **they are absorbing the discarded wall components of bacteria**, such as lipopolysaccharide (**LPS**) (Ashwood et al., 2007; Schneider, 2007; Achtschin and Sipahi, 2017). LPS has a certain look and a certain feel that we can use to our advantage. Our immune system has cell-based sensors all over the place to detect LPS, and upon detection, an inflammatory response is formulated and executed. Unfortunately, the more LPS exposure, the greater the focus and intensity of the inflammatory response (Richman and Rhodes, 2013)—with the distinct possibility that microparticles, in combination with LPS or other bacterial components, may mimic invasive bacteria (Ashwood et al., 2007). And to think, in our Western society, we are individually exposed to a trillion or more microparticles per day along with an increased exposure to LPS—adding to the reasons why the Western diet is an unhealthy diet, an unhealthy diet that leads to disease.

But it is not only the food we eat that supplies our gut with microparticles in great abundance, so does the air we breathe. With each respiration, particulate matter circulating in the air can become trapped in the mucus layer that lines our airway and lungs (Kish et al., 2013; Nogueira et al., 2012). But it doesn't just stay there. This mucus layer is in constant motion, moving mucus upward towards the throat where it is swallowed, along with entrapped microparticles (Kish et al., 2013; Nogueira et al., 2012). This normal housekeeping activity (upward mucus movement and swallowing), seldom noticed, supplies the gut with a considerable number of microparticles to deal with. In this manner, air pollution contributes to non-respiratory disease via microparticle exposure. Things can get serious. In addition to a negative effect on the gut, other adverse consequences can occur

> . . . including stroke, myocardial infarction [heart attack], arrythmia [abnormal heart rhythm], cardiac arrest, venous thrombosis [blood clot in veins], and lung cancer. (Kish et al., 2013)

The reason I am going into airborne microparticle exposure in our conversation is because the following conclusion has been reached: **"Ingestion of airborne particulate matter _alters the gut microbiome_ and induces acute and chronic inflammatory responses in the intestine."** (Kish et al., 2013, emphasis added) So, you can add airborne microparticle exposure to the list of things that are out to get you.

During my review of the issues, I was surprised to learn there was an association identified between air pollution and abdominal pain, as well as an increased risk of appendicitis (Kish et al., 2013) Something unseemly must be going on.

Since there are several things about microparticles that concern me, and since I believe you should be in the know, I will list my major concerns. Studies reveal:

- There is no GI barrier for inert particles with a diameter below 20 micrometers (Gatti, 2004)

- Microparticles can suppress Treg numbers (Bettini et al., 2017). Recall, Treg cells serve to restrain inflammation

- Microparticles can alter the microbiome (Kish et al., 2013; McClements and Xiao, 2017)

- Microparticles modify the expression of genes, at least 40 of which are found operational in the colon (Kish et al., 2013)

- Microparticle TiO2 fed to rats leads to a nearly 40% incidence of precancerous lesions in the colon (Bettini et al., 2017)

- Microparticles in food and from air pollution enter our water supply, compounding our exposure to microparticles (Kish et al., 2013)

- *"When a particle measures 20 µm or less, it can pass through the intestinal barrier and is likely to end up in the bloodstream."* (Gatti and Rivasi, 2002)

- Microparticles (several types) *"have antimicrobial properties and may therefore alter the balance of different bacterial species in the colon, potentially leading to adverse health effects."* (McClements and Xiao, 2017)

- The smaller the particle, the greater the inflammatory response (Zhang et al., 2012)

- *"TiO2 as nano-sized particles is more toxic than similarly composed, but larger sized particles."* (Nogueira et al., 2012)

- *"Nanoparticles that reach the colon may interact with colonic bacteria and alter their viability, thereby changing the relative proportions of different bacterial species."* (McClements and Xiao, 2017)

- Nanoparticles generate reactive oxygen species (ROS) in cells in which they accumulate, which *"may then cause damage to cell membranes, organelles, and the nucleus."* (McClements and Xiao, 2017) (Note: ROS causes what is known as oxidative stress.)

As to the last point mentioned above, *"Oxidative stress is thought to be a key mechanism responsible for adverse biological effects exerted by NPs [nanoparticles]."* (Skocaj et al., 2011) What does all this have to do with ulcerative colitis?

Free radicals are inflammatory process mediators capable of causing rupture through the tight junctions of the intestinal epithelial cells layer, thus increasing intestinal paracellular permeability and modifying both the structure and the function of these junctions of the intestinal epithelial cells. <u>*This might be an aggravating factor to*</u> **an already established inflammatory bowel disease**<u>*, or even be the primary causative agent triggering an inflammatory response.*</u> *The ability of these particles to generate ROS and induce oxidative stress has been proposed as a mechanism of their* <u>*toxicity.*</u> *These properties have been associated with the* **activation of inflammatory mediators, oxidative DNA damage and mutagenesis.**

Micro- and nanoparticles have been found in the colon and the blood of cancer patients and patients with Crohn's disease and

ulcerative colitis, *although they were absent in healthy individuals.*
(Achtschin and Sipahi, 2017, emphasis added)

Apparently, a diseased colon is less capable of defending against microparticles than a healthy one. Oh! If my memory serves me well, you have a diseased colon, one you are not particularly thrilled with at the moment.

Aside from the sorry state of your colon (and rectum), what should concern us all is the fate of our children and their precious rectums and colons. Because sweets have the highest concentrations of TiO_2, and children eat a lot more sweets than adults, children have the highest exposure to this particular food additive (Weir et al., 2012). Toothpaste is also a major TiO_2-exposure risk for children, precious little children who also come down with IBD in ever-increasing numbers (see Rompelberg et al., 2016). *"Toothpaste dominated the contribution to the dietary intake [of TiO_2] by young children (57%), followed by sweets and cookies."* (Rompelberg et al., 2016) Perhaps you should take candy and cookies away from your children and mail them to me for proper disposal. I will give you my address later.

> *It is noteworthy that the amount of TiO_2 nanoparticles consumed was 2–4 times higher for children than for adults, which may be due to the fact that products heavily consumed by children has some of the highest levels of TiO_2 nanoparticles, such as candies, gums, desserts, and beverages.* (McClements and Xiao, 2017)

Let's move on.

So where do we find all those microparticles? Besides the exposures from the air we breathe and the water we drink (Lomer et al., 2001; Kish et al., 2013), and the toothpaste we swallow, we are exposed to microparticles when we consume the following:

List of food items reported to contain added microparticles*

Mayonnaise (major source)
(Richman and Rhodes, 2013)

Salt
Hard-coated candy
Chewing gum
Artificial sweeteners
Marshmallows
Icing for cakes and donuts
Chocolate and malted drink
    powders
Low-fat or fat-free dressings
Tartar sauce
Horseradish sauce
Thousand Island dressing
Refined carbohydrates
Potato- and corn-based snacks
Pork sausages
(Lomer et al., 2004)

Cottage cheese

Mozzarella cheese
Horseradish cream and sauces
Lemon curd
Low-fat products such as skim milk
    and ice cream
(Skocaj et al., 2011)

Nutritional supplements
Candy
Powdered milk
Salt
(McClements and Xiao, 2017)

Candy bars
Bakery product (cake, pie,
    pastries, cookies, biscuits)
Coffee creamer
Soft, sports drinks, fruit drinks
Breakfast cereals
(Rompelberg et al., 2016)

*Not all manufacturers add micro- or nanoparticles to the named product

And leave it to pharmaceutical companies to add unnecessary microparticles to our medications, including TiO2 and silicates. But nothing surprises me anymore.

Pharmaceuticals reported to be formulated with microparticles*

Ibuprofen	Codeine phosphate
Mesalazine	Hormone replacement
Co-proxamol	Loperamide
Paracetamol	Fe (iron) and folic acid
Co-codamol	Ranitidine
Azathioprine	Budesonide
Cyclosporin	Aspirin
Lansoprazole	Diclofenac sodium
Azathioprine	Prednisolone
Erythromycin	

(Lomer et al., 2004)

*Dependent on manufacturer and formulation

As we close out this section, what are the takeaways? **First**, we need to recognize that micro- and nanoparticles represent a threat on many levels—and particularly a threat to those who are battling ulcerative colitis. Although they do not trigger *"IBD-related colitis,"* micro- and nanoparticles do favor *"the development of low-grade inflammation in the colon."* (Bettini et al., 2017) **Second**, micro- and nanoparticles, so commonplace, are next to impossible to completely avoid. **Third**, micro- and nanoparticles can be avoided to a relevant degree—but doing so takes deliberate measures to limit foods high in microparticles. **Fourth**, since toothpaste represents a major source of microparticles, an easy, first step would be avoid swallowing toothpaste by spitting and rinsing thoroughly after brushing. Alternatively, using a toothpaste (or baking soda) that does not contain microparticles may be a good option. Such measures are expected to substantially reduce micro- nanoparticle exposure. **Fifth**, preparing and eating home-made foods, made with natural ingredients that do not contain micro- or nanoparticles, will greatly lessen the exposure to these unhealthy additives. **Sixth**, we can't assume that food items are micro- or nanoparticle-free even if they are not listed on the list of ingredients, as there may be loopholes that exempt such listing. And **finally**, fast and confidence foods typically contain micro- or nanoparticles, so it may be wise to limit fast and convenience food consumption. Commonsense measures such as these may give you an edge in the battle against ulcerative colitis. And since yours is a battle that carries an elevated risk for colon cancer, limiting nanoparticles may also be helpful on this front (see Nogueira et al., 2012).

Combining all information presently available, we must assume that especially inflammatory conditions at the intestinal mucosa carry an increased risk of NP [nanoparticle] uptake. (Sinnecker et al., 2014)

Iron in excess

*Accumulating evidence indicates that **excess of unabsorbed iron that enters the colon lumen causes unwanted side effects** at the intestinal host–microbiota interface.*

Notably, accumulating evidence suggests that unabsorbed iron can stimulate growth and virulence of bacterial pathogens in the intestinal environment. **~Kortman et al., 2014, emphasis added**

When iron meets the inflamed intestinal mucosa it may increase ROS [reactive oxygen species, leading to oxidative stress] and thereby tissue damage, as demonstrated in animal models of IBD. **~Erichsen et al., 2005**

Oral iron supplementation anecdotally exacerbate inflammatory bowel disease and iron levels are elevated in the inflamed mucosa. **~Millar et al., 2000**

In my book on Crohn's, I spend a lot of time warning of the dangers of iron, and how consuming it in excess, so commonplace in our society, leads to disease. Excess iron exposure may have led to the very disease you have (Aamodt et al., 2008; Gisbert and Gomollón, 2008). And it certainly has the power to amplify the disease process you are experiencing (Barollo et al., 2004; Uritski et al., 2004). No one else seems to be telling you this story, so I guess it's up to me. (If only people would listen.) And why do I raise the alarm? Because iron feeds and strengthens the pathogens in the gut. It increases their numbers. It makes them more aggressive and more likely to offend. Furthermore, it can cause ongoing physical damage to intestinal mucosa.

> *Besides the effects of iron on the gut microbiota, which may cause a shift towards a more pathogenic profile and an increase in virulence of enteric pathogens, iron may also directly exert unfavorable effects on the gut epithelium most likely by the promotion of redox stress.* (Kortman et al., 2014)

Danger danger! (and I really mean this)

Don't get me wrong, we need dietary iron. But not in the amounts our society provides. Bacteria need iron, too—many of which are young, aspiring pathogens. Notably, *"Acquiring iron is a fundamental step in the development of a pathogen."* (Doherty, 2007) They like all the excess iron that we do not need. Excess iron availability promotes their growth, virulence, and strengthens their numbers (Aamodt et al., 2008; Radek 2010; Kortman et al., 2014). Iron excess is the gift of dysbiosis, favoring the growth of pathogenic bacteria.

> *Ultimately, iron use allows for greater microbial growth and an increased capacity of the bacteria to adhere and possibly disseminate to distal sites to cause infection.* (Radek, 2010)

> *Iron is an important factor for the growth of bacteria and their expression of virulence. When the level of iron increases, the*

*balance between the quantities of different bacteria species in the gut is altered, depending on their ability to compete for iron. **The interaction between bacteria and host tissue will also be altered when iron levels are enhanced, including the ability for the bacteria to express virulence.*** (Aamodt et al., 2008, emphasis added)

Leave it to our society to "decide" that we need more iron than we could possibly use. And so, we fortify. Danger danger!

*Because > 90% of dietary iron is not absorbed, oral supplementation <u>may elevate gastrointestinal iron concentration</u> and **amplify mucosal damage** in patients with inflammatory bowel disease.* (Uritski et al., 2004, emphasis added)

In a laboratory study, the researchers found that human intestinal cells with excess iron were more susceptible to attack by bacteria that caused infection of the small intestine. The study suggests that enriching breakfast foods and other foods with high doses of iron—a nutritional strategy that has been widely adopted to eliminate iron deficiency—could be causing other health problems.

The scientists found that cells containing high levels of iron were more easily invaded by the bacteria.

"Instead of fortifying everyone's diet with excess iron, we should diagnose iron deficiency and then provide supplemental iron only to those who need it." —Quoting Dr. Mark Failla (Ohio State Research News, 2001)

As I said, we need iron. Particularly, we need sufficient quantities of iron for transfer to the **200 billion** new red blood cells we make each day—each with a pressing need for iron (Hentze et al., 2004). To replace losses when red blood cells meet their maker (killed by design at a rate of **2–3 million each second**), we have sophisticated recycling mechanisms in play that capture the iron from the dead and dying and deliver it to the next generation of red blood cells, cells which we also create at the rate of **2–3 million each second** (Gasche et al., 2004). Unless bleeding is an issue, or an inflammatory disease process like IBD is present, we need only small amounts of iron in our diet—only about 1 to 2 mg/day (Hentze et al., 2004). Iron consumed in excess of our need, and above what we can absorb in the upper portions of the small intestine, accumulates in the colon and can be problematic, as the quotations I am sharing with you clearly indicate. Read them again and again. (You are free to tremble.)

Iron, of course, is at the heart of the hemoglobin molecule, the molecule hidden within the red blood cell that allows it to carry oxygen to the various parts of the body. Astonishingly, each red blood cell—a cell we cannot see with the naked eye—contains **270 million** molecules of hemoglobin (Wikipedia, 2018), allowing one single red blood cell to contain over **1 billion** atoms of iron! (Cassat and Skaar, 2013) Now that's a lot of iron, all packed into a tiny little cell.

Fortunately, we have systems in place that allow us to extract all the iron we need from our food—and the cells that perform this noble service are found primarily in the duodenum and upper jejunum, far, far away from the colon (Gasche, 2000; Kortman et al., 2014). These specialized iron-uptake cells are under tight regulatory control; and after extracting their fill of dietary or supplemental iron, they take a break for a few days, then things reset, and they resume iron uptake all over again (and the cycle repeats over and over again) (Papanikolaou and Pantopoulos, 2005).

The iron that does make it past the absorptive cells in the duodenum and jejunum have the potential to accumulate in the colon where it can stir up trouble. ***Trouble!*** The colon can absorb iron to *"a small extent,"* (Kortman et al., 2014), or perhaps in *"significant"* quantities (Chua et al., 2010), but it is hoping you are eating a lot of vegetables, legumes, whole grains, and taking supplements like tumeric and quercetin—all of which will bind iron, withhold it from bacteria, and keep it from contact with inflamed mucosa (Gasche et al., 2004; Guo et al., 2007; Weinberg and Miklossy, 2008; Jiao et al., 2009; Kortman et al., 2014). The colon is also hoping you will lay off all the red meat you are eating, at least in the excessive amounts you are probably accustomed to.

> **The Western diet is characteristically rich in sources of iron, especially red meat,** and UC has historically been more prevalent in Western countries.

> **The <u>potentially deleterious effects</u> of a high-iron diet on UC are attributed to the <u>accumulation of iron in the colonic lumen in high concentrations</u>,** a direct result of the tight regulation of body iron levels and the restriction of dietary iron absorption. (Seril et al., 2006, emphasis added)

At this point in the conversation, I should mention this: Your colon has one final item on its wish list. It is hoping you will come to your senses and reduce your exposure to iron in order to decrease its risk of cancer. The iron that arrives in the colon accumulates in the cells of the colon and damages their DNA (Seril et al., 2006; Chua et al., 2010). And, as I have mentioned previously, ulcerative colitis carries a substantial risk of colon cancer—with the longer you have the disease, the more elevated the risk (Chen et al., 2013). Combined with rectal cancer, colon cancer rates for ulcerative colitis patients are *"10-fold higher than in the normal population."* (Chua et al., 2010) Experimentally, *"Iron has been found to be a <u>complete</u> carcinogen and to* **induce tumors without other co-carcinogen treatment.**" (Liehr and Jones, 2001, emphasis added)

In the midst of all this iron, typically more than we need, anemia can still rear its ugly head. Leave it to you to come down with a disease often complicated by anemia. Indeed, approximately one out of three IBD patients have anemia (Gasche et al., 2004) Typically, *"The only way to lose iron is by menstrual and intestinal bleeding."* (Gasche et al., 2004) Actually, there are a few other ways to lose iron: Bleeding, as from trauma, and blood loss due to blood donation. But with respect to the ulcerative colitis patient, anemia is often due to blood loss from the diseased colon (Seril et al., 2006; Bayraktar and Bayraktar, 2010; Weiss, 2011). But the anemia in ulcerative colitis is not always due to blood loss or at least from blood loss alone (Oldenburg et al., 2001).

Anemia in ulcerative colitis can be intentional from a physiological standpoint, a result of the body's purposeful block on iron absorption, a block imposed on iron uptake cells. This is an *"immune-mediated"* strategy aimed *"at restricting the supply of the essential nutrient iron to pathogens."* (Nairz et al., 2010; Oldenburg et al., 2001). Inflammation is a big clue that bacteria are present, and on the move (Nairz et al., 2010; Oldenburg et al., 2001). The body is taking extraordinary measures to keep you safe by drastically limiting iron availability for pathogen acquisition. And often, anemia follows—due to the protective efforts the immune system employs to block iron absorption and keep iron away from bacteria bent on evil. And in our hour of need, iron supplementation is generally considered, and often employed, to correct the anemia that results from intentional iron-withholding efforts or from chronic blood loss. But regardless of the cause, with iron supplementation I see trouble ahead.

> *Oral iron supplementation renders high fecal iron concentrations. Since only a fraction of supplemented iron will be absorbed, virtually the entire dose winds up in the distal parts of the bowel. In an already inflamed bowel, this may reinforce the inflammation by catalyzing production of ROS [reactive oxygen species] . . ..* (Erichsen et al., 2003, emphasis added)

> *Moreover, iron and reactive oxygen species can amplify inflammation, increasing mucosal permeability, recruiting neutrophils, and activating NF-κB.* (Barollo et al., 2004, emphasis added)

Another mechanism by which iron may exert a proinflammatory effect is the activation of nuclear factor-kappa B (NF-κB), a transcription factor which regulates the expression of many genes involved in inflammatory responses. (Oldenburg et al., 2001)

I'm sure by now you have a few questions

Taken into account the harm that iron may inflict on the already inflamed intestinal mucosa, the question remains whether inflammatory bowel disease patients with anemia should be treated with iron supplements. **~Oldenburg et al., 2001**

Now that you are aware of the dangers of iron excess and how it can feed the pathogens in your life, as well as intensify the disease process you are experiencing, you probably have a few questions. Let's see if I can round up a few physicians and scientists to help you out. (I know where to look, and I have a feeling they can.)

Question 1: "Should I limit the consumption of red meat as a measure to reduce my exposure to iron?" **Answer:** *"Yes,"* according to these guys:

The Western diet is characteristically rich in sources of iron, especially red meat, and UC has historically been more prevalent in Western countries.

The potentially deleterious effects of a high-iron diet on UC are attributed to the accumulation of iron in the colonic lumen in high concentrations, a direct result of the tight regulation of body iron levels and the restriction of dietary iron absorption. (Seril et al., 2006, emphasis added)

Specifically, we observed a 14% increase in risk of UC for every one serving increase in weekly red meat intake. (Khalili et al., 2017, emphasis added)

Question 2: "If my anemia is symptomatic, should it be treated?"
Answer: *"I would certainly think so."*

> *. . . there is enough evidence to support the following statements: (a) anemia is very common in IBD, (b) anemia should be investigated with care because many factors can be responsible, (c) treatment of anemia results in clear improvement in the objective parameters of well-being especially in the quality of life . . ..* (Gisbert and Gomollón, 2008)

Question 3: "Should I use oral iron supplements to correct my anemia?" **Answer:** *"Maybe not."*

> *Unless the host response is impaired by severe iron deficiency, there is <u>rarely</u> an urgency to **supplement iron and it is likely to contribute little to host iron status** <u>due to the block on absorption associated with inflammation</u>.* (Doherty, 2007, emphasis added)

> *. . . oral iron replacement therapy is poorly tolerated and may even contribute to the inflammatory process and tissue pathology in patients with IBD.* (Werner et al., 2011)

Question 4: "Should I take high-dose iron supplementation to correct my anemia?" (Don't be silly!) **Answer:** *"For heaven's sake, No!"*

> *Oral iron supplementation renders high fecal iron concentrations. Since <u>only a fraction of supplemented iron will be absorbed, virtually the entire dose winds up in the distal parts of the bowel</u>. In an already inflamed bowel, <u>this may reinforce the inflammation</u> by catalyzing production of ROS [reactive oxygen species] . . ..* (Erichsen et al., 2003, emphasis added)

> *Although conventional wisdom dictates administration of 200 mg elemental iron daily for correction of IDA [iron deficiency anemia], there is no rationale for using such a high dose of oral iron. Iron absorption from the GI tract is <u>highly efficient but saturable</u>.*

Accordingly, Rimon et al demonstrated that oral iron preparations at **doses as low as 15 mg/d could be used to correct iron deficiency.** (Bayraktar UD, Bayraktar S, 2010, emphasis added)

Common misconception: When oral iron is administrated, high doses—higher than usual—should be prescribed as iron absorption is generally impaired in IBD patients. (Gisbert and Gomollón, 2008)

Question 5: "My doctor is pleased that I am following a diet high in iron to correct my anemia. Should he or she be pleased?" **Answer:** *"No! He or she should be trembling."*

The potentially deleterious effects of a high-iron diet on UC are attributed to the accumulation of iron in the colonic lumen in high concentrations, a direct result of the tight regulation of body iron levels and the restriction of iron absorption. (Seril et al., 2006)

Question 6: "Should I take vitamin C with my iron supplement to increase its absorption?" **Answer:** *"Probably not a good idea. Probably a bad idea. Perhaps a very bad idea."*

Co-supplementation of ferrous salts (iron) with vitamin C exacerbates oxidative stress in the gastrointestinal tract leading to ulceration in healthy individuals, exacerbation of chronic gastrointestinal inflammatory diseases and can lead to cancer. (Fisher and Naughton, 2004)

Question 7: "Should I take enteric-coated iron to reduce GI upset?" **Answer:** *"Not recommended."*

In general, enteric-coated formulations should be avoided, because they may release their iron content beyond the intestinal site of maximal iron absorption. (Gasche, 2000)

Question 8: "Should I ask my physician for intravenous iron to correct my anemia?" **Answer:** *"Perhaps, you should."*

Intravenous iron sucrose has a good safety profile and a 65–75% response within 4–8 weeks, which is paralleled by improvement in the quality of life. (Gasche et al., 2004)

Question 9: "Should I ask my physician for EPO, whatever the heck that is?" **Answer:** *"Sure, you can ask! He or she will know."*

The best way to treat anaemia of chronic disease is by curing the underlying disease and the administration of iron in such patients should be avoided. Recombinant erythropoietin [EPO] has been shown to raise haemoglobin levels in inflammatory bowel disease patients with anaemia refractory to treatment with iron . . .. (Oldenburg et al., 2001)

Intravenous iron sucrose has a good safety profile and a 65–75% response within 4–8 weeks, which is paralleled by improvement in the quality of life. Combination therapy with erythropoietin (Epo) leads to a faster and larger haemoglobin increase. (Gasche et al., 2004)

(Note: Erythropoietin is a hormone that stimulates red blood cell production.)

Question 10: "What else besides blood loss and the anemia due to inflammation should be considered as a cause of my anemia?" **Answer:** *"There are few things."*

In some cases, anemia may be drug induced (Mesalazine, sulfasalazine, azathioprine, mercaptopurine) or due to folate/vitamin B12 deficiency. (Bayraktar and Bayraktar, 2010)

In conclusion

This section has a simple take-home message: Be ever-so-careful when it comes to iron. Make no mistake about it. Work closely with a physician (one who clearly understands the issues) in all things iron.

Sulfur intake

One significant change in the diet in the 20th century in areas with high incidence of UC is the high intake of sulfur-containing food. ~**Korzenik, 2005**

Foods rich in sulphur compounds have been associated with UC disease symptoms. In addition, dietary sulphur compounds can increase the likelihood of subsequent relapse. Thus, a sulphur-rich diet may be a contributory factor in the development and/or maintenance of UC. ~**Khalil et al., 2014**

Dietary factors such as red and processed meat, protein, and alcohol, as well as sulfur and sulfate intake were positively associated with relapses [in ulcerative colitis]. ~**Tilg and Kaser, 2004, emphasis added**

"As an individual with ulcerative colitis, and not particularly happy about it, should I become serious about reducing the consumption of sulfur-containing foods?" Good question, you ask. Let's see if this section can help you make the decision.

If you were to live in rural Africa, a no-Western-diet zone, your dietary intake of sulphate is a mere 2.7 mmol/day. In contrast, those of us that follow the Western diet (and love every minute of it) may consume sulphate in excess of 16.6 mmol/day (Pitcher and Cummings, 1996). That's about 6 times the sulphates consumed by following the Western diet compared to a more natural diet. Could be a problem.

One problem with sulphates is that they promote the overgrowth of what are called sulphate-reducing bacteria (SRB), bacteria that are *"uniquely capable of reducing inorganic sulphate to hydrogen sulphide"* and are *"largely dependent on the availability of sulphate."* (Pitcher and Cummings, 1996) Of course, the overgrowth of one group of bacteria in the bowel falls under the heading "dysbiosis." Furthermore, one byproduct of SRB metabolism is **hydrogen sulphide** (otherwise known as hydrogen sulfide). Unfortuinately, hydrogen sulphide, is *"toxic, mutagenic and cancerogenic to epithelial intestinal cells."* (Kushkevych, 2014) Now, that could be a problem.

Although hydrogen sulfide does have some usefulness to the bowel, there are limits (Miller et al., 2012). Due to its toxicity, it has been implicated in the pathogenesis of the very disease you have.

> *Hydrogen sulfide is a luminally acting, bacterially derived cell poison that has been implicated in ulcerative colitis.* (Magee et al., 2000)

The damage incurred by hydrogen sulfide toxicity is *"mediated by free radicals."* (Rowan et al., 2009) From a previous discussion, we know that excess free-radical production is nothing but trouble. But there is more.

The damage incurred by hydrogen sulfide includes a dysfunction of the colonocyte—and does this by inhibiting the utilization of butyrate (Rowan et al., 2009; Khalil et al., 2014). Remember butyrate? It is the preferred fuel for this cell. Without it, the colonocyte lives on a starvation diet and lives a life of compromise (Rowan et al., 2009, Khalil et al., 2014). Butyrate deficiency is not a welcome sight for anyone wishing to recover from ulcerative colitis.

One thing that the ulcerative colitis patient may have going for him or her is the fact that the mainstay of ulcerative colitis therapy, 5-ASA (Asacol; Pentasa; sulfasalazine), inhibits hydrogen sulphide production by sulfide reducing bacteria (Rowan et al., 2009). However, this benefit provided by 5-ASA may not be enough to keep you out of trouble. Furthermore, there are sulfites in 5-ASA, possibly leading to *"sensitivity reactions"* observed with this class of drugs (Roediger et al., 1993) All things considered, perhaps dietary sulphur restriction is in order. Why complicate things with dietary excess of a substance known to be intimately involved in the disease process we call ulcerative colitis?

One last (troubling) thing that may result from excessive sulphate reducing bacteria concentrations is this: The excess hydrogen sulfide so produced, may *"contribute to unwanted T cell activation."* (Miller et al., 2012) Importantly, depending on sub-type and activation state, T cells are immune cells that actively and aggressively promote chronic intestinal inflammation (Jantchou et al., 2010).

So, is it any wonder,

> *The increased number of sulfate-reducing bacteria . . . can cause inflammatory bowel disease of humans and animals.* (Kushkevych, 2014)

"What then should I do?"

> *Roediger found elimination of sulphur-containing foods (eggs, cheese, whole milk, ice cream, mayonnaise, soy milk, mineral water, wine, cordials, nuts, cabbage, broccoli, cauliflower, Brussels sprouts) as well as decreased intake of red meat led to prolonged remission (0 relapses over 56 patient-months with an expected rate of 22.6% in four subjects).*
> ~Buchman, 2012

It is logical that an evil such as this (excess dietary sulphur) should be met with decisive action. Work with a physician here! If you get the green light on limiting sulphur-containing foods, there is a fairly simple formula to follow: The less sulphur-containing foods consumed, particularly with a focus on those with the highest levels, the less hydrogen sulfide will be produced, followed by a decline in the numbers of sulphate-reducing bacteria and at least some degree of dysbiosis resolution. Here is a list of some of the food items reported to be high in sulfur-containing compounds:

List of foods rich in sulfur-containing compounds *

Dried fruit; lemon, lime, grape, and sauerkraut juices; store-bought fresh sauces (all high in sulfites) (Simon, 1998)

Red meat
Cheese
Milk
Fish
Nuts
Eggs
Sausages
Commercial bread (preservatives)
Beer and other alcohol drinks
    (preservatives)
(Tilg and Kaser, 2004)

Ice cream
Mayonnaise
Mineral water
Wine
Cordials
Nuts
Cabbage
Broccoli
Cauliflower
Brussels sprouts
(Buchman, 2012)

Carrageenan [food additive]
(Gibson et al., 1991; Roediger et al., 1993)

*Examples only, not an exhaustive list. Some items listed are high in sulfur due to added preservatives.

It should be noted, from the above list, major sources of organic sulphur are the protein foods, particularly *"the sulphur amino acids (found in high protein foods such as red meat, cheese, milk, fish, nuts, and eggs)."* (Jowett et al., 2004) So, I would question the adoption of a diet high in animal protein. In one study, the dietary factor with the strongest risk of relapse in ulcerative colitis was *"a high intake of meat, particularly of red meat and processed meat."* (Jowett et al., 2004)

Are you beginning to see that we have another big problem on our hands, associated with the Western diet? That would be the flood of sulfur-containing foods, so readily consumed. You do need sulfur-containing foods in your life, yes you do, but not in the amounts we receive due to our devotion to the Western diet—particularly so for those of us suffering from intestinal inflammation. And of course, some foods are higher in sulfur than others, and should be regarded as a greater threat.

A high sulphur diet, either from sulphur amino acids [high in red meat] or sulphated additives, results in the generation of hydrogen sulphide and mucosal damage in the colon.

Red meat, for instance, is stated as a food to be avoided on a low sulphur amino acid diet and processed foods contain large amounts of sulphate as a food additive. (Jowett et al., 2004)

Given the problems that center around consuming red meat, it looks like we need to engage in yet another little conversation. Accordingly, I will introduce you to an evil that may stand directly in the way of remission in ulcerative colitis. And it is downright irritating.

Red meat

Heme, the iron porphyrin pigment, primarily found in red meat, poultry and fish is poorly absorbed in the small intestine. Approximately 90% of dietary heme transits to the colon, and is exploited by colonic bacteria as a growth factor.

Dietary heme directly injures colonic surface epithelium by generating cytotoxic and oxidative stress. ~Khalili et al., 2017, emphasis added

*. . . the **irritating** influence of heme is continuously present in the colon and not just a single "hit," meaning the **dietary heme can constantly modulate the severity of colitis.***

A diet high in red meat might be a risk factor for inflammatory bowel disease development. ~Schepens et al., 2011, emphasis added

Anything that directly damages the epithelial lining of the colon and affects the severity of colitis should probably command our attention.

I have mentioned the dangers of red meat before, particularly with respect to iron. Now, we will drill down a little deeper and see why red meat poses such a threat to you, the patient suffering from ulcerative colitis, and to me, an individual who has no interest at all in developing colon cancer, much less increasing my risk of ulcerative colitis.

Red meat is rich in what is called "heme." Heme is the molecule the red blood cell hides all its iron within. Iron, as we have previously discussed, should not be present in abundance in the colon. However, given the right circumstances, it arrives in the colon in large amounts, contained in the heme of red meat or contained in the heme of red blood cells that arrive within the colon from GI bleeding (Constante et al., 2017).

The meats high in heme are *"beef, veal, lamp, mutton, pork, and offal"* (Bastide et al., 2011). When I first read this, I didn't know exactly what an offal was. Is it cute? Is it furry? Is it cuddly? Is it similar to a gopher? No. An offal is none of these. It is the organ meats and the butcher block scraps (of who knows what) that wind up on the dinner plate. And while we're at it, let's not overlook the <u>processed</u> meats that are also high in heme: *"sausages, meat burgers, ham, bacon, and salami"* (Santarelli et al., 2010). They pose danger, too—perhaps even more danger due to the additives that, shall we say, have been added.

On the other hand, chicken also contains heme, but *"the heme content of red meat is 10-fold higher than that of white meat (such as chicken)."* (Bastide et al., 2011) Fish is also low in heme (Sesink et al., 1999). The low heme content of both chicken and fish is credited for the lack of association between these two food items and the risk of colon cancer (de Vogel et al., 2008; Ijssennagger et al., 2012).

Willingly and delightfully, on the Western diet we eat our fill of dietary heme. What happens next? The heme winds up within the colon where pathogenic bacteria catch a break. For the pathogen, it's another awesome day.

> Dietary heme is poorly absorbed in the small intestine, and approximately 90% of dietary heme proceeds to the colon where it can be used by colonic bacteria as a growth factor. (Ijssennagger et al., 2012)

> **Bacteria pathogens are particularly efficient at capturing heme and thriving in heme-rich environments.** (Constante et al., 2017, emphasis added)

As we have previously discussed, heme is loaded with iron. I'm sure you could use at least some of that iron, but so can pathogenic bacteria. And they can "extract" all they need from heme (Constante et al., 2017). In as much as heme is a growth factor for pathogens, heme also becomes a driver of dysbiosis (Ijssennagger et al., 2012; Constante et al., 2017). Heme also contains amino acids that are useful for bacterial growth (Constante et al., 2017) Now if you were a pathogen, you would be in favor of all the dietary heme we consume on the Western diet—the more, the better! For pathogens, it's a win-win. And they don't seem to care what happens to you.

> A variable proportion of heme and amino acids, contained in animal proteins, are **not absorbed by the small bowel and reach the colonic** lumen, where they are metabolized by the microflora. **This results in a number of end products, which include <u>hydrogen sulfide</u>, phenolic compounds, and amines and ammonia, some of which are potentially toxic to the colon.** (Jantchou et al., 2010)

Oh! We've discussed **hydrogen sulfide** before, just recently in fact. Recall, hydrogen sulfide is an unfortunate byproduct of sulfate-reducing bacteria, and it is toxic to the intestinal epithelial cell (Magee et al., 2000; Jowett et al., 2004; Kushkevych, 2014). And, if that wasn't bad enough, hydrogen sulfide damages, actually *"breaks,"* the mucus layer of protection (Ijssennagger et al., 2016).

> *Hydrogen sulfide, produced by sulfate-reducing bacteria (SRB) and some other bacteria, reduces disulfide bonds present in the mucus network, thereby breaking the mucus barrier.*

> *Inflammatory bowel disease (IBD) is characterized by decreased mucus barrier function, which may be due to increased sulfide production by altered microbial species present in IBD patients with active disease.*

> ***Lowering hydrogen sulfide concentrations in the gut lumen could represent an exciting potential therapeutic strategy for treating IBD.*** (Ijssennagger et al., 2016, emphasis added)

And if that wasn't enough evil in one meal, another poison created in a *"considerable amount"* during the cellular metabolism of heme is **hydrogen peroxide** (Gemelli et al., 2014). *"There is substantial evidence that hydrogen peroxide can have deleterious effects on the colon."* (Jacobs et al., 2009)

Hydrogen peroxide generated within the cell can damage the cells DNA and, among other negative things, can contribute to the production of proinflammatory cytokines (Gemelli et al., 2014). So, all I can say is "danger danger!"

But it's not as if we are defenseless. We do have an enzyme that degrades heme, called heme oxygenase-1 (HO-1) (Vijayan et al., 2010). *"HO-1 not only protects against oxidative stress and apoptosis [programed cell death], but has received a great deal of attention in recent years because of its potent anti-inflammatory functions."* (Vijayan et al., 2010) Indeed, the upregulation of this enzyme *"amplifies the effects of IL-10"*—a cytokine that restrains inflammation (if it can) (Chang et al., 2015). Interestingly, in a laboratory model of ulcerative colitis, 5-ASA drugs (Asacol; Pentasa; sulfasalazine) upregulate HO-1 (Chang et al., 2015)—yet another potential beneficial action offered by this class of drugs. However, while HO-1 is trying to save you from heme, this enzyme turns heme into the poisonous hydrogen peroxide molecule, and in a *"considerable amount,"* right inside the cell where it can do a lot of damage (Gemelli et al., 2014). The cell is not too happy. The cell is under threat. Listen closely. A cry for help can be heard.

Regardless of HO-1's role as a defense mechanism against heme, and regardless of its attractiveness as a therapeutic target in IBD, *"it seems questionable whether HO-1 induction is useful for treatment of established IBD, but rather might be useful as a preventive measure."* (Vijayan et al., 2010) Besides, it's probably already working overtime, as *"there has been no other enzyme described to date that is affected by so many stimuli of diverse nature as HO-1"* and it is already upregulated in the inflamed tissues of the colon (Zhu et al., 2011). So, it looks like we're left with reducing our consumption of red meat, and all the heme it contains, to avoid the ongoing damage it can inflict. But there are other defensive measures we can take.

Heme does have an antidote, and it is found in green vegetables (de Vogel et al., 2005; Ijssennagger et al., 2012). It is known as chlorophyll. Chlorophyll is high in spinach, and chlorophyll extract appears to be just as protective as spinach against the damage heme can cause (de Vogel et al., 2005). Chlorophyll seems to work because it is structurally similar to heme, and thereby may be able to compete with heme for metabolic degradation (de Vogel et al., 2005). Experimentally, when rats were fed chlorophyll along with heme, the fecal output of heme increased, as opposed to rats only consuming heme (de Vogel et al., 2005). The rats taking chlorophyll were pleased to learn that they were among those of us with a lower colon cancer risk. You should join us. *"Supplementation* of the heme diet with chlorophyll and spinach completely inhibited this heme-induced increase in cytotoxicity." (de Vogel et al., 2005)

Besides spinach and chlorophyll extract, this "antidote" can be found in other leafy green vegetables such as Swiss chard, beet greens, bok choy, green cabbage and collard greens. You can also find chlorophyll in celery, green beans, peas, and green bell peppers. And the list could go on.

Other heme "antidotes" include calcium, polyphenols (a class of beneficial, bioactive components found in fruits and vegetables), and vitamin C (Bastide et al., 2011). But please be careful with vitamin C, particularly taking the amounts commonly found in supplements, as it can act with available iron to exacerbate oxidative stress in the cells that line the colon, and can lead to ulceration and increased severity of GI inflammation as well as an increased risk of colon cancer. (see Fisher and Naughton, 2004) It should be noted that diets high in chlorophyll are also higher in calcium and polyphenols. The Western diet is low in all three of these defenders of colon health.

Should you take the plunge and substantially reduce your intake of red meat, you will be substantially reducing your intake of another dietary item that inflicts harm on the IBD patient and upon others as well. We'll discuss that next.

Omega-6 fatty acid excess

It is well recognized that long-chain omega-6 (n-6) and omega-3 (n-3) polyunsaturated fatty acids (PUFA) play important and opposing roles in the modulation of inflammation. Generally, n-6 PUFA promote inflammation, whereas n-3 PUFA have anti-inflammatory properties.

The worldwide trends of excessive n-6 PUFA and insufficient n-3 PUFA intake have been implicated in today's health epidemics. ~**Kaliannan et al., 2015**

. . . a high intake of the n-6 PUFA linoleic acid more than doubled the
risk of developing ulcerative colitis. ~Tjonneland et al., 2009,
emphasis added

The Western diet is a rich source of many things, many of which are good, many of which are harmful when consumed in excess. The excess of the omega-6 polyunsaturated fatty acids (**PUFA**), also called **n-6** or **v-6** fatty acids, serve as an outstanding example. The principle omega-6 fatty acid readily converts to arachidonic acid, a pro-inflammatory fatty acid (Tjonneland et al., 2009). This fatty acid is the cause of a whole lot of trouble when consumed in excess.

The richness in the omega-6 fatty acids in the Western diet, due to the consumption of the vegetable/seed cooking oils and the consumption of the meat of grain-fattened animals (Ghosh et al., 2013), increases the likelihood of developing ulcerative colitis and may be standing in the way of its resolution (Tjonneland et al., 2009; Brown et al., 2012). Linoleic acid is the principal omega-6 in the Western diet. We need it in our diet, as well as the other essential (necessary) omega-6 fatty acids, but not in excessive amounts.

A high dietary intake of n-6 PUFAs and their incorporation into colonic cell membranes would lead to a source of pro-inflammatory molecules which could predispose to ulcerative colitis. The essential n-6 PUFA fatty acid linoleic acid, is present in red meat (particularly beef and pork), cooking oils (especially corn and sunflower oils) and polyunsaturated margarines. (Tjonneland et al., 2009)

Reinforcing the significance of all this in the context of ulcerative colitis, one study revealed

*. . . excessive consumption of omega-6 PUFA increases ulcerative colitis by **30%***; *whereas consumption of docosahexaenoic acid, an omega-3 fatty acid, reduced the disease burden by **77%**.* (Brown et al., 2012, emphasis added)

In another study of ulcerative colitis patients, investigators found *"a high intake of total polyunsaturated fatty acids increased the risk of ulcerative colitis by 6.54 times."* (Tjonneland et al., 2009, emphasis added) An additional study found that individuals with the highest intake of DHA (a primary omega-3 fatty acid) demonstrated a whopping **83% decrease** in the risk of ulcerative colitis (John et al., 2010).

But why? Why does omega-6 excess lead to ulcerative colitis? And why is omega-6 excess able to stand in the way of its resolution? Five fundamental reasons readily come to mind.

First, linoleic acid, for example, can be transformed into metabolites that promote and sustain inflammation, metabolites found to be elevated in the colonic mucosa of patients in ulcerative colitis (Tjonneland et al., 2009). **Second**, omega-6 PUFA compete with the same enzymes that allow the omega-3s to be converted to the beneficial substances known as **protectins** and **resolvins**—important substances that should be available to restrain inflammation and help resolve it should it occur (Serhan et al., 2008). **Third**, *"an unbalanced diet containing increased n-6 PUFA has a suppressive effect on cellular defenses."* (Miura et al., 1998) **Fourth**, omega-6 fatty acids *"have been shown to up-regulate epithelial permeability and inflammation associated with mucosal damage."* (Kankaapää et al., 2001) **Finally**, in animal models, omega-6 rich diets *"induced the growth of microbes known to induce pro-inflammatory responses"* (Ghosh et al., 2013). This makes dietary omega-6 fatty acid excess a driver of dysbiosis, pure and simple. It is believed that this sort of thing happens in humans, too. In IBD patients, omega-6 PUFA-rich diets lead to an increase of Enterobacteriaceae, a family of bacteria associated with IBD (Ghosh et al., 2013).

The above listing is brief and elementary. This whole business of fatty acid-derived mediators of inflammation is so complex and at times confusing—in as much as some omega-6 metabolites can be useful in controlling and resolving inflammation in spite of their proinflammatory properties (Weylandt et al., 2007; Calder, 2009). That being said, there seems to be a major problem associated with omega-6 excess and ulcerative colitis, regarding its pathogenesis as well as its perpetuation. Rule of thumb: The more out of balance the ratio between the omega-6s and the omega-3s is, the more likely we get into trouble, ulcerative colitis or not, and the harder it is to get out of trouble, ulcerative colitis or not.

Recall, the enzymes that process the omega-6s are the same enzymes that process the omega-3s. Unfortunately, this scheme of things allows omega-6 excess to competitively reduce the creation of the omega-3 metabolites—potentially leading to a deficit of protectins, resolvins, and other anti-inflammatory modifiers of inflammation.

Besides acting as a substrate for protectin and resolvin synthesis, other benefits offered by the omega-3 metabolites include: **1)** reversing or *"antagonizing"* the negative effects of the omega-6s (Varnalidis et al., 2011; Ghosh et al., 2013); **2)** functioning as antioxidants (Hassanshahi and Masoumi, 2018; Varnalidis et al., 2011); **3)** suppressing inflammatory cytokine synthesis (Varnalidis et al., 2011); and **4)** reducing the expression of pro-inflammatory genes (Calder, 2012). You, the ulcerative colitis patient, are likely going to need some of these positive effects to achieve your goal of achieving and/or maintaining remission. You're likely going to need your omega-6/omega-3 ratio in better balance.

Estimates vary on what a healthy omega-6/omega-3 ratio should look like. The hunter-gatherer of old likely ate a diet that included nearly as many omega-3s as omega-6s, close to a 1:1 ratio (Kaliannan et al., 2015). The hunter-gatherer of old never heard of ulcerative colitis, and gastroenterologists were nowhere to be found. But as time went by, the omega-6/omega-3 ratio dramatically changed (and gastroenterologists popped up from out of nowhere). Today, thanks to the ease by which omega-6s can be obtained (they are everywhere!), the ratio is *"10:1" to "50:1"* (Kaliannan et al., 2015)! *"This shift in the n-6/n-3 ratio is thought to contribute to today's prevalence of chronic disease."* (Kaliannan et al.,

2015) Ulcerative colitis is a chronic disease. Omega-6 excess not only may lead to the disease, omega-6 excess may firmly stand in the way of achieving remission (Tjonneland et al., 2009; Brown et al., 2012; Ghosh et al., 2013). Take notice. Take action.

Increasing the intake of the omega-3s (fish, maybe an occasional fish oil supplement, and egg yolk) and increasing the intake of the omega-3 fatty acid **alpha-linolenic acid**, <u>which can be converted to other omega-3 fatty acids</u> is probably in order (John et al., 2010). Alpha-linolenic acid can be found in plants (nuts, avocado, flax seeds, tofu, spinach, etc.), and their consumption is another approach to raise omega-3 levels. But why bother when you follow a diet high in the omega-6s? Decreasing the intake of the omega-6s (seed/vegetable oils and the red meats) is yet another approach. But why bother when you follow a diet low in the omega-3s? Perhaps, a more sensible approach is to combine the above two approaches, with the goal of dramatically improving the omega-6/omega-3 ratio in favor of the omega-3s. To achieve this goal, fish oil supplementation may be of benefit. Maybe. But, may not be a wise course of action.

There are only a few studies demonstrating a positive outcome in using fish oil supplementation <u>as a therapy</u> for ulcerative colitis (systematically reviewed by Hassanshahi and Masoumi, 2018). Indeed, the majority of studies have *"failed to demonstrate a benefit in inducing or maintaining remission."* (Ananthakrishnan et al., 2014) Taking things one step further, this recommendation has been offered:

> *Overall, it does not appear that full fat diets should be avoided, however fat including diets rich in olive oil, dairy products and fish <u>but not fish oil pills</u> should be consumed while avoiding large intakes of vegetable oils rich in n-6 PUFA.* (Haskey and Gibson, 2017, emphasis added)

But why should fish oil supplementation be avoided as a therapy for ulcerative colitis? "It seems so ideal and warranted to control all the madness!" (You're beginning to talk a lot like me.) There are a few good reasons why it may be wise to avoid fish oil supplementation as a therapy for ulcerative colitis, as follows:

First, fish oils can suppress some immune responses, immune responses that you may need. *"Consumption of v-3 PUFA rich diets may have anti-inflammatory properties however this may prevent the body from mounting appropriate immune responses critical for host defense."* (Ghosh et al., 2013) **Second**, fish oils can shift the cytokine pattern from what is called the Th1 response to what is called the Th2 response. This can intensify the pattern of Th2 cytokine expression known to drive the inflammation occurring in ulcerative colitis. (Zhang et al., 2005). **Third**, *"paradoxically, fish oil appears to enhance TNF-α production in some subjects."* (Grimble et al., 2002) I'm sure I could find other reasons why fish oil supplementation is not particularly effective in ulcerative colitis, but we need to move on.

The issue of fish oil supplementation underscores the need to work with a physician to guide you in the choices you make, every step of the way. Fish oil supplementation may not be helpful, and it may actually be detrimental. But doing *something* is in order! The omega-6/omega-3 ratio should not be ignored. No, it should be addressed. Improving the omega-6/omega-3 ratio is clearly an appropriate action to take.

> . . . *elevating tissue n-3 PUFA status and lowering the n-6/n-3 PUFA ratio can improve the gut microbiota profile and suppress chronic low-grade inflammation provides two major implications of today's health problems.* (Kaliannan et al., 2015)

> *An increase in IBD incidence has been associated with increased dietary intake of v-6 PUFA in humans*, while IBD patients remain in remission longer when dietary intake of v-3 PUFA increases. (Ghosh et al., 2013)

What then can we do?

Looks like it would be wise to limit omega-6 consumption in as a measure to improve the omega-6/omega-3 ratio and gain an advantage in the battle against ulcerative colitis. This would require a reduction in the seed/vegetable oils (salad and cooking oils, margarine, shortening, etc), using butter and olive oil as a substitute, as well as limiting red meat (beef and pork) in favor of an increased consumption of white meat (chicken) and fish (Cordain et al., 2005; Tjonneland et al., 2009; Haskey and Gibson, 2017). This would also include reading product labels. Well, there goes most of the snack foods you adore! The goal in all this is to reduce the negative influence of the omega-6s and increase the positive influence of the omega-3 fatty acids. Each of the above interventions are basic, simple actions to take. You may not want to, but you may need to, should you want to achieve and maintain remission.

Alcohol consumption

*Alcohol consumption is a potential trigger for flare in Inflammatory Bowel Disease (IBD) because **of alcohol's pro-oxidant effects and its deleterious effects on gut barrier function.*** ~Swanson et al., 2010, **emphasis added**

Alcohol exposure can promote growth of Gram negative bacteria in the intestine which may result in the accumulation of endotoxin. ~**Purohit et al., 2008**

The iron content of some alcoholic beverages is high, particularly red wines and foreign beers. ~**Watts, 1988**

Are you beginning to see why alcohol could be a problem with respect to the pathogenesis and perpetuation of ulcerative colitis? Pro-oxidation! Dysbiosis! Gut barrier compromise! *Iron!* I see trouble ahead! But then again, I always see trouble ahead. And this time I see trouble ahead for approximately two billion people.

> It has been estimated that approximately 2 billion people worldwide drink alcohol on a daily basis, with more than 70 million people having a diagnosed alcohol use disorder (World Health Organization 2004). (Engen et al., 2015)

Alcohol is passed off as the gateway to happiness. It is not. (That would be chocolate.) Look around. Alcohol is a disaster for our society. So much harm. So much harm. *"Globally, alcohol use is the fifth leading risk factor for premature death and disability among people between the ages of 15 and 49 . . . and the third leading cause of preventable death in the United States."* (Engen et al., 2015) Sounds like a real enemy to me! You may like alcohol, but if you are an individual with ulcerative colitis, it is doubtful that alcohol is a friend.

> *Potentially modifiable dietary factors, such as a high meat or alcoholic beverage intake, have been identified that are associated with an increased likelihood of relapse for UC patients."* (Jowett et al., 2004)

> *. . . alcoholic drinks are rich sources of sulfur and sulfate, which increase the concentration of fecal hydrogen sulfide, which is toxic to colonocytes.* (Hsu et al., 2016)

If you run across a study concluding there is no statically significant association between alcohol consumption and ulcerative colitis, that's okay, you can move on. Pay little to no attention. Don't hang your hat on this one! A study such as this may be a study of other studies, studies that are flawed in ways that obscure reality. Ask yourself this: "If sulfates and iron are harmful if derived in excess from meat and other foods, why would they not be as harmful if derived in excess from alcohol?" Furthermore, many drinkers are smokers, and in as much as smoking suppresses the onset and symptoms of ulcerative colitis, not factoring this in, and not including the effects of second-hand smoking, may lead to erroneous conclusions regarding the risks posed by alcohol with respect to ulcerative colitis. (see Hsu et al., 2016; Swanson et al., 2010). I will move on. I think you get the point.

In addition to contributing to dysbiosis, *"alcohol consumption can disrupt gut barrier function and increase intestinal permeability."* (Hsu et al., 2016). This can allow harmful and hideous things to pass (Purohit et al., 2008). Trouble follows.

Although alcohol is risky business, you may get away with it. It seems to be a double-edged sword with respect to ulcerative colitis, in as much as there may be some benefits gained; while at the same time, danger is present.

> The results of the present and previous studies suggest **light alcohol drinking may have a protective effect against IBD**, whereas **moderate-to-heavy drinking increases the risk of IBD.**

> *Alcohol may exert a protective effect by inhibiting the systemic immune system and neutrophil migration. Furthermore, some antioxidants present in red wine, such as resveratrol, have anti-inflammatory properties, and thus, <u>light</u> alcohol drinking can potentially prevent the relapse of IBD. By contrast . . .* **alcohol consumption can disrupt gut barrier function and increase intestinal permeability,** *to which patients with IBD are particularly vulnerable.* (Hsu et al., 2016, emphasis added)

There also seems to be a dose-dependent relationship with respect to alcohol and its damaging effect on the colon.

> *Alcohol has been previously examined through a prospective detailed diet history in 191 patients with inactive UC over a one year period (Jowett et al., 2004). In that cohort, patients that had a relapse or disease flare over that year consumed 14 grams of*

alcohol daily compared to 10 grams daily in non-relapsers.
(Swanson et al., 2010)

Although you may get away with it, to me it seems both irresponsible and inadvisable to continue alcohol consumption to any relevant degree when you are doing everything you can to gain an edge in the battle against the greatest evil you have ever known.

Sodium excess

A specific factor that has changed in the Western diet over time is the increasing amount of sodium-containing salt intake. ~**Aguiar et al., 2018**

. . . increased salt intake can undermine the course and balance of the immune response by promoting the development of macrophages and T cells with proinflammatory functions. ~**Min and Fairchild, 2015, emphasis added**

Sodium chloride mediates the inflammatory effects of immune cells that are very important to IBD. ~**Guo et al., 2018**

More recently, studies indicated that salt has a crucial role in the development of inflammatory processes and augmentation of autoimmunity. ~**Abdoli, 2016, emphasis added**

Salt, the common name for sodium chloride (NaCl), is consumed in great excess in our society. This harms our society. It's beginning to look like excessive salt consumption can particularly harm the individual with ulcerative colitis.

Recently, it was uncovered that salt consumption, at levels occurring in the Western diet (and other diets as well), has a negative affect the immune system of the gut. *". . . salt, which due to its higher consumption in the western diet, has recently emerged to play a **game changing** role* *in the gut immune response."* (Goyal et al., 2017, emphasis added) Let's take a look at what this little game changer is all about.

We normally relate excess salt intake to diseases such as hypertension (high blood pressure), heart attack, and stroke. And we should take heed and limit our salt intake for these very reasons. What may surprise you: **Emerging data reveals that salt can inappropriately support and intensify the immune response occurring in ulcerative colitis and place remission further out of reach.** In the gut, it can provoke and sustain proinflammatory responses and suppress anti-inflammatory activities. *"Within the gastrointestinal track, increased exposure to dietary salt causes an increased inflammatory milieu [environment]."* (Hernandez et al., 2015)

High salt intake can do this in several ways. Here are two: **First**, it *"dampens regulatory functions,"* allowing inflammation to get out of control and stay out of control *"long-term"* (Min and Fairchild, 2015). **Second**, excess salt intake (think Western diet-level salt intake) expands the concentrations of Th17 cells within the inflamed regions of the colon (Khalili et al., 2016; Goyal et al., 2017). If these immune cells had nothing but good intentions, there would be no need for concern, but *"TH17 cells massively infiltrate the inflamed intestine in IBD patients, where they produce . . . cytokines, **triggering and amplifying** the inflammatory process."* (Gálvez, 2014, emphasis added)

I think we'd better become a little better acquainted with the immune cell called the Th17 cell. I'll be brief. We don't need to get bogged down here or get lost in the weeds.

T "helper" (Th) cells are a family of immune cells that are mobile and arrive in inflamed tissues in great numbers to "help" orchestrate immune responses (Gálvez, 2014). *"These cells regulate immune responses through their ability to differentiate into distinct classes of cell according to the nature of the offending pathogen."* (O'Shea and Jones, 2013) One member of the T cell family is the Th17 cell, a cell with the ability to defend against pathogenic bacteria by producing cytokines *"crucial"* for host defense (Gálvez, 2014). This could come in handy in a disease where bacteria are continually advancing and evoking an inflammatory response.

The Th17 cell can also respond to signals in the local environment where it lives and works—and prompted by the messages it receives, the T cell can transform itself into another T cell, like a Treg cell, a cell we depend on to restrain or *"dampen"* inflammation and promote healing (Gálvez, 2014, Guo et al., 2018). Surprisingly, despite its reputation for promoting inflammation and tissue damage, the Th17 cell can also promote *"tissue-protective effects,"* such as supporting the integrity of the tight junctions between intestinal epithelial cells and by stimulating mucus production (Gálvez, 2014). But guess what? Excess salt consumption messes with everything! All the good the Th17 cell can accomplish can be overshadowed by the harm sodium excess can cause. Sodium excess can intensify and dysregulate the Th17-driven, proinflammatory response in ulcerative colitis . . . perhaps so unnecessarily.

> *Not only does high sodium increase the inflammatory function of macrophages and T cells that are activated in response to infection and/or tissue trauma, but **high salt also neutralizes the inherent regulatory mechanisms that have evolved to limit the levels of immune-mediated inflammation and promote resolution of tissue injury.*** (Min and Fairchild, 2015, emphasis added)

In ulcerative colitis, the Th17 cell causes much harm, and is clearly out of control. *"Although Th17 cells play a protective role against certain extracellular pathogens, a dysregulated Th17 response can induce severe tissue inflammation and autoimmunity and can be dangerous to the host."* (Awasthi and Kuchroo, 2009, emphasis added) Furthermore, the inflammation associated with ulcerative colitis is *"sustained by the production of cytokines made by a distinct lineage of Th cells, termed the Th17 cells."* (Monteleone et al., 2009, emphasis added)

The game changer here is that we now know that the consumption of dietary salt in excess amplifies and dysregulates the Th17-mediated immune responses in the gut and, and at the same time, impairs the ability of Tregs to restrain and resolve gut inflammation. These are *major* discoveries! Studies in mice and men indicate that the negative effects of sodium excess apply to the gastrointestinal inflammation occurring in ulcerative colitis (Goyal et al., 2017). *"High dietary salt intake has recently been linked with induction of Th17 cells along with impairment of Treg cells."* (Dar et al., 2018, emphasis added) We can do something about this.

First, we can reduce our consumption of salt and foods high in salt (so many, so many). **Second**, we can increase our consumption of foods rich in potassium, as can be found in fruits and vegetables (Carrera-Bastos et al., 2011).

Potassium seems to be the antidote, at least in part, for sodium excess (Carrera-Bastos et al., 2011). Intriguingly, potassium also regulates the balance between Th17 and Treg cells (Khalili et al., 2016). And there appears to be *"an inverse relationship between dietary potassium and the risk of CD (Crohn's disease) and UC."* (Goyal et al., 2017) Although one study found a positive effect of potassium supplementation on ulcerative colitis patients, exhibited by lower disease scores, and attributed to the Th17 cell (Goyal et al., 2017), another study cautions against diets rich in potassium (and magnesium), reporting a potential increase in disease activity (Aguiar et al., 2018). Probably the first order of business here is to diet for success by reducing the consumption of foods rich in salt. When you do this, and simultaneously increase your intake of fruits and vegetables as so many physicians and scientists advise, you will automatically increase your intake of dietary potassium and change your sodium/potassium ratio. Reduced salt consumption and increased potassium intake are features common to many diets that demonstrate a remarkable degree of success in inducing and maintaining remission in ulcerative colitis.

A few loose ends to tie up before we move on and celebrate the fact that this rather lengthy chapter has thankfully come to an end.

It appears that sodium excess alters the microbiome, suppressing lactobacilli numbers and reducing the production of short chain fatty acids (think butyrate) (Willebrand and Kleinewietfeld, 2018; Wilck et al., 2017; Miranda et al., 2018). Perhaps unexpectedly, it has been discovered that butyrate helps control the Th17 cell, reducing its pathogenic potential in addition to supporting the anti-inflammatory activity of the Treg cell (Willebrand and Kleinewietfeld, 2018).

Along these lines, another interesting finding: The course of multiple sclerosis (MS), another Th17-driven disease process, becomes more severe when sodium intake is elevated (Hucke et al., 2016). This happens in both mice and men (Hucke et al., 2016; Abdoli, 2017; Toussirot et al., 2018). *". . . MS patients with medium or high salt intakes had 2.75- to 3.95-fold increases in MS activity than MS patients with low salt intake."* (Abdoli, 2017)

Underscoring the negative impact dietary salt excess has on inflammatory disease risk, the risk of rheumatoid arthritis doubles in individuals with high salt intake (Lucca and Hafler, 2015).

So, there you have it! Sodium excess is yet another enemy for you to confront. And now that you are in the know, we can move on.

Hidden danger (and a lot of it)

In our Western society, a lot of sodium is hidden in the common foods we eat. For example, **frozen pizza** may have between **370 to 730 mg of sodium <u>per slice</u>** and a fast-food **cheeseburger** may have between **710 mg and 1690 mg of sodium**. Add **French fries** to the cheeseburger, and the fast-food meal provides an <u>additional</u> **250 mg of sodium**. A **milkshake** added to the mix provides an addition **230 mg of sodium**. Are you beginning to see how easy it is to get a lot of sodium in a typical fast-food meal? One single meal, considered "normal" in our society, can easily provide more sodium than an individual should consume in one day!

A **fish sandwich** may contain up to **1,324 mg of sodium.** A **large taco** may provide you with **1,233 mg of sodium.** And I haven't even mentioned breakfast.

Two pancakes, with butter and syrup, provides **1,104 mg of sodium.** A single, 4-inch **buttermilk biscuit** provides nearly **600 mg of sodium,** and that doesn't include the butter and the gravy.

Soup is good food, or so we are told. A cup of **chicken noodle soup** may net you **1,106 mg of sodium.** A **vegetable soup** may offer you **1010 mg of sodium.** I could go on. I think I will.

A can of **pork and beans** will give you **1106 mg of sodium per cup.** A cup of **beef stew** provides **947 mg of sodium.** A cup of **chili con carne** provides **1007 mg of sodium.**

And why does all this matter? Excess sodium is proinflammatory, intensifying the Th17 response and suppressing the Treg function—not good news for the patient with ulcerative colitis. Do you really want an intensified Th17 response as well as depressed Treg function?

(The above statistics are largely based on data provided by the USDA.)

You need some help

The Cleveland Clinic has a great article entitled ***Sodium-Controlled Diet***. Check it out: https://my.clevelandclinic.org/health/articles/15426-sodium-controlled-diet. I will quote portions of the article, as follows:

> *The daily recommendation of sodium is 2,300 mg per day. However, some patients may be advised to eat lower amounts.*

General Guidelines

- *Eliminate the salt shaker.*

- Avoid using garlic salt, onion salt, MSG, meat tenderizers, broth mixes, Chinese food, soy sauce, teriyaki sauce, barbeque sauce, sauerkraut, olives, pickles, pickle relish, bacon bits, and croutons.

- Use fresh ingredients and/or foods with no added salt.

- For favorite recipes, you may need to use other ingredients and delete the salt added. Salt can be removed from any recipe except for those containing yeast.

- Try orange, lemon, lime, pineapple juice, or vinegar as a base for meat marinades or to add tart flavor.

- Avoid convenience foods such as canned soups, entrees, vegetables, pasta and rice mixes, frozen dinners, instant cereal and puddings, and gravy sauce mixes.

- Select frozen meals that contain around 600 mg sodium or less.

- Use fresh, frozen, no-added-salt canned vegetables, low-sodium soups, and low-sodium lunchmeats.

- Look for seasoning or spice blends with no salt, or try fresh herbs, onions, or garlic.

- Do not use a salt substitute unless you check with your doctor or dietitian first, due to potential drug or nutrient interactions.

- Be aware of and try to limit the "Salty Six" (American Heart Association), which include:

  o Breads, rolls, bagels, flour tortillas, and wraps.

  o Cold cuts and cured meats.

- *Pizza.*

- *Poultry (much poultry and other meats are injected with sodium. Check the Nutrition Facts for sodium content or read the package for a description of a solution, for example, "Fresh chicken in a 15% solution.")*

- *Soup.*

- *Sandwiches.*   (Cleveland Clinic, 2016)

The above reference also gives great advice on how to read food labels. This is an outstanding resource. Be sure to check it out.

DASH to the finish line

There are many books available on reduced sodium dieting. One popular diet, the DASH diet, is a great template to follow when reducing your sodium intake. This diet is good for another reason, too. It promotes a greater consumption of fruits and vegetables. *"DASH is a sodium-restricted (<2400 mg/d) diet rich in vegetables, fruits, whole grains, and low-fat dairy, and low in saturated fat, cholesterol, refined grains, and sweets."* (Hsu et al., 2017) Do your homework, then discuss sodium restriction with your physician. If sodium restriction is appropriate and approved, start reading labels and start reducing sodium intake. Regardless of the impact of sodium restriction on ulcerative colitis, sodium restriction is a good general health practice to follow.

Busted!

I found a great infographic on sodium I would like to draw your attention to, published by the good folks of the American Heart

Association, entitled *7 Salty Sodium Myths Busted*. You can access this infographic by searching for it by name, or using the following address:

http://www.heart.org/HEARTORG/HealthyLiving/HealthyEating/Hea
lthyDietGoals/7-Salty-Myths-BUSTED-
Infographic_UCM_456341_SubHomePage.jsp

Beware the chicken!

An excellent article written by Gina Roberts-Grey and published on the Huffington Post, is a must read. Who knew a lifeless chicken could be so dangerous . . . so unnecessarily? Here is an excerpt:

> **Beware the chicken** We often consider turkey and chicken healthy alternatives to red meat, but we should also be aware of their potentially high sodium content, which can be traced to the saltwater solution producers typically inject into poultry during processing. "This adds flavor and weight to the meat, and it plumps up the poultry," says Steve Hoad of Emma's Family Farm in Windsor, Maine, "although we process birds without salt or water added and they still taste very good."
>
> While boneless, skinless chicken breast not treated with saltwater typically carries 50 to 75 mg of sodium per 4-ounce serving, Hartley says, "enhanced chicken often delivers over 400 milligrams of sodium per serving."
>
> About a third of the fresh chicken found in supermarket cases has been synthetically saturated with saltwater, Hartley says. To spot (and avoid) the affected poultry, you've got to read the labels very carefully. Look for the phrase "Enhanced with up to 15 percent chicken broth" within the package's fine print, she advises, and be aware that poultry enhanced with saltwater can still be called "all natural" if the ingredients in the solution meet the U.S. Department of Agriculture's definition of "natural."

Read the entire article entitled *Too Much Salt? 5 Simple Ways to Slash the White Stuff in Your Diet* at:

https://www.huffingtonpost.com/2013/09/12/too-much-salt_n_3894986.html

Beware! What "they" do to food, although seemingly innocent, can cause harm.

Sounding the alarm (The videos of Dr. Greger)

To reinforce some of the things I am reporting on, I invite you to watch the following videos produced by **NutritionFacts.org**, an organization founded by Dr. Michael Greger, MD. The focus of NutritionFacts is on health issues common in our society, and to address these ills by promoting plant-based dieting.

I can't imagine a better resource on healthful living than Dr. Greger. We spoke of several topics in this chapter that he covers exceptionally well in the following three excellent video presentations. Watching them will reinforce several concepts we have covered in this chapter. Here are a few of the videos you should check out:

—**Butyrate**
https://nutritionfacts.org/video/bowel-wars-hydrogen-sulfide-vs-butyrate/

—**Ulcerative Colitis**
https://nutritionfacts.org/video/treating-ulcerative-colitis-with-diet/

—**Titanium dioxide**
https://nutritionfacts.org/video/titanium-dioxide-inflammatory-bowel-disease/

Bonus video:

—**Sodium and Autoimmune Disease: Rubbing Salt in the Wound?**
https://nutritionfacts.org/video/sodium-and-autoimmune-disease-
rubbing-salt-in-the-wound/

~References~

Aamodt G, Bukholm G, Jahnsen J, Moum B, Vatn MH, IBSEN Study Group. **The association between water supply and inflammatory bowel disease based on a 1990–1993 cohort study in southeastern Norway.** American journal of epidemiology. 2008 Sep 18;168(9):1065-72.

Abdoli A. **Salt and miscarriage: Is there a link?.** Medical hypotheses. 2016 Apr 1;89:58-62.

Abdoli A. **Hypothesis: High salt intake as an inflammation amplifier might be involved in the pathogenesis of neuropsychiatric disorders.** Clinical and Experimental Neuroimmunology. 2017 May;8(2):146-57.

Achtschin CG, Sipahi AM. **The role of titanium dioxide in the gut.** Nutrition & Food Science. 2017 May 8;47(3):432-42.

Ananthakrishnan AN, Khalili H, Konijeti GG, Higuchi LM, de Silva P, Fuchs CS, Willett WC, Richter JM, Chan AT. **Long-term intake of dietary fat and risk of ulcerative colitis and Crohn's'disease.** Gut. 2014 May 1;63(5):776-84.

Andersen V, Olsen A, Carbonnel F, Tjønneland A, Vogel U. **Diet and risk of inflammatory bowel disease.** Digestive and liver disease. 2012 Mar 1;44(3):185-94.

Ashwood P, Thompson RP, Powell JJ. **Fine particles that adsorb lipopolysaccharide via bridging calcium cations may mimic bacterial pathogenicity towards cells.** Experimental Biology and Medicine. 2007 Jan;232(1):107-17.

Aguiar SL, Miranda MC, Guimarães MA, Santiago HC, Queiroz CP, Cunha PD, Cara DC, Foureaux G, Ferreira AJ, Cardoso VN, Barros PA. **High-salt diet induces IL-17-dependent gut inflammation and exacerbates colitis in mice.** Frontiers in immunology. 2018 Jan 15;8:1969.

Awasthi A, Kuchroo VK. **Th17 cells: from precursors to players in inflammation and infection.** International immunology. 2009 Mar 4;21(5):489-98.

Barollo M, D'Incà R, Scarpa M, Medici V, Cardin R, Fries W, Angriman I, Sturniolo GC. **Effects of iron deprivation or chelation on DNA damage in** experimental colitis. International journal of colorectal disease. 2004 Sep 1;19(5):461-6.

Bastide NM, Pierre FH, Corpet D. **Heme iron from meat and risk of colorectal cancer: a meta-analysis and a review of the mechanisms involved.** Cancer prevention research. 2011 Jan 5:canprevres-0113.

Bayraktar UD, Bayraktar S. **Treatment of iron deficiency anemia associated with gastrointestinal tract diseases.** World Journal of Gastroenterology: WJG. 2010 Jun 14;16(22):2720.

Becker K, Schroecksnadel S, Geisler S, Carriere M, Gostner JM, Schennach H, Herlin N, Fuchs D. **TiO2 nanoparticles and bulk material stimulate human peripheral blood mononuclear cells.** Food and chemical toxicology. 2014 Mar 1;65:63-9.

Bettini S, Boutet-Robinet E, Cartier C, Coméra C, Gaultier E, Dupuy J, Naud N, Taché S, Grysan P, Reguer S, Thieriet N. **Food-grade TiO 2 impairs intestinal and systemic immune homeostasis, initiates preneoplastic lesions and promotes aberrant crypt development in the rat colon.** Scientific Reports. 2017 Jan 20;7:40373.

Bhattacharyya S, Borthakur A, Dudeja PK, Tobacman JK. **Carrageenan induces cell cycle arrest in human intestinal epithelial cells in vitro.** The Journal of nutrition. 2008 Mar 1;138(3):469-75.

Bhattacharyya S, Shumard T, Xie H, Dodda A, Varady KA, Feferman L, Halline AG, Goldstein JL, Hanauer SB, Tobacman JK. **A randomized trial of the effects of the no-carrageenan diet on ulcerative colitis disease activity.** Nutrition and healthy aging. 2017 Jan 1;4(2):181-92.

Brown K, DeCoffe D, Molcan E, Gibson DL. **Diet-induced dysbiosis of the intestinal microbiota and the effects on immunity and disease.** Nutrients. 2012 Aug;4(8):1095-119.

Buchman AL. **Is iron over-rated? Sulphates may be the more important compound in development of colitis in rodent models, and perhaps humans.** Gut. 2012 Feb 1;61(2):323-4.

Calder PC. **Polyunsaturated fatty acids and inflammatory processes: new twists in an old tale.** Biochimie. 2009 Jun 1;91(6):791-5.

Calder PC. **Omega-3 polyunsaturated fatty acids and inflammatory processes: nutrition or pharmacology?.** British journal of clinical pharmacology. 2012 Mar;75(3):645-62.

Carrera-Bastos P, Fontes-Villalba M, O'Keefe JH, Lindeberg S, Cordain L. **The western diet and lifestyle and diseases of civilization.** Res Rep Clin Cardiol. 2011 Mar 9;2(2):2-15.

Cassat JE, Skaar EP. **Iron in infection and immunity.** Cell host & microbe. 2013 May 15;13(5):509-19.

Chan YK, Estaki M, Gibson DL 2013. **Clinical Consequences of Diet-Induced Dysbiosis.** Annals of Nutrition and Metabolism 63(Suppl. 2):28–40.

Chang M, Xue J, Sharma V, Habtezion A. **Protective role of hemeoxygenase-1 in gastrointestinal diseases.** Cellular and molecular life sciences. 2015 Mar 1;72(6):1161-73.

Chassaing B, Koren O, Goodrich JK, Poole AC, Srinivasan S, Ley RE, Gewirtz AT. **Dietary emulsifiers impact the mouse gut microbiota promoting colitis and metabolic syndrome.** Nature. 2015 Mar;519(7541):92.

Chen X, Zhai X, Shi J, Liu WW, Tao H, Sun X, Kang Z. **Lactulose mediates suppression of dextran sodium sulfate-induced colon inflammation by increasing hydrogen production.** Digestive diseases and sciences. 2013 Jun 1;58(6):1560-8.

Chia CW, Shardell M, Tanaka T, Liu DD, Gravenstein KS, Simonsick EM, Egan JM, Ferrucci L. **Chronic low-calorie sweetener use and risk of abdominal obesity among older adults: a cohort study.** PloS one. 2016 Nov 23;11(11):e0167241.

Chua AC, Klopcic B, Lawrance IC, Olynyk JK, Trinder D. **Iron: an emerging factor in colorectal carcinogenesis.** World journal of gastroenterology: WJG. 2010 Feb 14;16(6):663.

Constante M, Fragoso G, Calvé A, Samba-Mondonga M, Santos MM. **Dietary heme induces gut dysbiosis, aggravates colitis, and potentiates the development of adenomas in mice.** Frontiers in microbiology. 2017 Sep 21;8:1809.

Cordain L, Eaton SB, Sebastian A, Mann N, Lindeberg S, Watkins BA, O'Keefe JH, Brand-Miller J. **Origins and evolution of the Western diet: health implications** for the 21st century. The American journal of clinical nutrition. 2005 Feb 1;81(2):341-54.

Csáki KF. Synthetic surfactant food additives can cause intestinal barrier dysfunction. Medical Hypotheses. 2011 May 1;76(5):676-81.

Dar HY, Singh A, Shukla P, Anupam R, Mondal RK, Mishra PK, Srivastava RK. High dietary salt intake correlates with modulated Th17-Treg cell balance resulting in enhanced bone loss and impaired bone-microarchitecture in male mice. Scientific reports. 2018 Feb 6;8(1):2503.

de Vogel J, Jonker-Termont DS, Van Lieshout EM, Katan MB, van der Meer R. Green vegetables, red meat and colon cancer: chlorophyll prevents the cytotoxic and hyperproliferative effects of haem in rat colon. Carcinogenesis. 2005 Feb 1;26(2):387-93.

de Vogel J, van-Eck WB, Sesink AL, Jonker-Termont DS, Kleibeuker J, van der Meer R. Dietary heme injures surface epithelium resulting in hyperproliferation, inhibition of apoptosis and crypt hyperplasia in rat colon. Carcinogenesis. 2008 Jan 3;29(2):398-403.

Doherty CP. Host-pathogen interactions: the role of iron. The Journal of nutrition. 2007 May 1;137(5):1341-4.

Engen PA, Green SJ, Voigt RM, Forsyth CB, Keshavarzian A. The gastrointestinal microbiome: alcohol effects on the composition of intestinal microbiota. Alcohol research: current reviews. 2015;37(2):223.

Erichsen K, Hausken T, Ulvik RJ, Svardal A, Berstad A, Berge RK. Ferrous fumarate deteriorated plasma antioxidant status in patients with Crohn disease. Scandinavian journal of gastroenterology. 2003 Jan 1;38(5):543-8.

Erichsen K, Ulvik RJ, Grimstad T, Berstad A, Berge RK, Hausken T. Effects of ferrous sulphate and non-ionic iron–polymaltose complex on markers of oxidative tissue damage in patients with inflammatory bowel disease. Alimentary pharmacology & therapeutics. 2005 Nov 1;22(9):831-8.

Evans SM, Ashwood P, Warley A, Berisha F, Thompson RP, Powell JJ. The role of dietary microparticles and calcium in apoptosis and interleukin-1β release of intestinal macrophages. Gastroenterology. 2002 Nov 1;123(5):1543-53.

Fisher AE, Naughton DP. Iron supplements: the quick fix with long-term consequences. Nutrition journal. 2004 Dec 1;3(1):2.

Fowler SP, Williams K, Resendez RG, Hunt KJ, Hazuda HP, Stern MP. **Fueling the obesity epidemic? Artificially sweetened beverage use and long-term weight gain.** Obesity. 2008 Aug 1;16(8):1894-900.

Gálvez J. **Role of Th17 cells in the pathogenesis of human IBD.** ISRN inflammation. 2014 Mar 25;2014.

Gasche C. **Anemia in IBD: the overlooked villain. Inflammatory bowel diseases.** 2000 May 1;6(2):142-50.

Gasche C, Lomer MC, Cavill I, Weiss G. **Iron, anaemia, and inflammatory bowel diseases.** Gut. 2004 Aug 1;53(8):1190-7.

Gatti AM. **Biocompatibility of micro-and nano-particles in the colon. Part II.** Biomaterials. 2004 Feb 1;25(3):385-92.

Gatti AM, Rivasi F. **Biocompatibility of micro-and nanoparticles. Part I: in liver and kidney.** Biomaterials. 2002 Jun 1;23(11):2381-7.

Gemelli C, Dongmo BM, Ferrarini F, Grande A, Corsi L. **Cytotoxic effect of hemin in colonic epithelial cell line: Involvement of 18 kDa translocator protein (TSPO).** Life sciences. 2014 Jun 27;107(1-2):14-20.

Ghosh S, DeCoffe D, Brown K, Rajendiran E, Estaki M, Dai C, Yip A, Gibson DL. **Fish oil attenuates omega-6 polyunsaturated fatty acid-induced dysbiosis and infectious colitis but impairs LPS dephosphorylation activity causing sepsis.** PloS one. 2013 Feb 6;8(2):e55468.

Gibson GR, Cummings JH, Macfarlane GT. **Growth and activities of sulphate-reducing bacteria in gut contents of healthy subjects and patients with ulcerative colitis.** FEMS Microbiology Letters. 1991 Dec 1;86(2):103-11.

Gisbert JP, Gomollón F. **Common misconceptions in the diagnosis and management of anemia in inflammatory bowel disease.** American Journal of Gastroenterology. 2008 May 1;103(5):1299-307.

Goyal S, Rampal R, Kedia S, Mahajan S, Bopanna S, Yadav DP, Jain S, Singh AK, Wari MN, Makharia G, Awasthi A. **Urinary potassium is a potential biomarker of disease activity in Ulcerative colitis and displays in vitro immunotolerant role.** Scientific reports. 2017 Dec 22;7(1):18068.

Grimble RF, Howell WM, O'R'illy G, Turner SJ, Markovic O, Hirrell S, East JM, Calder PC. **The ability of fish oil to suppress tumor necrosis factor α** production by peripheral blood mononuclear cells in healthy men is associated with polymorphisms in genes that influence tumor necrosis factor α production. The American journal of clinical nutrition. 2002 Aug 1;76(2):454-9.

Guo M, Perez C, Wei Y, Rapoza E, Su G, Bou-Abdallah F, Chasteen ND. **Iron-binding properties of plant phenolics and cranberry's' bio-effects.** Dalton Transactions. 2007(43):4951-61.

Guo HX, Ye N, Yan P, Qiu MY, Zhang J, Shen ZG, He HY, Tian ZQ, Li HL, Li JT. **Sodium chloride exacerbates dextran sulfate sodium-induced colitis by tuning proinflammatory and antiinflammatory lamina propria mononuclear cells through p38/MAPK pathway in mice.** World journal of gastroenterology. 2018 Apr 28;24(16):1779.

Hamer HM, Jonkers DM, Venema K, Vanhoutvin SA, Troost FJ, Brummer RJ. **The role of butyrate on colonic function.** Alimentary pharmacology & therapeutics. 2008 Jan 1;27(2):104-19.

Haskey N, Gibson DL. **An examination of diet for the maintenance of remission in inflammatory bowel disease.** Nutrients. 2017 Mar 10;9(3):259.

Hassanshahi N, Masoumi SJ. **The Effect of Omega-3 Fatty Acids in Ulcerative Colitis: A Systematic Review.** International Journal of Nutrition Sciences. 2018 Apr 9.

Hentze MW, Muckenthaler MU, Andrews NC. **Balancing acts: molecular control of mammalian iron metabolism.** Cell. 2004 Apr 30;117(3):285-97.

Hernandez AL, Kitz A, Wu C, Lowther DE, Rodriguez DM, Vudattu N, Deng S, Herold KC, Kuchroo VK, Kleinewietfeld M, Hafler DA. **Sodium chloride inhibits the suppressive function of FOXP3+ regulatory T cells.** The Journal of clinical investigation. 2015 Nov 2;125(11):4212-22.

Hsu TY, Shih HM, Wang YC, Lin LC, He GY, Chen CY, Kao CH, Chen CH, Chen WK, Yang TY. **Effect of alcoholic intoxication on the risk of inflammatory bowel disease: a nationwide retrospective cohort study.** PloS one. 2016 Nov 1;11(11):e0165411.

Hsu CC, Ness E, Kowdley KV. **Nutritional Approaches to Achieve Weight Loss in Nonalcoholic Fatty Liver Disease.** Advances in Nutrition. 2017 Mar 10;8(2):253-65.

Hucke S, Wiendl H, Klotz L. **Implications of dietary salt intake for multiple sclerosis pathogenesis.** Multiple Sclerosis Journal. 2016 Feb;22(2):133-9.

Ijssennagger N, Derrien M, van Doorn GM, Rijnierse A, van den Bogert B, Müller M, Dekker J, Kleerebezem M, van der Meer R. **Dietary heme alters microbiota and mucosa of mouse colon without functional changes in host-microbe cross-talk.** PloS one. 2012 Dec 11;7(12):e49868.

Ijssennagger N, van der Meer R, van Mil SW. **Sulfide as a mucus barrier-breaker in inflammatory bowel disease?.** Trends in molecular medicine. 2016 Mar 1;22(3):190-9.

Jacobs DM, Gaudier E, Duynhoven JV, Vaughan EE. **Non-digestible food ingredients, colonic microbiota and the impact on gut health and immunity: a role for metabolomics.** Current drug metabolism. 2009 Jan 1;10(1):41-54.

Jantchou P, Morois S, Clavel-Chapelon F, Boutron-Ruault MC, Carbonnel F. **Animal protein intake and risk of inflammatory bowel disease: The E3N prospective study.** The American journal of gastroenterology. 2010 Oct;105(10):2195.

Jiao Y, Wilkinson IV J, Di X, Wang W, Hatcher H, Kock ND, D'Agostino Jr R, et al 2009 **Curcumin, a Cancer Chemopreventive and Chemotherapeutic Agent, Is a Biologically Active Iron Chelator.** Blood; January 8; 113(2):462–9.

John S, Luben R, Shrestha SS, Welch A, Khaw KT, Hart AR. **Dietary n-3 polyunsaturated fatty acids and the aetiology of ulcerative colitis: a UK prospective cohort study.** European journal of gastroenterology & hepatology. 2010 May 1;22(5):602-6.

Jowett SJ, Seal CJ, Pearce MS, Phillips E, Gregory W, Barton JR, Welfare MR 2004 **Influence of Dietary Factors on the Clinical Course of Ulcerative Colitis: A Prospective Cohort Study.** Gut 53:1479–1484.

Kaliannan K, Wang B, Li XY, Kim KJ, Kang JX. **A host-microbiome interaction mediates the opposing effects of omega-6 and omega-3 fatty acids on metabolic endotoxemia.** Scientific reports. 2015 Jun 11;5:11276.

Kankaanpää PE, Salminen SJ, Isolauri E, Lee YK 2001 **The Influence of Polyunsaturated Fatty Acids on Probiotic Growth and Adhesion.** FEMS Microbiology Letters 194:149–153.

Kell DB, Pretorius E. **On the translocation of bacteria and their lipopolysaccharides between blood and peripheral locations in chronic, inflammatory diseases: the central roles of LPS and LPS-induced cell death.** Integrative Biology. 2015;7(11):1339-77.

Khalil NA, Walton GE, Gibson GR, Tuohy KM, Andrews SC. **In vitro batch cultures of gut microbiota from healthy and ulcerative colitis (UC) subjects suggest that sulphate-reducing bacteria levels are raised in UC and by a protein-rich diet.** International journal of food sciences and nutrition. 2014 Feb 1;65(1):79-88.

Khalili H, de Silva PS, Ananthakrishnan AN, Lochhead P, Joshi A, Garber JJ, Richter JR, Sauk J, Chan AT. **Dietary iron and heme iron consumption, genetic susceptibility, and risk of Crohn's'disease and ulcerative colitis. Inflammatory bowel diseases.** 2017 Jun 9;23(7):1088-95.

Khalili H, Malik S, Ananthakrishnan AN, Garber JJ, Higuchi LM, Joshi A, Peloquin J, Richter JM, Stewart KO, Curhan GC, Awasthi A. **Identification and characterization of a novel association between dietary potassium and risk of Crohn's disease and ulcerative colitis.** Frontiers in immunology. 2016 Dec 7;7:554.

Kish L, Hotte N, Kaplan GG, Vincent R, Tso R, Gänzle M, Rioux KP, Thiesen A, Barkema HW, Wine E, Madsen KL. **Environmental particulate matter induces murine intestinal inflammatory responses and alters the gut microbiome.** PloS one. 2013 Apr 24;8(4):e62220.

Kortman GA, Raffatellu M, Swinkels DW, Tjalsma H. **Nutritional iron turned inside out: intestinal stress from a gut microbial perspective.** FEMS microbiology reviews. 2014 Nov 1;38(6):1202-34.

Korzenik JR. **Past and current theories of etiology of IBD: toothpaste, worms, and refrigerators.** Journal of clinical gastroenterology. 2005 Apr 1;39(4):S59-65.

Kushkevych IV. **Etiological role of sulfate-reducing bacteria in the development of inflammatory bowel diseases and ulcerative colitis.** Am. J. Infect. Dis. Microbiol. 2014;2:63-73.

Lerner A, Matthias T. **Changes in intestinal tight junction permeability associated with industrial food additives explain the rising incidence of autoimmune disease.** Autoimmunity reviews. 2015 Jun 1;14(6):479-89.

Liehr JG, Jones J. **Role of iron in estrogen-induced cancer.** Current medicinal chemistry. 2001 Jun 1;8(7):839-49.

Lomer MC, Harvey RS, Evans SM, Thompson RP, Powell JJ. **Efficacy and tolerability of a low microparticle diet in a double blind, randomized, pilot study in Crohn's'disease.** European journal of gastroenterology & hepatology. 2001 Feb 1;13(2):101-6.

Lomer MC, Hutchinson C, Volkert S, Greenfield SM, Catterall A, Thompson RP, Powell JJ. **Dietary sources of inorganic microparticles and their intake in healthy subjects and patients with Crohn's'disease.** British Journal of Nutrition. 2004 Dec;92(6):947-55.

Lucca LE, Hafler DA. **Sodium-activated macrophages: the salt mine expands.** Cell research. 2015 Aug;25(8):885.

Magee EA, Richardson CJ, Hughes R, Cummings JH 2000 **Contribution of Dietary Protein to Sulfide Production in the Large Intestine: An in vitro and a Controlled Feeding Study in Humans.** Am J Clin Nutr 72:1488–1494.

Martino JV, Van Limbergen J, Cahill LE. **The role of carrageenan and carboxymethylcellulose in the development of intestinal inflammation.** Frontiers in pediatrics. 2017 May 1;5:96.

McClements DJ, Xiao H. **Is nano safe in foods? Establishing the factors impacting the gastrointestinal fate and toxicity of organic and inorganic food-grade nanoparticles.** npj Science of Food. 2017 Nov 20;1(1):6.

Michielan A, D'Incà R. **Intestinal permeability in inflammatory bowel disease: pathogenesis, clinical evaluation, and therapy of leaky gut.** Mediators of inflammation. 2015;2015.

Millar AD, Rampton DS, Blake DR. **Effects of iron and iron chelation in vitro on mucosal oxidant activity in ulcerative colitis.** Alimentary Pharmacology and Therapeutics. 2000 Sep 1;14(9):1163-8.

Miller TW, Wang EA, Gould S, Stein EV, Kaur S, Lim L, Amarnath S, Fowler DH, Roberts DD. **Hydrogen sulfide is an endogenous potentiator of T cell activation.** Journal of Biological Chemistry. 2012 Feb 3;287(6):4211-21.

Min B, Fairchild RL. **Over-salting ruins the balance of the immune menu.** The Journal of clinical investigation. 2015 Nov 2;125(11):4002-4.

Miranda PM, De Palma G, Serkis V, Lu J, Louis-Auguste MP, McCarville JL, Verdu EF, Collins SM, Bercik P. **High salt diet exacerbates colitis in mice by decreasing Lactobacillus levels and butyrate production.** Microbiome. 2018 Dec;6(1):57.

Miura S, Tsuzuki Y, Hokair R, Ishii H 1998 **Modulation of Intestinal Immune System by Dietary Fat Intake: Relevance to Crohn's Disease.** Journal of Gastroenterology and Hepatology 13:1183–1190.

Monteleone I, Pallone F, Monteleone G. **Interleukin-23 and Th17 cells in the control of gut inflammation.** Mediators of inflammation. 2009;2009.

Nairz M, Schroll A, Sonnweber T, Weiss G. **The struggle for iron–a metal at the host–pathogen interface.** Cellular microbiology. 2010 Dec;12(12):1691-702.

Nickerson KP, McDonald C. **Crohn's'disease-associated adherent-invasive Escherichia coli adhesion is enhanced by exposure to the ubiquitous dietary polysaccharide maltodextrin.** PLos One. 2012 Dec 12;7(12):e52132.

Nickerson KP, Chanin R, McDonald C. **Deregulation of intestinal anti-microbial defense by the dietary additive, maltodextrin.** Gut microbes. 2015 Jan 2;6(1):78-83.

Nogueira CM, de Azevedo WM, Dagli ML, Toma SH, de Arruda Leite AZ, Lordello ML, Nishitokukado I, Ortiz-Agostinho CL, Duarte MI, Ferreira MA, Sipahi AM. **Titanium dioxide induced inflammation in the small intestine.** World journal of gastroenterology: WJG. 2012 Sep 14;18(34):4729.

Ohio State Research News 2001 **Excess Iron Intake Increases Risk of Intestinal Infections, Study Suggests.** http://researchnews.osu.edu/archive/iron.htm

Oldenburg B, Koningsberger JC, Van Berge Henegouwen GP, Van Asbeck BS, Marx JJ. **Iron and inflammatory bowel disease.** Alimentary pharmacology & therapeutics. 2001 Apr;15(4):429-38.

O'Shea JJ, Jones RG. **Autoimmunity: rubbing salt in the wound.** Nature. 2013 Apr;496(7446):437-9.

Papanikolaou G, Pantopoulos K. **Iron metabolism and toxicity.** Toxicology and applied pharmacology. 2005 Jan 15;202(2):199-211.

Payne AN, Chassard C, Lacroix C. **Gut microbial adaptation to dietary consumption of fructose, artificial sweeteners and sugar alcohols:**

implications for host–microbe interactions contributing to obesity. Obesity reviews. 2012 Sep 1;13(9):799-809.

Pitcher MC, Cummings JH. **Hydrogen sulphide: a bacterial toxin in ulcerative colitis?.** Gut. 1996 Jul;39(1):1.

Powell JJ, Harvey RS, Thompson RP. **Microparticles in Crohn's'disease—has the dust settled?.** Gut. 1996 Aug;39(2):340.

Powell JJ, Thoree V, Pele LC. **Dietary microparticles and their impact on tolerance and immune responsiveness of the gastrointestinal tract.** British Journal of Nutrition. 2007 Oct;98(S1):S59-63.

Purohit V, Bode JC, Bode C, Brenner DA, Choudhry MA, Hamilton F, Kang YJ, Keshavarzian A, Rao R, Sartor RB, Swanson C. **Alcohol, intestinal bacterial growth, intestinal permeability to endotoxin, and medical consequences: summary of a symposium.** Alcohol. 2008 Aug 1;42(5):349-61.

Qin X. **What made Canada become a country with the highest incidence of inflammatory bowel disease: Could sucralose be the culprit?.** Canadian Journal of Gastroenterology and Hepatology. 2011;25(9):511-.

Radek KA. **Antimicrobial anxiety: the impact of stress on antimicrobial immunity.** Journal of leukocyte biology. 2010 Aug;88(2):263-77.

Richman E, Rhodes JM. **Review article: evidence-based dietary advice for patients with inflammatory bowel disease.** Alimentary pharmacology & therapeutics. 2013 Nov 1;38(10):1156-71.

Roberts CL, Keita ÅV, Duncan SH, O'Kennedy N, Söderholm JD, Rhodes JM, Campbell BJ. **Translocation of Crohn's disease Escherichia coli across M-cells: contrasting effects of soluble plant fibres and emulsifiers.** Gut. 2010 Oct 1;59(10):1331-9.

Rodriguez-Palacios A, Harding A, Menghini P, Himmelman C, Retuerto M, Nickerson KP, Lam M, Croniger CM, McLean MH, Durum SK, Pizarro TT. **The artificial sweetener splenda promotes gut proteobacteria, dysbiosis, and myeloperoxidase reactivity in Crohn's disease–like ileitis.** Inflammatory bowel diseases. 2018 Mar 15;24(5):1005-20.

Roediger WE, Duncan A, Kapaniris O, Millard S. **Reducing sulfur compounds of the colon impair colonocyte nutrition: implications for ulcerative colitis.** Gastroenterology. 1993 Mar 1;104(3):802-9.

Rompelberg C, Heringa MB, van Donkersgoed G, Drijvers J, Roos A, Westenbrink S, Peters R, van Bemmel G, Brand W, Oomen AG. **Oral intake of added titanium dioxide and its nanofraction from food products, food supplements and toothpaste by the Dutch population.** Nanotoxicology. 2016 Nov 25;10(10):1404-14.

Rowan FE, Docherty NG, Coffey JC, O'c'nnell PR. **Sulphate-reducing bacteria and hydrogen sulphide in the aetiology of ulcerative colitis.** British Journal of Surgery. 2009 Feb 1;96(2):151-8.

Ruemmele FM. **Role of diet in inflammatory bowel disease.** Annals of Nutrition and Metabolism. 2016;68(Suppl. 1):32-41.

Santarelli RL, Vendeuvre JL, Naud N, Taché S, Guéraud F, Viau M, Genot C, Corpet DE, Pierre FH. **Meat processing and colon carcinogenesis: cooked, nitrite-treated, and oxidized high-heme cured meat promotes mucin-depleted foci in rats.** Cancer Prevention Research. 2010 Jun 8:1940-6207.

Schepens MA, Vink C, Schonewille AJ, Dijkstra G, van der Meer R, Bovee-Oudenhoven IM. **Dietary heme adversely affects experimental colitis in rats, despite heat-shock protein induction.** Nutrition. 2011 May 1;27(5):590-7.

Schneider JC. **Can microparticles contribute to inflammatory bowel disease: innocuous or inflammatory?.** Experimental biology and medicine (Maywood, NJ). 2007 Jan;232(1):1.

Schneider H, Braun A, Füllekrug J, Stremmel W, Ehehalt R. **Lipid based therapy for ulcerative colitis—modulation of intestinal mucus membrane phospholipids as a tool to influence inflammation.** International journal of molecular sciences. 2010 Oct;11(10):4149-64.

Schulzke JD, Ploeger S, Amasheh M, Fromm A, Zeissig S, Troeger H, Richter J, Bojarski C, Schumann M, Fromm M. **Epithelial tight junctions in intestinal inflammation.** Annals of the New York Academy of Sciences. 2009 May 1;1165(1):294-300.

Serhan CN, Chiang N, Van Dyke TE. **Resolving inflammation: dual anti-inflammatory and pro-resolution lipid mediators.** Nature Reviews Immunology. 2008 May;8(5):349.

Seril DN, Liao J, West AB, Yang GY. **High-iron diet: foe or feat in ulcerative colitis and ulcerative colitis-associated carcinogenesis.** Journal of clinical gastroenterology. 2006 May 1;40(5):391-7.

Sesink AL, Termont DS, Kleibeuker JH, Van der Meer R. **Red meat and colon cancer: the cytotoxic and hyperproliferative effects of dietary heme.** Cancer research. 1999 Nov 15;59(22):5704-9.

Simon RA 1998 **Update on Sulfite Sensitivity.** Allergy 53 (Suppl) 46:78–79.

Sinnecker H, Krause T, Koelling S, Lautenschläger I, Frey A. **The gut wall provides an effective barrier against nanoparticle uptake.** Beilstein journal of nanotechnology. 2014;5:2092.

Skocaj M, Filipic M, Petkovic J, Novak S. **Titanium dioxide in our everyday life; is it safe?.** Radiology and oncology. 2011 Dec 1;45(4):227-47.

Suez J, Korem T, Zeevi D, Zilberman-Schapira G, Thaiss CA, Maza O, Israeli D, Zmora N, Gilad S, Weinberger A, Kuperman Y. **Artificial sweeteners induce glucose intolerance by altering the gut microbiota.** Nature. 2014 Oct;514(7521):181.

Swanson GR, Sedghi S, Farhadi A, Keshavarzian A. **Pattern of alcohol consumption and its effect on gastrointestinal symptoms in inflammatory bowel disease.** Alcohol. 2010 May 1;44(3):223-8.

Swidsinski A, Loening-Baucke V, Herber A. **Mucosal flora in Crohn's disease and ulcerative colitis-an overview.** J Physiol Pharmacol. 2009 Dec 1;60(Suppl 6):61-71.

Tailford LE, Crost EH, Kavanaugh D, Juge N. **Mucin glycan foraging in the human gut microbiome.** Frontiers in genetics. 2015 Mar 19;6:81.

Tilg H, Kaser A. **Diet and relapsing ulcerative colitis: take off the meat?.** Gut. 2004 Oct 1;53(10):1399-401.

Tjonneland, A.; Olsen, A.; Overvad, K.; Bergmann, M. M.; Boeing, H.; Nagel, G.; Linseisen, J.; Hallmans, G.; Palmqvist, R. and Sjodin, H., et al. **Linoleic acid, a dietary n-6 polyunsaturated fatty acid, and the aetiology of ulcerative colitis: a nested case–control study within a European prospective cohort study.** Gut. 2009 Dec 1;58(12):1606-11.

Tobacman JK. **Review of harmful gastrointestinal effects of carrageenan in animal experiments.** Environmental health perspectives. 2001 Oct;109(10):983.

Toussirot E, Béreau M, Vauchy C, Saas P. **Could Sodium Chloride be an Environmental Trigger for Immune-Mediated Diseases? An Overview of the Experimental and Clinical Evidence.** Frontiers in physiology. 2018;9.

Uritski R, Barshack I, Bilkis I, Ghebremeskel K, Reifen R. **Dietary iron affects inflammatory status in a rat model of colitis.** The Journal of nutrition. 2004 Sep 1;134(9):2251-5.

Varnalidis I, Ioannidis O, Karamanavi E, Ampas Z, Poutahidis T, Taitzoglou I, Paraskevas G, Botsios D. **Omega 3 fatty acids supplementation has an ameliorative effect in experimental ulcerative colitis despite increased colonic neutrophil infiltration.** Revista Espanola de Enfermedades Digestivas. 2011 Oct 1;103(10):511.

Vijayan V, Mueller S, Baumgart-Vogt E, Immenschuh S. **Heme oxygenase-1 as a therapeutic target in inflammatory disorders of the gastrointestinal tract.** World journal of gastroenterology: WJG. 2010 Jul 7;16(25):3112.

Watts DL. **The nutritional relationships of iron.** Journal of Orthomolecular Medicine. 1988 Jan 1;3(3):110-6.

Weinberg ED, Miklossy J. **Iron withholding: a defense against disease.** Journal of Alzheimer's'Disease. 2008 Jan 1;13(4):451-63.

Weir A, Westerhoff P, Fabricius L, Hristovski K, Von Goetz N. **Titanium dioxide nanoparticles in food and personal care products.** Environmental science & technology. 2012 Feb 8;46(4):2242-50.

Weiss G. **Iron in the inflamed gut: another pro-inflammatory hit?.** Gut. 2011 Mar 1;60(3):287-8.

Werner T, Wagner SJ, Martínez I, Walter J, Chang JS, Clavel T, Kisling S, Schuemann K, Haller D. **Depletion of luminal iron alters the gut microbiota and prevents Crohn's'disease-like ileitis.** Gut. 2011 Mar 1;60(3):325-33.

Weylandt KH, Kang JX, Wiedenmann B, Baumgart DC. **Lipoxins and resolvins in inflammatory bowel disease.** Inflammatory bowel diseases. 2007 Jan 29;13(6):797-9.

Wikipedia 2018 **Red Blood Cell.** https://en.wikipedia.org/wiki/Red_blood_cell

Wilck N, Matus MG, Kearney SM, Olesen SW, Forslund K, Bartolomaeus H, Haase S, Mähler A, Balogh A, Markó L, Vvedenskaya O. **Salt-responsive gut commensal modulates TH 17 axis and disease.** Nature. 2017 Nov;551(7682): 585.

Willebrand R, Kleinewietfeld M. **The role of salt for immune cell function and disease.** Immunology. 2018 Feb 21.

Yang Y, Owyang C, Wu GD. **East Meets West: the increasing incidence of inflammatory bowel disease in Asia as a paradigm for environmental effects on the pathogenesis of immune-mediated disease.** Gastroenterology. 2016 Dec 1;151(6):e1-5.

Yokel RA, MacPhail RC. **Engineered nanomaterials: exposures, hazards, and risk prevention.** Journal of Occupational Medicine and Toxicology. 2011 Dec;6(1):7.

Zhang P, Smith R, Chapkin RS, McMurray DN. **Dietary (n-3) polyunsaturated fatty acids modulate murine Th1/Th2 balance toward the Th2 pole by suppression of Th1 development.** The Journal of nutrition. 2005 Jul 1;135(7): 1745-51.

Zhang R, Bai Y, Zhang B, Chen L, Yan B. **The potential health risk of titania nanoparticles.** Journal of hazardous materials. 2012 Apr 15;211:404-13.

Zhu X, Fan WG, Li DP, Kung H, Lin MC. **Heme oxygenase-1 system and gastrointestinal inflammation: a short review.** World Journal of Gastroenterology: WJG. 2011 Oct 14;17(38):4283.

Chapter 10

Not so fast!

The Western diet pattern is dominated by increased consumption of refined sugar, omega-6 polyunsaturated fats and fast food, combined with a diet deficient in fruit and vegetables, and fiber.

Fast food intake, defined as more than once a week, was <u>significantly</u> associated with the risk of UC [ulcerative colitis]. *~Haskey and Gibson,* **2017, emphasis added**

*The Western diet is characterized by a high intake of saturated and omega-6 fatty acids, reduced omega-3 fat intake, an <u>overuse of salt</u>, and too much refined sugar. Most are aware that this type of eating, if not in moderation, can damage the heart, kidneys, and waistlines; however, it is becoming increasingly clear that **the modern diet also damages the immune system.** ~Myles, 2014, emphasis added*

It is said that regular consumption of fast food increases the risk of ulcerative colitis. It is said that consuming the Western diet increases the risk of ulcerative colitis. What is said is true. And what should be appreciated here is this: **Fast food is a more intense experience with the Western diet. With fast food you go from bad to worse.** In this chapter we will explore the reasons why both fast food and the Western diet damages the immune system, increases the risk of ulcerative colitis, and promotes its persistence. I'd like to pick up where we left off in the last chapter. Consider this:

Salt (sodium chloride, NaCl) intake varies vastly around the world, ranging from less than 1 g/day in some indigenous populations to more than 20 g/day in the Western world and Japan.

*The sodium content of processed foods and 'fast food' preferentially consumed in the developed societies can be more than **100 times** higher in comparison to similar homemade meals.*
(Manzel et al., 2014)

Did you just hear what I just heard? ***"100 times!"*** *Oh, my!* From an immunological standpoint, this degree of sodium consumption can only be dreadful. And what should be appreciated here is this: **The Western diet of processed and 'fast' foods is a more intense experience with sodium.** Once again, I see trouble ahead. Let's take a few moments to review and expand on the problem of sodium excess.

Sodium excess revisited

In addition, a high-salt diet (HSD) can alter the composition of the intestinal microbiome and thereby additionally influence T helper 17 (TH17) cell differentiation and function. **~Wilck et al., 2019**

In the last chapter we learned that excessive sodium consumption **1)** unfavorably alters the microbiome, **2)** unbalances the immune system in the gut, **3)** intensifies Th17 cell-mediated inflammation, and **4)** suppresses the anti-inflammatory activity and numbers of anti-inflammatory Treg cells—all factors implicated in the initiation and progression of ulcerative colitis. The sodium excess found in our prepared foods and our fast foods promotes immune system dysregulation, the nature of which simply *cannot* be helpful to the individual who is struggling with ulcerative colitis.

Those of us who eat largely of prepared and fast foods are generally not eating largely of foods low in sodium and high in potassium. For us, our diet is a high sodium and low potassium diet. And with a lower potassium consumption, the problem of sodium excess is intensified. Recall from the previous chapter, potassium helps regulate the balance between the Th17 and the Treg cell (Khalili et al., 2016). In this context, studies have identified *"an inverse relationship between dietary potassium and the risk of CD (Crohn's disease) and UC."* (Goyal et al., 2017) Clearly, one of the harmful features of the Western diet is excess of sodium consumption in context with insufficient potassium intake, as one could obtain from a diet abundant in fruits and vegetables (Carrera-Bastos et al., 2011). Are you beginning to see why experts want you to consume more fruits and vegetables and less of the other stuff? Among other things, what they want is for you to consume less sodium and more potassium.

It is recommended that we keep our daily sodium intake at less than **2,300 mg/day,** with some recommendations on the order of **1,500 mg/day** or less (AHA, 2018). In contrast, on the Western diet an individual is likely to consume **3,400 mg/day** or more (CDC, 2016), with approximately **71%** of our sodium intake derived from processed and restaurant foods (CDC, 2018). *71%!*

Those who strongly recommend that you lower your intake of sodium, do so because they want you to reduce your risk of hypertension, stroke, cardiovascular disease, renal failure, misery, and untimely death. I would like you to reduce your sodium intake so you have a better chance of getting well. But, as with all things, discuss your intention to reduce sodium intake with your physician. You could probably use some guidance here, so you don't run into trouble. For instance, if you are losing a lot of sodium due to diarrhea, you may need a daily sodium intake higher than an individual not plagued with this problem. Furthermore, IBD patients are prone to disturbances in sodium chloride and potassium balance, so careful consideration of sodium restriction is undoubtedly warranted (Barkas et al., 2013).

I've covered dietary sodium excess well enough that I feel confident you have been sufficiently warned of the danger and are fully aware of the need to involve your physician in any sodium- or potassium-related interventions you are considering. Now we can move on. And what do I see?

More trouble ahead

Reduced consumption of fruits and possibly vegetables, resulting in a reduced overall intake of fiber, with high intake of meats, fast foods and trans-fatty acids appears to be associated with an overall increase in the risk of developing IBD. ~**Haskey and Gibson, 2017**

In this regard, consumption of the so-called "Western" diet is associated with increased risk for IBD. Westernized diet is characterized by a high content of proteins (derived from fatty domesticated and processed meats), saturated fats, refined grains, sugar, alcohol, salt and corn-derived fructose syrup, with an associated reduced consumption of fruits and vegetables. ~**Statovci et al., 2017**

There are other dangers in the Western and fast food diet that are relevant to ulcerative colitis, things that can increase the risk, things that are likely to make matters worse. A diet high in fat is one such danger. It fattens you and harms you in other ways, too. It is highly likely that high-fat dieting makes ulcerative colitis worse, as we shall see in short order. One thing we know for certain, it can expand the waistline!

It is well documented that "fast food" with high fat and salt content at relatively low cost is a major cause of the obesity epidemic in Western societies. (Poutahidis et al., 2013)

In this chapter on trouble, next we'll turn our attention to the problem of excessive fat consumption.

High-fat dieting

> *. . . a high-fat diet alters the structure of the microbiome even in the absence of obesity.* ~**Manzel et al., 2014**

> *Epidemiological and clinical studies reveal that higher-fat diets are associated with a **2.5-fold** increased risk of colitis in young adults.* ~**Gulhane et al., 2016, emphasis added**

> *Consuming a Western diet, high in fat (**particularly saturated fat**), is enough to induce endotoxemia in healthy subjects.* ~**Knight-Sepulveda et al., 2015, emphasis added**

> *Also, **a direct correlation of colonic cytokine levels with saturated fatty acids (SFA) was identified in patients with UC.*** ~Statovci et al., 2017

> *. . . it is clear that **a portion of ingested fats enters the human colon each day**. Increased consumption of dietary fats on a Western diet likely saturates the ability of small intestine to emulsify and absorb all dietary lipids, thus allowing a considerable fraction to avoid absorption and reach the colon. This conclusion is supported by multiple studies which showed that a high-fat diet leads to significant alterations in gut microbial communities in both humans and animals.* ~**Agans et al., 2018, emphasis added**

The Western diet, including the fast foods we love to death (quite literally), is a high-fat diet, high in saturated fat and high in other fats as well, particularly the omega-6 PUFAs. But since we have discussed the omegs-6s at length in the last chapter, we'll move on and address the problem of excessive saturated fat consumption.

Although saturated fats can be of vegetable origin (coconut oil, palm oil, and others), the Western diet and its fast foods is a diet rich in saturated fat of animal origin. One reason for the excess is this: The animals we consume are farmed and fattened with grain before harvest—therefore not lean, but rather they are enriched with saturated fat as well as enriched with the omegs-6 fatty acids (Cordain et al., 2005; Haskey and Gibson, 2017).

There are a few of things that make excess saturated fat consumption a big problem in the context of ulcerative colitis. Saturated fat, in excess, alters the bacterial composition of the bowel, making it pro-inflammatory (Statovci et al., 2017). Furthermore, the heme and other proteins consumed, <u>along with</u> saturated fat, further contributes to dysbiosis (Statovci et al., 2017). Saturated fat, in excess, also promotes leaky gut, *"allowing harmful substances to leak from the gut into the blood stream and contribute to immune dysfunction that worsens infection control."* (Myles et al., 2014) Surprisingly, **saturated fat molecules can mimic bacteria**, and can therefore evoke an inflammatory response (Myles et al., 2014). "What, pray tell, is *this* all about?"

To answer your question, I'll begin with this:

> *One of the first-line weapons the immune system deploys against infection are molecules called Toll-like receptors (TLR). While complex in its workings, when the immune system comes across a potential invader these receptors are designed to evaluate if it is bacterial, viral, or fungal.* (Myles et al., 2014)

Continuing . . . *"One of the TLR weapons, **TLR4**, is designed to sense bacteria"* and **this sensor can be inappropriately stimulated by saturated fat, generating *"inappropriate signaling."*** (Myles et al., 2014, emphasis added) This *"abnormal signaling"* <u>may</u> result in a *"misguided attack upon saturated fat when it is perceived as a bacterial invader."* (Myles et al., 2014) This misguided attack can lead to a cascade of events that contributes to immune system dysregulation (Myles et al., 2014). Importantly, TLR4 is expressed in the colonocyte (Fukata et al., 2007), which may allow saturated fat to not only initiate and perpetuate an inflammatory response in the colon but misguide it as well.

As with just about everything, there is more to the story. It has been discovered that a bacterial component of the cell wall of Gram-negative bacteria, called **lipopolysaccharide (LPS)**, is largely composed of two saturated fatty acids, palmitic and steric fatty acids (Myles et al., 2014), which may be why **LPS has a high affinity for the molecules that carry dietary fat, including saturated fat, through the gut wall and into the circulation** (Piya et al., 2013).

From my perspective: From an immunological standpoint, humans can and do tolerate excessive saturated fat consumption quite well, day in and day out—but it takes a lot of anti-inflammatory prowess to deal with the challenge. Healthy individuals can pull this off, at least for a while. In contrast, it stands to reason that an individual genetically predisposed to or already dealing with ulcerative colitis will likely be at greater risk of harm from a diet high in saturated fat compared to an individual not predisposed to or already suffering from this disease. And for the ulcerative colitis patient, I see more of the same—inflammation and more inflammation, and inflammation resistant to resolution.

> *Consuming the Western diet, _high in fat_ (**particularly saturated fat**), is enough to induce endotoxemia in healthy subjects. These results suggest that even in a healthy state, this diet may be causing a leaky gut with increased permeability and changes in the microbiota, resulting in systemic low-level inflammation.* (Knight-Sepulveda et al., 2015, emphasis added)

Ponder this: Since a diet high in saturated fat can cause endotoxemia (bacterial components like LPS within the bloodstream), leaky gut, and low-level inflammation, even in healthy people, imagine what it could do to you, an individual compromised by ulcerative colitis. It could make matters worse. And while you are at it, imagine what it would be like to be well again. Oh, wouldn't that be nice?

Protein excess

> *The Western dietary pattern [high fat, high n-6 polyunsaturated fatty acids [PUFAs], high meat, low fruits and vegetables] is associated with an increased IBD risk and also with exacerbated colitis [red meat, dietary fats].* *In addition, an increased incidence of **IBD has been associated with diets high in animal protein.***

> *Red meat is also a hallmark of the Western diet pattern.* *Its consumption is associated with an increased IBD risk . . ..* **~Marion-Letellier et al., 2016, emphasis added**

> **High protein intake was associated with a <u>3.3-fold increased risk</u> of IBD,** *suggesting a diet high in animal protein is a major risk factor for the development of IBD.* **~Haskey and Gibson, 2017, emphasis added**

We've examined the dangers of red meat before—all the heme, all the iron, all the sulfur, and all the flavor that keeps you coming back for more. Since we have discussed all the heme, all the iron, all the sulfur, and all the flavor previously, we can now focus on another problem associated with the Western/fast food diet, we can focus on the problem of protein excess—another hallmark of the Western diet (Manzel et al., 2014). *"With the traditional Western diet, the average American consumes about double the protein her or his body needs."* (Physicians Committee for Responsible Medicine, date not specified)

A diet high in protein is definitely on the harmful side (Russell et al., 2011). It is said that *"protein-rich diets increase the activity of bacterial enzymes . . . which produce toxic metabolites that trigger inflammatory responses."* (Brown et al., 2012) Unfortunately, high protein dieting is often employed as a strategy for losing weight (Russell et al., 2011). Hey! Why bother with high protein dieting when you can lose weight with ulcerative colitis! However, I don't recommend ulcerative colitis as a weight loss strategy. It is simply not worth it. Costly, too! But I do recommend you pay attention to this:

Protein fermentation mainly occurs in the distal colon, when carbohydrates get depleted[,] and results in the production of potentially toxic metabolites such as ammonia, amines, phenols and sulfides.

*In addition, some important bowel diseases such as colorectal cancer (CRC) and ulcerative colitis appear most often in the **distal colon, which is the <u>primary site</u> of protein fermentation.*** (Windey et al. 2012)

The proteins in meat can easily reach the colon, undigested. And, following fermentation by bacteria, are transformed into harmful products that can cause inflammation and potentially lead to colon cancer (Russell et al., 2011; Windey et al., 2012). What should be appreciated here is this: **The Western and fast food diet is a protein-fermentation diet.** So is it any wonder, *". . . high protein intake, specifically animal protein (meat, not dairy products) was positively associated with an increased risk of IBD."* (Haskey and Gibson, 2017) However, dairy, due to its high calcium content, may protect against the negative effects of excessive protein ingestion (Windey et al., 2012). So, with dairy, we catch a break. There are other defenses, too, namely fruits, vegetables, and pre- pro-biotics and symbiotics, that may protect against the negative effect of excessive protein ingestion (Windey et al., 2012). Obviously, another strategy to employ in this regard is to simply reduce the intake of protein from animal sources. And when you do this, you are significantly restricting the sulfur-rich amino acids that lead to excess sulfite exposure and the generation of hydrogen sulfate in excess, both known to inflict mucosal damage in the colon (Roediger, 2008; Magee et al., 2005; Windey et al., 2012).

There may be a case to be made that the ulcerative colitis patient needs a high-protein intake to aid healing. However,

. . . an excessive amount of dietary protein may result in an increased intestinal production of potentially deleterious bacterial

metabolites. This could possibly affect epithelial repair as several of these metabolites are known to inhibit colonic epithelial cell respiration, cell proliferation, and/or to affect barrier function. (Vidal-Lletjós et al., 2017)

Let's see what we can learn from the following case report. Since the subject of this report is a Japanese gentleman, I'll give him the popular Japanese name, Yuto.

Case report: Yuto

Yuto was 38 at the time he decided he was large enough. For a male, five foot five inches, a weight of 160 pounds was simply too much to accept, representing a probable 20 to 30-pound degree of overweightfullness. (Did I just create a new word?) For Yuto, it was time to diet.

The report detailing Yuto's experience, recently published in a reputable medical journal, is a little shy on detail, but it was reported that the diet Yuto followed was a high protein/low carbohydrate diet patterned after the Atkins diet. Accordingly, *"He decreased his white rice consumption to approximately one-third and consumed meat every day and minced or processed meat 3 to 5 servings per week."* (Chiba et al., 2016)

On the diet, Yuto achieved a 13-pound weight loss within a period of approximately 3 months; and continued the high protein/low carbohydrate diet as a way of life, ostensibly to effect further weight loss. So far so good. But things were about to change.

A little over a year after starting the diet, Yuto began to experience an occasional bloody stool. This went on for a month or so, then "occasional" gave way to "daily." The bloody-stool issue continued for several months before Yuto received appropriate medical attention and was given the diagnosis of ulcerative colitis, some 15 months after starting his high protein/low carbohydrate diet.

Did I mention Yuto was a physician? Perhaps, as a physician, he was fully aware of the dangers of drug therapy, even the first line, "safer" therapy for ulcerative colitis, 5-ASA (Asacol; Pentasa; sulfasalazine). For whatever reason, Yuto opted not to take this route. His ulcerative colitis was considered mild, so perhaps it would just go away and maybe the risks posed by drug therapy, even 5-ASA, was considered unacceptable at the time. Perhaps he knew

> . . . patients administered 5-ASA or its derivatives suffer several serious adverse conditions, such as anorexia, dyspepsia, nausea/ vomiting, hemolysis, neutropenia, agranulocytosis, folate malabsorption, reversible, male infertility, and neuropathy. (Wu et al., 2009)

And he certainly he must have known

> Treatment with mesalamine-containing drugs is the gold standard for treatment of mild-to-moderate UC, but the results found with this treatment are far from satisfactory. (Sood et al., 2009)

According to the report, Yuto was aware of a dietary alternative to drug therapy. And approximately four months after his ulcerative colitis diagnosis, and many bloody stools later, Yuto entered an impatient treatment program specializing in the treatment of IBD using a plant-based, semi-vegetarian diet.

The program's director and associates write: *"We recognize IBD as a lifestyle-related disease mediated mainly by a westernized diet."* (Chiba et al., 2016) To give us further insight into the rationale for the plant-based, semi-vegetarian diet, the authors continue:

> The greatest environmental factor for IBD is diet-associated microflora. Diets rich in animal protein and animal fat cause a decrease in beneficial bacteria in the intestine. Prebiotics, foods

that increase beneficial bacteria in the gut, are mostly extracts of plants. Therefore, a semi-vegetarian diet was designed to combat dietary westernization. (Chiba et al., 2016)

With respect to the diet, basically

Our semi-vegetarian diet is a lacto-ovo-vegetarian diet [allowing dairy products and eggs] with an additional serving of fish once a week and meat once every 2 weeks. This semi-vegetarian diet is primarily a plant-based diet. Contemporary meals are far from a semi-vegetarian diet. Dietary intervention to restore dysbiosis in gut microflora is essential in the treatment of IBD. (Chiba et al., 2016)

Now back to Yuto. At some point in time during his 11-day inpatient program, Yuto's ulcerative colitis went into remission, doing so with diet alone. ***Diet alone!*** Bloody stools were no more. His remission lasted 11 months, until faint blood was noticed in his stool, occurring every other day. This suggested that his ulcerative colitis had returned, and prompted both a confession and a promise. Yuto confessed *"He had been too busy to maintain a plant-based diet but would try to restore his diet to a sound plant-based diet."*

You can read Yuto's story in its entirety by going online and locating the following paper:

Chiba M, Tsuda S, Komatsu M, Tozawa H, Takayama Y. **Onset of ulcerative colitis during a low-carbohydrate weight-loss diet and treatment with a plant-based diet: a case report.** The Permanente Journal. 2016;20(1):80.

What can we learn from this case report? Three things clearly stand out: **1)** The Western diet, with all the heme, all the iron, all the sulfur, all the saturated fat, and all the flavor would appear to be a trigger for ulcerative colitis and a driver for its persistence, consistent with the conclusions of the experts. **2)** A diet of abundant prebiotics, as per high dietary intake of fruits and vegetables, and very low in animal protein and fat, can be an effective treatment for ulcerative colitis. And **3)** drugs are not always necessary in the treatment of this disease. Certainly, this case report is a window into the possibilities of treating ulcerative colitis with a dietary practice that counters the evils of the Western diet—and doing so by restricting exposure to both saturated fat and animal protein.

Now as far as an individual obtaining enough protein on a semi-vegetarian, plant-based diet, don't worry at all. If you do things right, you can get all the protein you need from plant sources, and with the inclusion of milk products and eggs, there *is* no problem (see Physicians Committee for Responsible Medicine, date not specified).

Omega-6 excess revisited

> *Epidemiologic studies have shown an increased prevalence of IBD that correlates with increased animal fat and n-6 PUFA intake.* ~**Wiese et al., 2016**

> *Dietary n-6 PUFA, in particular linoleic acid, have been implicated in the etiology of IBD. Dietary n-6 PUFAs are essential fatty acids present in high amounts in red meat, cooking oils (safflower and corn oil) and margarines.* ~**Haskey and Gibson, 2017**

Need I remind you of the dangers of omega-6 PUFA excess? You're kinda forgetful, so I guess I do. I'll be brief.

So, here's the deal: Excess consumption of the omega-6 PUFAs favors the development and persistence of ulcerative colitis. This excess can be countered with decreased consumption of the omega-6s, but also by an increased consumption of the omega-3s (Varnalidis et al., 2011; Ghosh et al., 2013). Studies have shown that, in similarity with saturated fat, the omega-6s are proinflammatory, whereas the omega-3s are anti-inflammatory, even to the point of inhibiting NF-κB (Wiese et al., 2016). Remember NF-κB? NF-κB is *"a transcription factor which regulates the expression of many genes involved in inflammatory responses"*

(Oldenburg et al., 2001), and *"appears to be a central factor in virtually all inflammatory modulatory genes."* (Neish, 2002)

Recalling our little discussion on saturated fat and TLR4, TLR4 is a sensor for bacteria that can be inappropriately stimulated by saturated fat. Surprisingly, the *"n-3 PUFAs can __inhibit__ TLR4 signaling and the subsequent gene transcription of pro-inflammatory mediators . . .."* (Statovci et al., 2017, emphasis added) *This* could come in handy! *This* could calm things down! On the other hand, omega-6 excess, in concert with the omega-3 deficiency propagated by the Western diet, appears to be standing directly in the way. To place things into perspective,

> *. . . excessive consumption of omega-6 PUFA increases ulcerative colitis by **30%**; whereas consumption of docosahexaenoic acid, an omega-3 fatty acid, reduced the disease burden by **77%**.* (Brown et al., 2012, emphasis added)

Sulfate excess

> *A high sulphur diet, either from sulphur amino acids [high in red meat] or sulphated additives, results in the generation of hydrogen sulphide and mucosal damage in the colon.*
>
> *Red meat, for instance is stated as a food to be avoided on a low sulphur amino acid diet and processed foods contain large amounts of sulphate as a food additive.* **~Jowett et al., 2004**

Of course, excess consumption of red meat and the practice of preserving foods with sulfur compounds, common practices in the Western/fast food diet, increase the risk of ulcerative colitis and promotes its persistence. To keep things brief, I refer you to the previous chapter should you feel the need to review.

Dietary fiber deficiency

The Western diet practice is notoriously low in dietary fiber, reported to be **50%** lower than a diet should be (see Bengmark, 2010; Slavin, 2013). Since I devoted an entire chapter to dietary fiber, I will only take the time here to point out the following:

> *Incidentally, a recent study emphasized the importance of dietary fibers in maintaining the mucus layer by showing that **fiber-deprived microbiota use the colonic mucus layer as an alternative fuel source.*** (de Groot et al., 2017, emphasis added)

What should be appreciated here is this: **The Western/fast food diet is a mucus layer-depletion diet.** (God help us and spare us from disease!) It is far better for you that your gut bacteria eat dietary fiber rather than, in their desperation, eat (degrade) your mucus layer of defense. *This* is reason enough to forsake the Western/fast food diet and adopt a diet that is plant-based and mucus layer friendly.

Refined sugar

> *Westernized diet is characterized by a high content of proteins (derived from fatty domesticated and processed meats), saturated fats, refined grains, **sugar**, alcohol, salt and **corn-derived fructose syrup**, with an associated reduced consumption of fruits and vegetables.* **~Statovci et al., 2017**

> *. . . increased consumption of sugar and soft drinks with low vegetable intake was positively associated with UC risk.* **~Haskey and Gibson, 2017**

Excessive refined sugar consumption has been identified by many investigators as a risk factor for ulcerative colitis. However, not everyone has found such an association. Indeed, Middle Eastern populations consume far more than their fair share of refined sugar, yet their incidence of IBD is lower than in Western populations (Hou, 2010). So, here is your opening! Go ahead and eat all those surgery foods you have fallen deeply in love with.

Well, maybe not. So many of our sugary foods contain various additives known to cause harm. So, caution is advised. Perhaps it is the carrageenan, the mono- and diglycerides, the maltodextrin, the microparticles, and other food additives typically added to our sweets that cause the most harm, rather than their sugar content, in and of itself. Furthermore, creating foods containing both sugar and saturated fat, a common practice in Western populations, may make for a particularly harmful combination.

So, when it comes to sugar and ulcerative colitis, the jury may still be out. But there seems to be enough evidence after all to help us make a few important decisions.

> . . . total sugar intake, also elevated in Western diets, appeared to have no effect in IBD risk in a prospective cohort. However, a more recent prospective analysis of dietary patterns demonstrated that a diet marked by high sugar and soft drink consumption **plus low vegetable intake** was associated with increased UC risk for patients more than 2 years after dietary assessment was completed. (Dolan and Chang, 2017, emphasis added)

I suppose, when you are eating the sugary foods—and that would include foods sweetened with corn-derived fructose (otherwise known as high-fructose corn syrup or HFCS)—you are not eating your vegetables, at least not at the levels to keep you out of trouble. I get it! Sweets are a lot more fun to eat than Brussel sprouts. Yet, in this indirect way—by replacing the fruits and vegetables we should be eating—the sugary foods we find in the Western diet undoubtedly become a risk factor for ulcerative colitis. And, like so many other risk factors, sugary foods are likely not to be particularly helpful to those who are in the heat of the battle against the disease.

Food additives

Food additives are common in the Western diet, and animal and ex-vivo studies have suggested a detrimental effect of certain food additives, including polysorbate-80, carboxymethylcellulose, maltodextrin, carrageenan, and microparticles.

Moreover, artificial sweeteners and dietary emulsifiers adversely affect the gut microbiota and promote inflammatory responses. **~Yang et al., 2016**

Since I have mentioned emulsifyers, microparticles, and artificial sweeteners previously, and at great length, I will only mention them in passing. Emulsifyers, microparticles, and artificial sweeteners are harmful. Try to avoid. Danger danger! And there you have it! Now we can move on.

Next, I will introduce something new to the conversation. We can consider the potential impact **dietary aluminum** plays in the initiation and progression of ulcerative colitis. I'll begin with this:

Dietary exposure to aluminum (a cofactor for immune stimulation required in many vaccines) from food grown in aluminum-rich soil at industrial sites, or in the form of leavening products or additives in processed cake mixes, cheeses, cream powders or frozen dough, preservatives, food coloring, from cookware, or in cola drinks can potentially increase inflammation, at the very least in animal models of IBD. (Mutlu and Gor, 2008)

Surprisingly, there does not appear to be a lot of information on dietary aluminum and the risk and progression of ulcerative colitis, as this topic has barely been explored (de Chambrun et al., 2014). In view of the above quotation, perhaps greater efforts should be made to investigate aluminum and its effects on ulcerative colitis, both its pathogenesis and its persistence. As for me, I sense danger. That's what I do. (But I do so for good reason.)

We obtain a lot of information on disease risk and progression from animal models of IBD. According to a recent study of mice with colitis, aluminum <u>given in doses similar to what ordinarily occurs to humans in our society</u>, disease activity was enhanced and the healing progress impaired (de Chambrun et al., 2014). Sounds like a problem to me! Sounds like danger to me. Sounds like the effect of aluminum on disease activity in ulcerative colitis should be aggressively studied and not basically ignored.

Humans ordinarily consume some aluminum in food and water each day, but the Western diet makes sure we get a lot of it. It is **"estimated that Americans ingest >95 mg aluminum per day."** (de Chambrun et al., 2014, emphasis added) And wouldn't you know, in Western societies, aluminum is a frequently encountered food additive.

> *A main route of exposure to aluminum for the general population is through food and water. The decline in the use of unprocessed foods and the increased consumption of **cakes, pastries, and sugar-rich foods characterizing 'food westernization'** has resulted in an increased ingestion of aluminum, which exceeds the tolerable weekly intake of **7 mg kg^{-1} per week** in a significant proportion of the European and North American populations. For many years, exposure to aluminum was suggested to favor an abnormal immune response in different diseases, including autoimmune conditions. However, despite this known toxicity and a potential gut interaction, aluminum and its effect on intestinal homeostasis and inflammation have not been investigated so far, particularly in the physiopathology of IBD. (de Chambrun et al., 2014, emphasis added)*

Listen a little more to what these investigators have to say. (You have nothing better to do.)

In humans, the principal route of entry of aluminum is the ingestion of food or water containing aluminum. Oral bioavailability of aluminum is estimated to be <1%. Aluminum accumulates in the skeletal system and the brain, and a link with diseases such as osteomalacia and encephalopathy, Alzheimer and Parkinson's diseases have been reported. The low percentage of oral bioavailability of aluminum is actually misleading. In fact, **after oral administration, 40% of the ingested dose <u>accumulates within the intestinal mucosa, which makes the gut the main storage organ for aluminum in the body</u>.** (de Chambrun et al., 2014)

My belief: It's time, past time, to pay attention to the role of aluminum in the initiation and progression of ulcerative colitis. And the danger is ever present.

Indeed, it was estimated by a US food additives survey that most Americans ingest from 0.01 to 1.4 mg total aluminum per kg body weight per day. In the same study, is was estimated that ~5% of Americans ingested **>95 mg aluminum per day** *. . . as additives in commercially processed foods and beverages.* (de Chambrun et al., 2014)

No one can say I didn't warn you of the danger. And in a moment, no one can say I didn't warn you of frozen pizza. *"Cheese in a serving of* **frozen pizzas had up to 14mg of Al** *[aluminum], from basic sodium aluminum phosphate; whereas, the same amount of cheese in a ready-to-eat restaurant pizza provided 0.02–0.09 mg."* (Saiyed and Yokel, 2005, emphasis added)

And when all is said and done, no one can say I didn't warn you of pancakes and waffles. *". . .* **pancake/waffle mixes and frozen products,** *and* **ready-to-eat pancakes** *provided the most Al of the foods tested;* **up to 180 mg/serving.**" (Saiyed and Yokel, 2005, emphasis added)

It seems likely, the ingestion of dietary aluminum, <u>intentionally added to our foods</u>, is out to harm you and out to harm me—but you the most, for you have a disease negatively impacted by the things they do to food.

And of course, there is iron

> *The Western diet is characteristically rich in sources of iron, especially red meat, and UC has historically been more prevalent in Western countries.*
>
> *The <u>potentially deleterious effects of a high-iron diet on UC are attributed to the</u> **accumulation of iron in the colonic lumen in high concentrations**, a direct result of the tight regulation of body iron levels and the restriction of dietary iron absorption.* ~**Seril et al., 2006, emphasis added**

The above should be warning enough of the danger of red meat, a food so generously provided by the Western diet. Apart from red meat consumption, however, there are other warnings that should be issued, also related to excessive dietary iron exposure.

> *. . . high dietary iron intake, <u>independent of red meat consumption,</u> was specifically associated with an **increased risk of cancer** of the proximal colon.*
>
> *Unabsorbed dietary iron enters the colon and in conjunction with intraluminal bacteria may . . . generate hydrogen peroxide and hydroxyl radicals at the mucosal surface. **Hydrogen peroxide or iron may also enter colonocytes and increase the risk of <u>DNA damage</u>** in a manner similar to that described for immune cells, thus increasing the risk of a mutation, either as an initiating event or later in the adenoma-carcinoma sequence.* ~**Lund et al., 1999, emphasis added**

Now can you see why I make such a fuss over iron? Dietary iron, when consumed in excess from any source, can lead to not only the initiation and perpetuation of ulcerative colitis, but also can lead to colorectal cancer. Excess iron consumption should be a target in the battle against ulcerative colitis. There is no other conclusion that can be reached.

What about dairy? What about eggs?

> . . . high intake, specifically animal protein (meat, **not dairy** products) was positively associated with an increased risk of IBD.

> Overall, the consumption of dairy products is <u>not</u> a risk factor for IBD. ~**Haskey and Gibson, 2017, emphasis added**

> High total protein intake, specifically animal protein, was associated with risk of IBD. Regarding sources of animal protein, high consumption of meat and fish but **not of eggs or dairy products** was associated with IBD risk. ~**Andersen et al., 2012, emphasis added**

Many ulcerative colitis patients feel the need to avoid dairy. Reportedly, **1 in 5** ulcerative colitis patients benefit from the removal of milk and cheese from their diet (Richman and Rhodes, 2013). However, there is so much good in dairy, I hope you don't need to avoid it.

A few observations to share regarding this issue before we move on: **First**, and obviously, avoid dairy if it does not agree with you. **Second**, you can sort this all out with an elimination diet, a diet that restricts, then reintroduces a suspect food to determine reactivity. **Third**, it may be advisable to at least limit dairy as a measure to limit your intake of saturated fat. Non-fat milk solves this problem. **Finally**, it may be that a single element may be the offender. For example, you may be lactose intolerant, and simply by drinking lactose-free milk, you can avoid GI upset and take advantage of all the good milk has to offer. It seems that at least some authorities would like you to drink milk if it can be tolerated.

> Because of their calcium content, dairy products are especially recommended for these patients [IBD patients] and milk should only be restricted in the case lactose intolerance, substituted by other

fermented products (yoghurts and cheese) or calcium-enriched soya-based products. (Lucendo and De Rezende, 2009)

Now with respect to eggs, I see little evidence in the research literature that eggs should be restricted in the diet of the typical ulcerative colitis patient. And apparently, egg consumption does not stand out as an ulcerative colitis risk factor (Andersen et al. 2012). However, because of its high sulfur content (Jowett et al., 2004), perhaps eggs should be limited when following a dietary strategy that seeks to restrict sulfur. On the other hand, you do need adequate sulfur in your diet, so egg consumption may help meet this need, particularly if you plan to restrict dietary sulfur by eliminating a wide range of sulfur-rich foods.

Processed and highly refined foods

Heavily processed foods are a staple of the urban Western world where IBD runs rampant. Limiting such foods may decrease exposure to complex antigens [immune system stimulating molecules], expected to numerous ingredients and nutritionally empty additives and preservatives. ~Mutlu and Gor, 2008

*The consensus of previous studies on diet and UC pointed to the modern, processed, **highly refined**, Western diets as being damaging.* ~Magee et al., 2005, emphasis added

When you refine a food component and go on to manufacture a food item using this refined component, you wind up creating a food that lacks many nutritional components necessary to support health and resistance to disease. That's how things work. So, in our great wisdom, we add artificial vitamins and we add minerals back in to replace the ones we just removed. We call ourselves *"Modern."* But we don't stop there. We go the extra mile. So, in our great wisdom, we add iron to our creation—and in obscene amounts—totally unaware (or not) that some people will be harmed. Crazy world, I know. But there is more to the story. Not every nutrient removed during processing is returned.

For example, soluble fibers are likely not returned, and therefore do not end up into someone's colon to be transformed into butyrate and other compounds necessary for colon health and protection against disease. We've covered the importance of soluble fibers before, so I won't need to repeat myself here. But I will mention this:

When we follow a diet of Western, processed foods, we are limiting our consumption of other valuable nutrients besides vitamins, minerals, and fiber. One class of nutrients, removed and seldom returned, are called polyphenols, but that's a story for another time.

What should be appreciated here is this: **The Western/fast food diet is a diet of missing things, valuable things, things that should be added back into your life.**

There is nothing you can eat . . . *Nothing!*

There, I've gone and done it! I've taken every food imaginable off the table, leaving you with basically nothing to eat. But I'm not the only one that appears to want you to starve to death. (Of course, I'm joking. Or am I?) Others believe there are dangers in the food we eat and want you, the IBD patient, to limit or avoid a wide variety of foods. For example, **The American Dietetic Association** offers the IBD patient the following recommendations (restrictions):

- **Dairy:** Avoid whole milk, half-and half, cream and sour cream, yogurt with berries, orange or lemon rind, or nuts, and ice cream with the exception of low-fat or nonfat ice cream

- **Meat and protein foods:** Avoid fried meats, sausage, bacon, luncheon meats like bologna and salami, hot dogs, tough or chewy cuts of meat, fried eggs, dried beans, peas, and nuts including chunky peanut butter

- **Grains and breads:** Avoid whole-grain breads, rolls, crackers or pasta, brown and wild rice, whole grain cereals, and foods made with seeds or nuts

- **Vegetables:** <u>Avoid</u> beets, broccoli, Brussels sprouts, cabbage, sauerkraut, cauliflower, corn, greens leafy vegetables, lima beans, mushrooms, okra, onions, parsnips, peppers, potato skins and winter squash

- **Fruits:** <u>Avoid</u> raw fruits with the exception of peeled apples, ripe bananas and melon, canned berries and cherries, dried fruits including raisins, and prune juice

- **Fats and oils:** <u>Avoid</u> fat and oil intakes greater than eight teaspoons/day

- **Beverages:** <u>Avoid</u> caffeine containing beverages including coffee, tea, cola and some sport drinks, alcoholic. Sweet fruit juices, soft drinks, or other beverages made with sugar or corn syrup should be avoided if they make diarrhea worse

- **Sugar alcohols:** <u>Avoid</u> sorbitol, mannitol and xylitol, as they can cause diarrhea, and can be found in sugarless gums and candies, and some medications

(Reference: Brown et al., 2011)

It should be noted that some of the above recommendations apply more to Crohn's disease with strictures, and not to the average ulcerative colitis patient. Nevertheless, there is a lot that may apply.

Recognizing junk food

Junk food is a hallmark of the Western, manufactured and fast food diet. The following quotation will be helpful, serving as a "rule of thumb" when it comes to choosing healthier foods. And I quote,

Junk food, like many other things, can often be known only when you see it. One can spot what might be junk food by looking at a food label, including that it has little nutritional value and has:

- *35% of calories from fat (except for low-fat milk), > 10% of calories from saturated fats, Any trans fat.*

- *>35% of calories from sugar, unless it is made with 100% fruit and no added sugar.*

- *> 200 calories per servings for snacks.*

- *> 200 mg per serving for sodium (salt) for snacks.*

- *> 480 mg per serving for sodium (salt) for initial meal.*

Also the ingredients list of the food can be checked to spot many forms of junk food. ***In general, if one of the first two ingredients is either oil or a form of sugar, then it is likely a junk food. The presence of <u>high fructose corn syrup</u> in the ingredients is also often a tip-off to a food being a junk food.*** (Ashakiran and Deepthi, 2012, emphasis added)

I can give you another tip: If it is a manufactured food item, wrapped in a pretty package, be wary. Read the fine print. You will typically find a food loaded with one or several artificial ingredients and additives that can harm. Recognizing a junk food means noticing the emulsifyers, microparticles, the iron, the sodium content, even the aluminum added to what may otherwise be a reasonably good food choice.

~References~

Agans R, Gordon A, Kramer DL, Perez-Burillo S, Rufián-Henares JA, Paliy O. **Dietary fatty acids sustain the growth of the human gut microbiota.** Appl. Environ. Microbiol.. 2018 Nov 1;84(21):e01525-18.

AHA, 2018 **How much sodium should I eat per day?** https://www.heart.org/en/healthy-living/healthy-eating/eat-smart/sodium/how-much-sodium-should-i-eat-per-da

Andersen V, Olsen A, Carbonnel F, Tjønneland A, Vogel U. **Diet and risk of inflammatory bowel disease.** Digestive and liver disease. 2012 Mar 1;44(3):185-94.

Ashakiran, Deepthi R. **Fast foods and their impact on health.** Journal of Krishna Institute of Medical Sciences University. 2012 Jul 1;1(2):7-15.

Barkas F, Liberopoulos E, Kei A, Elisaf M. **Electrolyte and acid-base disorders in inflammatory bowel disease.** Annals of Gastroenterology: Quarterly Publication of the Hellenic Society of Gastroenterology. 2013;26(1):23.

Bengmark S. **Pre-, Pro-, Synbiotics and Human Health.** FOOD TECHNOL BIOTECH. 2010;48(4):464-75.

Brown AC, Rampertab SD, Mullin GE. **Existing dietary guidelines for Crohn's disease and ulcerative colitis.** Expert review of gastroenterology & hepatology. 2011 Jun 1;5(3):411-25.

Brown K, DeCoffe D, Molcan E, Gibson DL. **Diet-induced dysbiosis of the intestinal microbiota and the effects on immunity and disease.** Nutrients. 2012 Aug;4(8):1095-119.

Carrera-Bastos P, Fontes-Villalba M, O'K'efe JH, Lindeberg S, Cordain L. **The western diet and lifestyle and diseases of civilization.** Research Reports in Clinical Cardiology. 2011 Mar 9;2:15-35.

CDC: **World Salt Awareness Week.** Page last updated: Mar 2016 https://www.cdc.gov/features/sodium/index.html

CDC: **Salt.** Page last updated: Jun11, 2018 https://www.cdc.gov/salt/index.htm

Chiba M, Tsuda S, Komatsu M, Tozawa H, Takayama Y. **Onset of ulcerative colitis during a low-carbohydrate weight-loss diet and treatment with a plant-based diet: a case report.** The Permanente Journal. 2016;20(1):80.

Cordain L, Eaton SB, Sebastian A, Mann N, Lindeberg S, Watkins BA, O'Keefe JH, Brand-Miller J. **Origins and evolution of the Western diet: health implications for the 21st century.** The American journal of clinical nutrition. 2005 Feb 1;81(2):341-54.

de Chambrun GP, Body-Malapel M, Frey-Wagner I, Djouina M, Deknuydt F, Atrott K, Esquerre N, Altare F, Neut C, Arrieta MC, Kanneganti TD. **Aluminum enhances inflammation and decreases mucosal healing in experimental colitis in mice.** Mucosal immunology. 2014 May;7(3):589.

de Groot PF, Frissen MN, de Clercq NC, Nieuwdorp M. **Fecal microbiota transplantation in metabolic syndrome: history, present and future.** Gut Microbes. 2017 May 4;8(3):253-67.

Dolan KT, Chang EB. **Diet, gut microbes, and the pathogenesis of inflammatory bowel diseases.** Molecular nutrition & food research. 2017 Jan;61(1):1600129.

Erridge C, Samani NJ. **Saturated fatty acids do not directly stimulate Toll-like receptor signaling.** Arteriosclerosis, thrombosis, and vascular biology. 2009 Nov 1;29(11):1944-9.

Fukata M, Chen A, Vamadevan AS, Cohen J, Breglio K, Krishnareddy S, Hsu D, Xu R, Harpaz N, Dannenberg AJ, Subbaramaiah K. **Toll-like receptor-4 promotes the development of colitis-associated colorectal tumors.** Gastroenterology. 2007 Dec 1;133(6):1869-.

Gasche C, Berstad A, Befrits R, Beglinger C, Dignass A, Erichsen K, Gomollon F, Hjortswang H, Koutroubakis I, Kulnigg S, Oldenburg B. **Guidelines on the diagnosis and management of iron deficiency and anemia in inflammatory bowel diseases#.** Inflammatory bowel diseases. 2007 Nov 1;13(12):1545-53.

Ghosh S, DeCoffe D, Brown K, Rajendiran E, Estaki M, Dai C, Yip A, Gibson DL. **Fish oil attenuates omega-6 polyunsaturated fatty acid-induced dysbiosis and infectious colitis but impairs LPS dephosphorylation activity causing sepsis.** PloS one. 2013 Feb 6;8(2):e55468.

Goyal S, Rampal R, Kedia S, Mahajan S, Bopanna S, Yadav DP, Jain S, Singh AK, Wari MN, Makharia G, Awasthi A. **Urinary potassium is a potential biomarker** of disease activity in Ulcerative colitis and displays in vitro immunotolerant role. Scientific reports. 2017 Dec 22;7(1):18068.

Gulhane M, Murray L, Lourie R, Tong H, Sheng YH, Wang R, Kang A, Schreiber V, Wong KY, Magor G, Denman S. **High fat diets induce colonic epithelial cell stress and inflammation that is reversed by IL-22.** Scientific reports. 2016 Jun 28;6:28990.

Haskey N, Gibson DL. **An examination of diet for the maintenance of remission in inflammatory bowel disease.** Nutrients. 2017 Mar 10;9(3):259.

Hou JK. **Diet, nutrition and inflammatory bowel disease.** Clinical Practice. 2010 Mar 1;7(2):179.

Jowett SL, Seal CJ, Pearce MS, Phillips E, Gregory W, Barton JR, Welfare MR. **Influence of dietary factors on the clinical course of ulcerative colitis: a prospective cohort study.** Gut. 2004 Oct 1;53(10):1479-84.

Khalili H, Malik S, Ananthakrishnan AN, Garber JJ, Higuchi LM, Joshi A, Peloquin J, Richter JM, Stewart KO, Curhan GC, Awasthi A. **Identification and characterization of a novel association between dietary potassium and risk of Crohn's disease and ulcerative colitis.** Frontiers in immunology. 2016 Dec 7;7:554.

Knight-Sepulveda K, Kais S, Santaolalla R, Abreu MT. **Diet and inflammatory bowel disease.** Gastroenterology & hepatology. 2015 Aug;11(8):511.

Lucendo AJ, De Rezende LC. **Importance of nutrition in inflammatory bowel disease.** World journal of gastroenterology: WJG. 2009 May 7;15(17):2081.

Lund EK, Wharf SG, Fairweather-Tait SJ, Johnson IT. **Oral ferrous sulfate supplements increase the free radical–generating capacity of feces from healthy volunteers.** The American journal of clinical nutrition. 1999 Feb 1;69(2):250-5.

Magee EA, Edmond LM, Tasker SM, Kong SC, Curno R, Cummings JH. **Associations between diet and disease activity in ulcerative colitis patients using a novel method of data analysis.** Nutrition Journal. 2005 Dec;4(1):7.

Manzel A, Muller DN, Hafler DA, Erdman SE, Linker RA, Kleinewietfeld M. **Role of "Western diet" in inflammatory autoimmune diseases.** Current allergy and asthma reports. 2014 Jan 1;14(1):404.

Marion-Letellier R, Savoye G, Ghosh S. **IBD: in food we trust.** Journal of Crohn's'and Colitis. 2016 May 17;10(11):1351-61.

Mutlu EA, Gor N. **To diet or not if you have inflammatory bowel disease.** Expert review of gastroenterology & hepatology. 2008 Oct 1;2(5):613-6.

Myles IA. **Fast food fever: reviewing the impacts of the Western diet on immunity.** Nutrition journal. 2014 Dec;13(1):61.

Neish AS. **The gut microflora and intestinal epithelial cells: a continuing dialogue.** Microbes and Infection. 2002 Mar 1;4(3):309-17.

Oldenburg B, Koningsberger JC, Van Berge Henegouwen GP, Van Asbeck BS, Marx JJ. **Iron and inflammatory bowel disease. Alimentary pharmacology & therapeutics.** 2001 Apr;15(4):429-38.

Physicians Committee for Responsible Medicine. **Protein.** https://www.pcrm.org/good-nutrition/nutrition-information/protein

Piya MK, **Harte AL, McTernan PG. Metabolic endotoxaemia: is it more than just a gut feeling?.** Current opinion in lipidology. 2013 Feb 1;24(1):78-85.

Poutahidis T, Kleinewietfeld M, Smillie C, Levkovich T, Perrotta A, Bhela S, Varian BJ, Ibrahim YM, Lakritz JR, Kearney SM, Chatzigiagkos A. **Microbial reprogramming inhibits Western diet-associated obesity.** PloS one. 2013 Jul 10;8(7):e68596.

Richman E, Rhodes JM. **Review article: evidence-based dietary advice for patients with inflammatory bowel disease.** Alimentary pharmacology & therapeutics. 2013 Nov 1;38(10):1156-71.

Roediger WE 2008 **Nitric oxide from dysbiotic bacterial respiration of nitrate in the pathogenesis and as a target for therapy of ulcerative colitis.** Alimentary pharmacology & therapeutics. Apr 1; 27(7):531-541.

Russell WR, Gratz SW, Duncan SH, Holtrop G, Ince J, Scobbie L, Duncan G, Johnstone AM, Lobley GE, Wallace RJ, Duthie GG. **High-protein, reduced-carbohydrate weight-loss diets promote metabolite profiles likely to be detrimental to colonic health.** The American journal of clinical nutrition. 2011 Mar 9;93(5):1062-72.

Saiyed SM, Yokel RA. **Aluminium content of some foods and food products in the USA, with aluminium food additives.** Food additives and contaminants. 2005 Mar 1;22(3):234-44.

Seril DN, Liao J, West AB, Yang G-Y 2006 **High-Iron Diet: Foe of Feat in Ulcerative Colitis and Ulcerative Colitis-Associated Carcinogenesis.** J Clin Gastroenterol; May/June; 40(5):391–397.

Slavin J. **Fiber and prebiotics: mechanisms and health benefits.** Nutrients. 2013 Apr 22;5(4):1417-35.

Statovci D, Aguilera M, MacSharry J, Melgar S. **The impact of Western diet and nutrients on the microbiota and immune response at mucosal interfaces.** Frontiers in immunology. 2017 Jul 28;8:838.

Sood A, Midha V, Makharia GK, Ahuja V, Singal D, Goswami P, Tandon RK. **The probiotic preparation, VSL# 3 induces remission in patients with mild-to-moderately active ulcerative colitis.** Clinical Gastroenterology and Hepatology. 2009 Nov 1;7(11):1202-9.

Varnalidis I, Ioannidis O, Karamanavi E, Ampas Z, Poutahidis T, Taitzoglou I, Paraskevas G, Botsios D. **Omega 3 fatty acids supplementation has an ameliorative effect in experimental ulcerative colitis despite increased colonic neutrophil infiltration.** Revista Espanola de Enfermedades Digestivas. 2011 Oct 1;103(10):511.

Vidal-Lletjós S, Beaumont M, Tomé D, Benamouzig R, Blachier F, Lan A. **Dietary Protein and Amino Acid Supplementation in Inflammatory Bowel Disease Course: What Impact on the Colonic Mucosa?.** Nutrients. 2017 Mar 21;9(3):310.

Wiese DM, Horst SN, Brown CT, Allaman MM, Hodges ME, Slaughter JC, Druce JP, Beaulieu DB, Schwartz DA, Wilson KT, Coburn LA. **Serum fatty acids are correlated with inflammatory cytokines in ulcerative colitis.** PloS one. 2016 May 26;11(5):e0156387.

Wilck N, Balogh A, Markó L, Bartolomaeus H, Müller DN. **The role of sodium in modulating immune cell function.** Nature Reviews Nephrology. 2019 Jun 25:1.

Windey K, De Preter V, Verbeke K. **Relevance of protein fermentation to gut health.** Molecular nutrition & food research. 2012 Jan 1;56(1):184-96.

Wu SL, Chen JC, Li CC, Lo HY, Ho TY, Hsiang CY. **Vanillin improves and prevents trinitrobenzene sulfonic acid-induced colitis in mice.** Journal of Pharmacology and Experimental Therapeutics. 2009 Aug 1;330(2):370-6.

Yang Y, Owyang C, Wu GD. **East Meets West: the increasing incidence of inflammatory bowel disease in Asia as a paradigm for environmental effects on the pathogenesis of immune-mediated disease.** Gastroenterology. 2016 Dec 1;151(6):e1-5.

Chapter 11

Why diets work

*Experimental studies indicate that **commonly used food ingredients can alter the intestinal barrier,** thereby causing intestinal inflammation.*

Dietary elements that negatively affect the intestinal epithelia may trigger <u>a pro-inflammatory state that precedes the development of IBD</u>.
~Ruemmele, 2016, emphasis added

*. . . treatment of inflammatory bowel disease is far from ideal in both its effectiveness and potential risks of complications. By comparison, **diet therapy has the potential to be safe, lifelong and relatively cheap.***
~Mutlu and Gor, 2008, emphasis added

I n the last chapter I laid out a case against the Western diet, perhaps a good case. This chapter ushers in the diet therapy portion of the book, where I make the case, perhaps a great case, for the use of diet in the battle against ulcerative colitis. And I mean *really* use diet, not play around with diet.

When I hear a report of someone who achieved remission in ulcerative colitis by faithfully following this diet or that diet, I have no problem believing, for I know the power of diet. **If the diet is other than the Western diet, it is likely to be a diet with features that favor remission in ulcerative colitis.** Of course, the better the design, the more effective a diet can be.

So, what should a diet for ulcerative colitis look like? Previous chapters provide us clues. Evidence is strong, a diet with the best opportunity for success in ulcerative colitis will likely have at least some of the following features:

- Low in red meat

- Low in protein

- Low in dietary iron, all sources

- Low in sulfur

- Low in saturated fat

- Low in omega-6 polyunsaturated fatty acids

- Low in food additives such as emulsifyers, microparticles, artificial sweeteners, and aluminum

- Low in sodium and sufficient in potassium

- High in prebiotics such as soluble fibers and/or resistant starch

- Low in . . . (to be announced)

So, what are we left with? I'll tell you what we're left with. **For a diet with the best opportunity for success in the battle against ulcerative colitis, we are left with a plant-based diet, low in processed and manufactured foods. It's that simple!** And in the design and execution of such a dietary plan, the following suggestions should probably be heeded:

We argue that, first of all, we need to fix the food. We need to provide a better and more updated answer to the question: What should we eat? The question appears to have a rather simple answer provided by our evolutionary history: **Eat mostly whole foods.** *This approach corresponds with findings from a wide range of nutritional studies where whole foods are consistently associated with good health.* (Zinöcker et al., 2018, emphasis added)

In addition, I recommend that patients eat fresh foods, meaning that they should go to the grocery store, <u>buy ingredients, and prepare their own food</u>, as opposed to buying food that is prepackaged and processed. (Lewis, 2016, emphasis added)

So, let's dive right in, knife and fork in hand, and see what diet can do for the individual with ulcerative colitis. **And it may be that a <u>diet pattern</u> has the most to offer, rather than the practice of avoiding a certain class of foods or making every effort to avoid foods containing this or that sinister additive or diabolical ingredient.** However, regardless of the diet pattern employed, it would probably be wise to limit or avoid the evils we have discussed in the previous two chapters. In the next chapter we'll start with the diet pattern I consider the best of the best. And it won't be the Western diet, that I can assure you.

But if you want to just show up and take a drug, that's ok, do what you want. But keep in mind, drug therapy alone may not succeed. This route ignores so many things that may give you an edge in the battle and direct you toward remission.

*As the medical professionals taking care of patients with UC [ulcerative colitis], we have to admit that our treatment concepts have not been very successful. Ongoing disease activity is present in ~ **50%** of all patients with UC, colectomy rates remain high, and impaired quality of life, sick leave and disability pensions are higher in patients with UC than in the general population.* (Ochsenkühn and D'Haens, 2011)

Do you want more of this thing we call ulcerative colitis? I doubt it. Perhaps it would be wise to take a good hard look at what diet has to offer. (Which is plenty.)

Let's go back two pages and briefly review the first six items on my bullet point list, then we'll return here and pick up where we left off.

If one were to adopt a plant-based diet, these six items in the list are largely taken out of the equation. Greatly restricting red meat—which provides <u>excess</u> protein, iron, sulfur, omega-6 FFA and saturated fat—solves so many problems right off the bat, problems associated with the initiation and progression of ulcerative colitis. Substantially reducing or eliminating red meat and adopting a plant-based diet—as a dietary approach to treat ulcerative colitis—is undoubtedly **Job One**, in as much as *". . . high intakes of meat and margarine correlate with increased UC incidence and high meat also correlates with increased likelihood of relapse."* (Richman and Rhodes, 2013, emphasis added) And I'll share with you a dirty little secret: **Meat is more than meat.**

Due to processing techniques, even <u>minimally</u> processing, meat products and other food items, like chopped vegetables, become "enriched" by bacteria and their body parts (Zinöcker et al., 2018). Nothing out of the ordinary here. This is business as usual, and <u>not related to food spoilage</u>—but occurs to a greater extent in processed foods compared to home food preparation and cooking (Zinöcker et al., 2018). *"But doesn't heat kill the bacteria in processed food, making it safe to eat?"* I'll give you that. But even then, in a food considered safe from a bacterial-contamination standpoint, the <u>body parts of the dead remain</u>, body parts like the aforementioned bacterial cell-wall component, **LPS (endotoxin)**. Surprisingly, **one single bacterium may be composed of approximately 1,000,000 molecules of endotoxin!** (see Mani et al., 2013) Of course, we have defenses against all this endotoxin. One defense, of course, is to limit the consumption of the foods high in endotoxin. Another defense is an intact, tight intestinal barrier

(Champion et al., 2013). But with intestinal hyperpermeability, we run into trouble.

So, there you are, sitting down to a meal that includes red or processed meat. Are you aware you are sitting down to a meal loaded with LPS, a highly proinflammatory molecule? Apparently not. You have not put down your knife and fork. And I see no frightened look is on your face. On the other hand, if you were sitting down to a meal of *"fresh, unprocessed meats, fruits or vegetables,"* LPS consumption would not be occurring to any relevant degree (Herieka et al., 2016). More bad news. Cheese, ice cream, and chocolate may contain significant amounts of these immune stimulating, body parts of the dead (Zinöcker et al., 2018). Even processed vegetables can harbor significant amounts of LPS (Erridge, 2011). **Bottom line: The Western diet of processed foods, is a diet of excessive LPS exposure.** Perhaps we should call the Western diet **The Endotoxemia Diet**. And just like the Western diet as a whole, endotoxemia is not benign, the consequences can be serious.

Excessive exposure to LPS, leading to endotoxemia, is one of the reasons why we have obesity, fatty liver disease, diabetes type 2, Alzheimer's disease, and autoimmune diseases such as rheumatoid arthritis (Ahola et al., 2017; Lyte et al., 2016; Lorenz et al., 2013). And for you, the ulcerative colitis patient, endotoxemia is likely to be a way of life, likely to be part of the package, likely to be part of the disease process you find so disagreeable (Champion et al., 2013; Fukui, 2016; Rojo et al., 2006). Indeed, *"LPS plays an important role in the inflammatory process of inflammatory bowel disease (IBD)."* (Zhou et al., 2018, emphasis added) Furthermore,

> *Elevated intestinal permeability has been directly demonstrated in both CD and UC, with both significantly higher than controls and CD higher than UC. This leakiness leads to issues such as diarrhea as well as significant increases in bacterial antigen exposure in the bloodstream. It has been reported that **circulating endotoxin is***

elevated in IBD patients and correlates with disease severity.
(Champion et al., 2013, emphasis added)

Why compound the problem with additional, guaranteed, Western diet-strength LPS exposure? The Western diet makes it all so easy.

In a study using eight healthy subjects, placed on the **Western diet** for one month, demonstrated a *"**71% increase** in plasma levels of endotoxin activity (endotoxemia)"* and, after one month off the Western diet, the same subjects were placed on *"a prudent-style diet"* for one month, whereupon they subsequently demonstrated a ***31% reduction*** in endotoxin activity compared to their baseline status (Pendyala et al., 2012). **Wow! What a lesson!** Furthermore, in healthy subjects, a single, small intravenous dose of LPS promptly increased intestinal permeability (O'Dwyer et al., 1988), underscoring both the relevancy of this issue to the conversation and the negative influence endotoxemia has on intestinal permeability. *". . . as recent studies have demonstrated, an **endotoxin challenge** is able to promote neutrophil recruitment from circulation into the gut mucosa, **causing increased intestinal permeability**."* (Rojo et al., 2006, emphasis added)

What should be appreciated here in our discussion of diet vs. ulcerative colitis is this: **Just by limiting one item, processed meat, one can limit exposure to the evils inherent in meat, including exposure to the proinflammatory body parts of the dead that come along for the ride.** And if the meat you are eating has been minced (think hamburger), the increased surface area created by this process allows bacteria a greater opportunity to thrive on a temporary basis, and create more LPS in the process (Erridge, 2011). Heat kills the bacteria, kills them dead, but does not destroy the LPS left behind (Erridge, 2011). Food for thought.

Endotoxemia is not just a story about meat and processed, LPS-laden foods, it is also about high-fat dieting.

Chronic high-fat diets can affect the composition of gut microbiota, increase the incorporation of LPS into chylomicrons [fat containing transfer formations] and compromise gut mucosal integrity, which can result in the entry of pathogenic agents from, the intestinal lumen into the blood stream.

. . . excessive fat intake is considered to be one of the triggering factors that increase LPS in the circulatory system. (Moreira et al., 2012)

I've shared this with you before: "*Consuming a Western diet, high in fat (**particularly saturated fat**), is enough to induce endotoxemia in healthy subjects.*" (Knight-Sepulveda et al., 2015, emphasis added) Indeed, "***a person eating three high-SFA [saturated fatty acid] meals each day may encounter endotoxin levels that <u>remain perpetually high</u>, since refeeding may increase the levels.***" (Harte et al., 2012, emphasis added) Furthermore, "***The higher the fat content of a diet was, the higher the increase in plasma LPS levels.***" (Moreira et al., 2012, emphasis added) There are consequences. LPS is a potent stimulator of inflammation, "*highly pro-inflammatory*" (Ghoshal et al., 2009). A plant-based diet helps take the LPS pressure off an inflammatory process that is, for this and for other reasons, so out of control.

And while the warning goes out against saturated fat in particular, it does not go out against all fat. There are "healthy" fats that seem to protect against LPS translocation. The monosaturated fatty acids (think olive oil and avocado) and the omega-3 fatty acids (think oils from the fat of fatty fish) serve as examples. (see Kaliannan et al., 2015; Lyte et al., 2016; Ahola et al., 2017) On the other hand, similar to saturated fat, excess omega-6 fatty acid consumption promotes endotoxemia (Kaliannan et al., 2015). So, consider yourself forewarned.

Just a little more on endotoxemia, then we will attend to some unfinished business.

Not only does the ulcerative colitis patient <u>likely</u> have a problem with endotoxemia, his or her first-degree relatives can also demonstrate increased levels of endotoxin, indicating a genetic predisposition to improperly handling LPS (Amati et al., 2003). Endotoxin (LPS) is known to trigger pro-inflammatory signaling cascades involving TNF-α, and as such may play a pathogenic role in the development of ulcerative colitis (Amati et al., 2003), as endotoxemia can lead to increased intestinal permeability (Moreira et al., 2012). It is probably unknown to what degree ongoing endotoxemia impacts the ulcerative colitis patient, but what the research has revealed should justify placing endotoxemia on the list of unhelpful things.

Now on to our unfinished business. Recall, I did not complete the bullet point list on the second page of this chapter. I will do it now.

A diet with the best opportunity for success in ulcerative colitis will likely be

- **Low in fat . . . period**

You have read this before: *"Epidemiological and clinical studies reveal that **higher-fat diets are associated with a 2.5-fold increased risk of colitis in young adults**."* (Gulhane et al., 2016, emphasis added) And perhaps one reason for this is:

> *Excessive fat intake may favor an increase in circulatory LPS, leading to metabolic endotoxemia. Therefore, **<u>excessive</u> fat intake is considered to be one of the triggering factors that increase LPS in the circulatory system**.* (Moreira et al., 2012, emphasis added)

And now you know one of the reasons why a diet high in fat, particularly saturated fat, is harmful. A diet high in fat allows endotoxin to slip past the front lines and enter the blood stream. A diet high in saturated and polyunsaturated fats promotes endotoxemia. And there are other reasons for limiting fat intake in a diet that favors remission in ulcerative colitis.

*It is well-known that HFD [high fat diet] leads **to increased intestinal permeability** by several mechanisms, including changes in the expression of tight junction proteins . . ..*

*Our study shows HFD prologues and **aggravates the inflammatory manifestations of chronic ulcerative colitis**, thereby increasing the pro-inflammatory status of adipose [fat] tissue.* (Teixeira et al., 2011, emphasis added)

*Our data shows that a long term HFD leads to an **increase in colonic inflammation particularly in the distal colon**.* (Gulhane et al., 2016, emphasis added)

Take heed. Strongly consider a diet that reduces your exposure to LPS. Strongly consider a diet that limits the fats that are known to be harmful when consumed in excess. If a low-fat diet is in your future, consider making it a low-fat, plant-based diet to improve your chances of success.

With this chapter, I hope I have done a good, perhaps excellent job of setting the stage for the next chapter, in which we will discuss what I believe is the best of the best when it comes to a dietary approach to ulcerative colitis. It is the diet Yoto followed. It is the diet that allowed him to promptly go into remission—a testament to its power and its potential in the battle against ulcerative colitis. It tastes pretty good, too.

Remember SBI?

Recall our discussion on SBI in *Chapter 6*, here I give you another reason to request this form of treatment. The immunoglobins in SBI bind endotoxin (LPS), preventing their translocation through the intestinal mucosa (Van Arsdall et al., 2016). Take a few minutes to review *Chapter 6*, take a deep breath, make a doctor's appointment, and use the opportunity created to ask your gastroenterologist the following question: "Now tell me again, why have I not been placed on SBI?"

What are low endotoxemic foods? (You won't find red meat on this list)

> . . . we observed that dietary patterns, reflecting food choices that are generally considered healthy, were associated with lower LSP activity. Amongst some of the food items included in these dietary patterns, were fish, fresh vegetables, fruits and berries, yoghurt, pasta and rice, and poultry. (Ahola et al., 2017)

A case against milk

Many authorities advise the ulcerative colitis patient not to remove dairy products from their diet. (see Haskey and Gibson, 2017). However, according to one trial involving 77 IBD patients, 1 in 5 seemed to benefit from eliminating milk and cheese (Richman and Rhodes, 2013). What's going on? Two things come to mind.

The ulcerative colitis patient may also have **lactose intolerance**, unmasked or magnified by the disease process. There could also be a true allergy to specific components in milk and could thus contribute to the disease process. If eliminating dairy helps, strongly consider you are **intolerant or allergic** to milk and/or other dairy products, such as cheese and ice cream. An elimination diet may help identify this problem. We'll discuss the Elimination Diet a bit later. An additional drawback of milk is its high level of the amino acid cysteine, *"which can be used as an efficient source for the **generation of hydrogen sulfide (H2S) by sulfate-reducing bacteria (SRB)."** (Lewis and Abreu, 2017) "Furthermore, a diet high in milk fat (saturated fat) **alters the microbiome**, with an increase in a sulfite-reducing pathobiont* *[bacterium with pathogenic potential] Bilophila wadsworthia."* (Lewis and Abreu, 2017) Of course, we recognize both hydrogen sulfide and altered microbiome as harmful in the context of ulcerative colitis. One last consideration: Dairy products are **FODMAPS** (discussed in *Chapter 8*). Drastically limiting FODMAPS may improve your symptoms, particularly if your ulcerative colitis is acting a lot like irritable bowel syndrome. In essence, the low-FODMAP diet is an elimination diet. With this diet you are provided with an opportunity to withhold certain foods, then reintroduce a suspect food, like milk, to see if intolerance can be detected. Besides, you are not supposed to remain on the low-FODMAP diet for an extended period of time, so a controlled reintroduction of FODMAPS is necessary and can help identify food intolerances. Such foods should probably be avoided, as they can increase the severity of ulcerative colitis (Judaki et al., 2014). Now with respect to milk: I hope you are not among the 1 in 5, as there is so much good in dairy, like transforming growth factor $\beta1$—a growth factor that *"has been reported to improve intestinal tight-junction function."* (Kotler et al., 2013) Accordingly, one of the benefits of milk may be its capacity to limit leaky gut.

~References~

Ahola AJ, Lassenius MI, Forsblom C, Harjutsalo V, Lehto M, Groop PH. **Dietary patterns reflecting healthy food choices are associated with lower serum LPS activity.** Scientific reports. 2017 Jul 26;7(1):6511.

Amati L, Caradonna L, Leandro G, Magrone T, Minenna M, Faleo G, Pellegrino NM, Jirillo E, Caccavo D. **Immune abnormalities and endotoxemia in patients with ulcerative colitis and in their first degree relatives: attempts at neutralizing endotoxin-mediated effects.** Current pharmaceutical design. 2003 Sep 1;9(24):1937-45.

Champion K, Chiu L, Ferbas J, Pepe M. **Endotoxin neutralization as a biomonitor for inflammatory bowel disease.** PloS one. 2013 Jun 24;8(6):e67736.

Erridge C. **Stimulants of Toll-like receptor (TLR)-2 and TLR-4 are abundant in certain minimally-processed vegetables.** Food and chemical toxicology. 2011 Jun 1;49(6):1464-7.

Fukui H. **Increased intestinal permeability and decreased barrier function: does it really influence the risk of inflammation?.** Inflammatory Intestinal Diseases. 2016;1(3):135-45.

Ghoshal S, Witta J, Zhong J, De Villiers W, Eckhardt E. **Chylomicrons promote intestinal absorption of lipopolysaccharides.** Journal of lipid research. 2009 Jan 1;50(1):90-7.

Gulhane M, Murray L, Lourie R, Tong H, Sheng YH, Wang R, Kang A, Schreiber V, Wong KY, Magor G, Denman S. **High fat diets induce colonic epithelial cell stress and inflammation that is reversed by IL-22. Scientific reports.** 2016 Jun 28;6:28990.

Harte AL, Varma MC, Tripathi G, McGee KC, Al-Daghri NM, Al-Attas OS, Sabico S, O'Hare JP, Ceriello A, Saravanan P, Kumar S. **High fat intake leads to acute postprandial exposure to circulating endotoxin in type 2 diabetic subjects.** Diabetes care. 2012 Feb 1;35(2):375-82.

Haskey N, Gibson DL. **An examination of diet for the maintenance of remission in inflammatory bowel disease.** Nutrients. 2017 Mar 10;9(3):259.

Herieka M, Faraj TA, Erridge C. **Reduced dietary intake of pro-inflammatory Toll-like receptor stimulants favourably modifies markers of cardiometabolic risk in healthy men.** Nutrition, Metabolism and Cardiovascular Diseases. 2016 Mar 1;26(3):194-200.

Judaki A, Hafeziahmadi M, Yousefi A, Havasian MR, Panahi J, Sayehmiri K, Alizadeh S. **Evaluation of dairy allergy among ulcerative colitis patients.** Bioinformation. 2014;10(11):693.

Kaliannan K, Wang B, Li XY, Kim KJ, Kang JX. **A host-microbiome interaction mediates the opposing effects of omega-6 and omega-3 fatty acids on metabolic endotoxemia.** Scientific reports. 2015 Jun 11;5:11276.

Knight-Sepulveda K, Kais S, Santaolalla R, Abreu MT. **Diet and inflammatory bowel disease.** Gastroenterology & hepatology. 2015 Aug;11(8):511.

Kotler BM, Kerstetter JE, Insogna KL. **Claudins, dietary milk proteins, and intestinal barrier regulation.** Nutrition reviews. 2013 Jan 1;71(1):60-5.

Lan B, Yang F, Lu D, Lin Z. **Specific immunotherapy plus Clostridium butyricum alleviates ulcerative colitis in patients with food allergy.** Scientific reports. 2016 May 11;6:25587.

Lewis JD. **The role of diet in inflammatory bowel disease.** Gastroenterology & hepatology. 2016 Jan;12(1):51.

Lewis JD, Abreu MT. **Diet as a trigger or therapy for inflammatory bowel diseases.** Gastroenterology. 2017 Jan 1;152(2):398-414.

Lorenz W, Buhrmann C, Mobasheri A, Lueders C, Shakibaei M. **Bacterial lipopolysaccharides form procollagen-endotoxin complexes that trigger cartilage inflammation and degeneration: implications for the development of rheumatoid arthritis.** Arthritis research & therapy. 2013 Oct;15(5):R111.

Lyte JM, Gabler NK, Hollis JH. **Postprandial serum endotoxin in healthy humans is modulated by dietary fat in a randomized, controlled, cross-over study.** Lipids in health and disease. 2016 Dec;15(1):186.

Mani V, Hollis JH, Gabler NK. **Dietary oil composition differentially modulates intestinal endotoxin transport and postprandial endotoxemia.** Nutrition & metabolism. 2013 Dec;10(1):6.

Moreira AP, Texeira TF, Ferreira AB, Peluzio MD, Alfenas RD. **Influence of a high-fat diet on gut microbiota, intestinal permeability and metabolic endotoxaemia.** British Journal of Nutrition. 2012 Sep;108(5):801-9.

Mutlu EA, Gor N. **To diet or not if you have inflammatory bowel disease.** Expert review of gastroenterology & hepatology. 2008 Oct 1;2(5):613-6.

Ochsenkühn T, D'Hens G. **Current misunderstandings in the management of ulcerative colitis.** Gut. 2011 Jan 1:gut-2010.

O'Dwyer ST, Michie HR, Ziegler TR, Revhaug A, Smith RJ, Wilmore DW. **A single dose of endotoxin increases intestinal permeability in healthy humans.** Archives of Surgery. 1988 Dec 1;123(12):1459-64.

Pendyala S, Walker JM, Holt PR. **A high-fat diet is associated with endotoxemia that originates from the gut.** Gastroenterology. 2012 May 1;142(5):1100-1.

Richman E, Rhodes JM. **Evidence-based dietary advice for patients with inflammatory bowel disease.** Alimentary pharmacology & therapeutics. 2013 Nov 1;38(10):1156-71.

Rojo ÓP, Román AL, Arbizu EA, de la Hera Martínez A, Sevillano ER, Martínez AA. **Serum lipopolysaccharide-binding protein in endotoxemic patients with inflammatory bowel disease.** Inflammatory bowel diseases. 2006 Dec 19;13(3):269-77.

Ruemmele FM. **Role of diet in inflammatory bowel disease.** Annals of Nutrition and Metabolism. 2016;68(Suppl. 1):32-41.

Teixeira LG, Leonel AJ, Aguilar EC, Batista NV, Alves AC, Coimbra CC, Ferreira AV, de Faria AM, Cara DC, Leite JI. **The combination of high-fat diet-induced obesity and chronic ulcerative colitis reciprocally exacerbates adipose tissue and colon inflammation.** Lipids in health and disease. 2011 Dec;10(1):204.

Van Arsdall M, Haque I, Liu Y, Rhoads JM. **Is There a Role for the Enteral Administration of Serum-Derived Immunoglobulins in Human Gastrointestinal Disease and Pediatric Critical Care Nutrition?.** Advances in Nutrition. 2016 May 9;7(3):535-43.

Zhou SY, Gillilland M, Wu X, Leelasinjaroen P, Zhang G, Zhou H, Ye B, Lu Y, Owyang C. **FODMAP diet modulates visceral nociception by lipopolysaccharide-mediated intestinal inflammation and barrier dysfunction.** The Journal of clinical investigation. 2018 Jan 2;128(1):267-80.

Zinöcker MK, Lindseth IA. **The Western Diet–Microbiome-Host Interaction and Its Role in Metabolic Disease.** Nutrients. 2018 Mar 17;10(3):365.

Chapter 12

The Semi-Vegetarian Diet

We consider the lack of a suitable diet is the biggest issue faced in current treatment of IBD [so we did something about it]. **~Chiba et al., 2018**

Plant-based foods, such as fruit, vegetables, and whole grains, which contain significant amounts of bioactive phytochemicals, may provide desirable health benefits beyond basic nutrition to reduce the risk of chronic diseases. **~Liu, 2003**

A healthy, plant-based diet includes plant foods in their whole form, especially vegetables, fruits, legumes, seeds, and nuts. It limits animal products and total fat intake. It aims to maximize consumption of nutrient-dense plant foods while minimizing processed foods, oils, and animal foods. In addition, it encourages a large quantity of vegetables (cooked or raw), fruits, beans, peas, lentils, seeds, and nuts and is generally lower in fat.

Thus it is recommended to consume a diet rich in colorful fruits and vegetables for optimized health and wellness, and potential disease prevention. **~Poe, 2017**

W e met Yuto in *Chapter 10*. The success he achieved in his personal battle against ulcerative colitis was accomplished by forsaking the Western diet and adopting a plant-based diet . . . and it worked! Others, too, have achieved success in their battle against ulcerative colitis by substantially restricting or eliminating animal products and adopting a plant-based diet. There are many reasons why a plant-based diet favors remission in ulcerative colitis. We'll discuss it all in this chapter.

The formal use of a semi-vegetarian diet as a therapy for IBD, both Crohn's and ulcerative colitis, began in Japan in 2003 by a team of gastroenterologists who learned a lesson or two from history and were willing to step outside the box. Since time travel allows us a unique opportunity to learn how we got from Point A to Point B, let's go back in time to the middle of the last century (Point A) and visit Japan to see what we can learn about the role diet plays in the initiation and perpetuation of ulcerative colitis.

It's the early 1950s. The War is over. Westernization is on the horizon but has not yet taken hold to any great extent. The Japanese people are, for the most part, eating a very simple plant-based diet with not a Twinkie in sight. IBD is surprisingly rare. But this would all change. As of 2014, some sixty years later, Japan has at least 140,000 individuals with ulcerative colitis—a **100-fold increase** in the incidence of this disease compared to the 1950s (Kanai et al., 2014). Why? And what is this thing called Westernization?

Westernization is, of course, changes in fashion and the availability of silly TV shows, but it is also something else. It includes dietary changes, as well. Dietary Westernization in Japan meant that the dietary practices of the past would be replaced by modern, Western-style dietary practices, practices that include increased meat consumption, increased consumption of saturated and polyunsaturated fat, as well as a dramatic decrease in the consumption of soluble fibers. This profound change in diet was and is the perfect storm, allowing modern, Western diseases to gain a serious foothold. IBD serves as an example. So, what should be appreciated here is this: **The Western Diet is The Perfect Storm Diet**.

Westernization in Japan started well before World War II but was not widespread in the population. The story goes something like this:

Until about 150 years ago, Japan was officially sealed off from the outside world. Most Japanese individuals had no contact with

Western people or Western dietary habits, and ate traditional Japanese foods. After the end of the Edo era in 1868, the new Japanese government opened the country to Westerners and began diplomatic and cultural contract with many Western countries. Concurrently, the Japanese government promoted a Western lifestyle, including Western diets, housing, clothes, and culture. However, only a small proportion of Japanese people, known as the favored classes, could afford Western foods, while the vast majority continued to eat frugal Japanese foods for an additional 100 years. A typical Japanese diet at that time was a simple vegetarian meal composed of unthreshed rice mixed with barley, miso soup with root vegetables and/or tofu, small grilled fermented fish, and fermented pickled vegetables. Fermentation was essential to preserve foods in the absence of cooling systems. After the end of World War II in 1945, democracy emerged in Japan, with many people choosing Westernization. Annual reports by the Japanese Health, Labor and Welfare Ministry have shown rapid increased intake of sugar-rich carbonated beverages, fat- and carbohydrate-rich Western snacks (e.g., potato chips), and animal protein and fat, and a concurrent rapid decrease in the intake of dietary fiber. (Kanai et al., 2014, emphasis added)

All this Westernization led to unexpected consequences. An astonishing, **100-fold increase** in the incidence of ulcerative colitis in Japan is a case in point. A simple, plant-based diet offered protection against this evil. Give a population more red meat than it needs, more protein than it needs, more iron than it needs, more sulfur than it needs, more saturated fat than it needs, more omega-6 fatty acids then it needs, more food additives than it needs, and a lot less dietary fiber than it needs, and what do you get? You get more ulcerative colitis than a population needs. Thank you, Western diet.

Perhaps with a return to a plant-based diet, we can turn back time. This was the conclusion reached by a group of Japanese gastroenterologists. They put thought into action and developed a plan, a simple plan. Let's listen in on their thoughts.

Diets rich in animal protein and animal fat cause a decrease in beneficial bacteria in the intestine. . . . we regard IBD as a lifestyle-related disease that is mediated by mainly a westernized diet.

Therefore, we designed a diet that hopefully increases the number of beneficial bacteria. Limited foods are known to increase beneficial bacteria; green tea and unrefined brown rice. However, most prebiotics are extracts from plants. Therefore we thought that a vegetarian diet would be suitable for IBD. Considering that excessive restriction of foods can be less acceptable, a semi vegetarian diet (SVD) has been provided to IBD patients in our hospital since 2003. SVD, which is rich in dietary fiber, is quite opposite to conventional low-residue diets in IBD. (Chiba et al., 2010)

The plan was to return to the simple days and the simple ways—a time when a simple, plant-based diet ruled—and turn it into a simple therapy for IBD. And, initially combined with drug therapy (as needed), the results were impressive indeed. For Crohn's, in a study of 16 patients who followed the plant-based diet, the sustained remission rate was 100% at year one and 92% at year two, (Chiba et al., 2010). For ulcerative colitis, one recent study of 60 patients who followed the plant-based diet reported a relapse rate of only 2%, one-year post initiation of therapy (Chiba et al., 2018). At two years, the relapse rate was at 4%. At five years, the relapse rate was 19%. To be fair, in this study many individuals required standard medications to help maintain remission. But still, *"These relapse rates are far better than those previously reported."* (Chiba et al., 2018)

I am struck by the simplicity of The Semi-Vegetarian Diet, and that something so simple has the power to defeat something so complex. Basically,

The diet was lacto-ovo vegetarian, in which eggs and milk were allowed with small portions of meat offered once every two weeks and fish weekly. (Haskey and Gibson, 2017)

How simple is this? Very simple. And the diet comes with a pyramid—a sure sign the diet is legit and should be taken very seriously. You can find the pyramid online, in the paper written by Chiba et al., 2010. But since you have no intention of putting down this book any time soon, I'll go ahead and describe it to you now.

At the tip-top portion of the pyramid is meat. You are allowed a limited amount of meat, once every 2 weeks. (Yes, you can do it.) The next portion of the pyramid allows a limited portion of fish once a week—easy! The rest of the pyramid is fairly straightforward and chock-full of plants—hence a plant-based diet. The diet allows milk, eggs, and yogurt, in addition to fruits, vegetables, brown rice, legumes (beans), and potatoes. Basically, The Semi-Vegetarian Diet is a lacto-ovo vegetarian diet, with a little meat thrown in to satisfy the needs of the carnivore within. Of course, there are other restrictions and there are specific recommendations, as follows:

Foods that have been shown to be a risk factor for IBD in or outside Japan including sweets, bread, cheese, margarine, fast foods, carbonated beverages, and juices, were discouraged. Healthy habits were encouraged; no smoking, regular physical activity, moderate to no use of alcohol, regularity of meals, and not eating between meals. (Chiba et al., 2010)

Admittedly, this diet (and lifestyle constraints), seems harsh and so undoable, but it is not all that bad—particularly when you consider how harsh ulcerative colitis can be, how unacceptable ulcerative colitis is, and how desperately you are searching to find a way out.

Since The Semi-Vegetarian Diet is largely a vegetarian diet, you can get tons of menu ideas from books, magazines, and online, from those who promote vegetarianism or veganism as a way of life. Gather information. Formulate a plan. Make a day-to-day menu so you stay on track. Get approval from your physician. Then, eat yourself out of a jam.

So, in the spirit of The Semi-Vegetarian Diet, here are my simple rules: Follow a lacto-ovo-vegetarian diet, choosing foods easily found in our culture. Occasionally—very occasionally—allow yourself a little meat (maybe no meat at all—you're lovin' the casseroles!). Limit the use of sweets, bread, cheese, etc. Make healthy lifestyle choices, as previously recommended. Fast foods and convenience foods are to be avoided as much as possible. This diet is doable. You eat meat . . . rarely. You eat wholesome plant-based foods at every meal. You live a wholesome life. You limit the foods that are known to be a risk factor for ulcerative colitis. How does remission sound? You can do this! If needed, enlist the services of a dietitian to design a diet plan especially for you, constructed around the principles discussed in this and previous chapters.

Before we move on, we should examine the reasons why The Semi-Vegetarian Diet works. It's all rather simple, really.

One of the primary reasons offered to explain the diet is its **abundance of dietary fiber** (Chiba, et al., 2010). Recall, dietary fibers feed good bacteria and suppress the numbers of potentially pathogenic bacteria, thereby helping to alleviate dysbiosis, a persistent driver of intestinal inflammation. Besides all the fiber, there are other reasons for the success of The Semi-Vegetarian Diet.

Being a diet very **low in animal protein**, there is **less toxic heme exposure**, **less heme driven dysbiosis**, **less sulfur exposure**, **less LPS exposure**, and **less hydrogen peroxide generation** for the intestinal barrier and immune system to cope with. Allow me to repeat the following series of quotations from *Chapter 9.* (Thanks!)

> *Heme, the iron porphyrin pigment, primarily found in red meat, poultry and fish is poorly absorbed in the small intestine.* **Approximately <u>90%</u> of dietary heme transits to the colon, and is exploited by colonic bacteria as a growth factor.**

Dietary heme directly injures colonic surface epithelium by *generating cytotoxic and oxidative stress.* (Khalili et al., 2017, emphasis added)

*. . . the **irritating** influence of heme is continuously present in the colon and not just a single "hit," meaning the **dietary heme can constantly modulate the severity of colitis**.*

A diet high in red meat might be a risk factor for inflammatory bowel disease development. (Schepens et al., 2011, emphasis added)

Additionally, The Semi-Vegetarian Diet **reduces exposure to iron**. Recall, iron consumed in excess, has a negative impact on the colon. And I repeat:

The Western diet is characteristically rich in sources of iron, especially red meat, and UC has historically been more prevalent in Western countries.

*The potentially deleterious effects of a high-iron diet on UC are attributed to the **accumulation of iron in the colonic lumen in high concentrations**, a direct result of the tight regulation of body iron levels and the restriction of dietary iron absorption.* (Seril et al., 2006, emphasis added)

The Semi-Vegetarian Diet is also a diet **low in pro-inflammatory fats**—the saturated fats and the omega-6 fatty acids that are particularly high in meat and particularly high in harm. Recall,

*Consuming a Western diet, high in fat (**particularly saturated fat**), is enough to induce endotoxemia in healthy subjects.* (Knight-Sepulveda et al., 2015, emphasis added)

Also, a direct correlation of colonic cytokine levels with saturated fatty acids (SFA) was identified in patients with UC. (Statovci et al., 2017)

*. . . excessive consumption of omega-6 PUFA **increases ulcerative colitis by 30%**; whereas consumption of docosahexaenoic acid, an omega-3 fatty acid, **reduced the disease burden by 77%.*** (Brown et al., 2012, emphasis added)

And it is not just the omega-6 fatty acids in meat that lead to the consumption of the omega-6s in excess. Beware of salad dressings. Beware of factory-prepared entrees, even homemade foods, foods that typically contain vegetable oils high in the omega-6s as a major component.

And I could go on and on, but I think I've made my point about the evils of the Western diet and the virtues and advantages of The Semi-Vegetarian Diet. In my view, The Semi-Vegetarian Diet *is* the diet with the best chance for remission in ulcerative colitis. But, undoubtedly, you can screw things up. (I know you all too well.)

One mistake vegetarians typically make is excess consumption of sodium. Fortunately, their high intake of potassium offsets this. But it is still a problem. The best defense against sodium excess is to consume less factor-made foods like canned soup, canned vegetables, frozen entrees, and other prepared foods containing substantial levels of sodium. This is important!

More recently, studies indicated that salt has a crucial role in the development of inflammatory processes and augmentation of autoimmunity. (Abdoli, 2016)

*Not only does high sodium increase the inflammatory function of macrophages and T cells that are activated in response to infection and/or tissue trauma, but **high salt also neutralizes the inherent regulatory mechanisms that have evolved to limit the*** *levels of immune-mediated inflammation and promote resolution of tissue injury.* (Min and Fairchild, 2015, emphasis added)

Another cause for concern: Many prepared foods contain additives like emulsifyers, microparticles, artificial sweeteners, and aluminum.

Food additives are common in the Western diet, and animal and ex-vivo studies have suggested a detrimental effect of certain food additives, including polysorbate-80, carboxymethylcellulose, maltodextrin, carrageenan, and microparticles.

Moreover, artificial sweeteners and dietary emulsifiers adversely affect the gut microbiota and promote inflammatory responses. (Yang et al., 2016)

And don't forget about sulfur additives.

A high sulphur diet, either from sulphur amino acids [high in red meat] or sulphated additives, results in the generation of hydrogen sulphide and mucosal damage in the colon.

Red meat, for instance, is stated as a food to be avoided on a low sulphur amino acid diet and processed foods contain large amounts of sulphate as a food additive. (Jowett et al., 2004)

Word to the wise: Do what you can to limit the food additives known to harm, to allow The Semi-Vegetarian Diet a greater chance for success.

Finally, be sure to add alcohol to the list of things to avoid while on the diet (and possibly avoid forever).

*Similarly, a high alcohol intake was associated with an increased risk of relapse and <u>many alcoholic drinks contain large amounts of sulphates as additives</u>. A high sulphur diet, either from **sulphur amino acids** or sulphate additives, results in the generation of* *hydrogen sulphide and mucosal damage in the colon.* (Jowett et al., 2004, emphasis added)

That's about it! Time to move on.

There is another diet we can learn a lot from. It may be an acceptable alternative to The Semi-Vegetarian Diet. It is called The Mediterranean Diet. That's coming up, in the next chapter.

It happens so fast!

It seems far-fetched that an ulcerative colitis patient can go rapidly into remission with a plant-based diet. But it does happen. In fact, it happens quite regularly with The Semi-Vegetarian Diet. Yuto went into remission in a matter of days, off the Western diet and on the diet that I call the best of the best. The secret to the success of The Semi-Vegetarian Diet may be its ability to promptly resolve dysbiosis.

Surprisingly, dysbiosis, a driver of inflammation in ulcerative colitis, can be corrected in a matter of days.

> *Human studies have shown that the microbiota rapidly adapts to short-term dietary changes toward a plant-based or animal-based nutrition.* (Willebrand and Kleinewietfeld, 2018)

> *Within 4 d [days] of eating a specific dietary component, the human intestinal flora composition will change significantly.* (Zhang et al., 2016)

> *Interestingly, the human microbiome adapts very quickly to a diet. Changing diet for five consecutive days to a plant-based or animal-based diet is sufficient to alter the microbiome composition.* (Hucke et al., 2016)

Knowing what I know, I find it easy to believe rapid results can be achieved by something as simple, *as transformational*, as The Semi-Vegetarian Diet. The diet is a microbiome make-over! And, as such, the new bacteria that are now in charge exert their collective influence, and inflammation is brought under control. The colon gets the break it was longing for. Pro-resolution programs are set in motion. Someone gets to live a normal life.

Methionine restriction

While studying The Semi-Vegetarian Diet, searching for clues to its effectiveness, I noticed something about this diet that may contribute to its success. The Semi-Vegetarian Diet is low in the amino acid methionine. Vegetarian diets do contain methionine, all an individual really needs, but an animal-based diet contains a whole lot more, perhaps more than an individual really needs. And the excess methionine consumed in an animal-based diet may come with a price. This excess may contribute to leaky gut.

Experimentally, it has been discovered that restricting methionine decreases intestinal permeability (Ramalingam et al., 2010). While studying specific tissues, cultured to mimic the colon epithelia,

> . . . we observed that MR [methionine restriction] alters TJ [tight junction] structure and composition, decreases TJ permeability, and thereby enhances epithelial barrier function. This is one of extremely few modalities known to be able to induce improved barrier function, in contrast to a growing list of pathogenic agents capable of causing TJ leak. (Ramalingam et al., 2010)

This finding was confirmed using rats as test subjects.

> Here we report for the first time that rats fed on an MR [methionine-restricted] diet for a brief period (4 wk) showed improved TJ [tight junction] barrier function due to an alter TJ protein expression pattern. (Ramalingam et al., 2010)

In another study, using mice,

. . . our results indicate that MR [methionine restriction] can be used as a potent immunomodulatory and anti-inflammatory modulator, and the MR diet should be considered as an adjuvant diet for animal models and human patients with IBD. (Liu et al., 2017)

I think there is something here that speaks to the efficacy of The Semi-Vegetarian Diet.

An excellent resource, listing the methionine content of various foods, can be found online, entitled:

–Methionine- Restricted Diet... Who needs it?
https://www.brendadavisrd.com/methionine-restricted-diet/

~References~

Abdoli A. **Salt and miscarriage: Is there a link?.** Medical hypotheses. 2016 Apr 1;89:58-62.

Brown K, DeCoffe D, Molcan E, Gibson DL. **Diet-induced dysbiosis of the intestinal microbiota and the effects on immunity and disease.** Nutrients. 2012 Aug;4(8):1095-119.

Chiba M, Abe T, Tsuda H, Sugawara T, Tsuda S, Tozawa H, Fujiwara K, Imai H. **Lifestyle-related disease in Crohn's disease: relapse prevention by a semi-vegetarian diet.** World Journal of Gastroenterology: WJG. 2010 May 28;16(20):2484.

Chiba M, Nakane K, Tsuji T, Tsuda S, Ishii H, Ohno H, Watanabe K, Ito M, Komatsu M, Yamada K, Sugawara T. **Relapse prevention in ulcerative colitis by plant-based diet through educational hospitalization: A single-group trial.** The Permanente Journal. 2018;22.

Haskey N, Gibson DL. **An examination of diet for the maintenance of remission in inflammatory bowel disease.** Nutrients. 2017 Mar 10;9(3):259.

Hucke S, Wiendl H, Klotz L. Implications of dietary salt intake for multiple sclerosis pathogenesis. Multiple Sclerosis Journal. 2016 Feb;22(2):133-9.

Jowett SL, Seal CJ, Pearce MS, Phillips E, Gregory W, Barton JR, Welfare MR. **Influence of dietary factors on the clinical course of ulcerative colitis: a prospective cohort study.** Gut. 2004 Oct 1;53(10):1479-84.

Kanai T, Matsuoka K, Naganuma M, Hayashi A, Hisamatsu T. **Diet, microbiota, and inflammatory bowel disease: lessons from Japanese foods.** The Korean journal of internal medicine. 2014 Jul;29(4):409.

Khalili H, Malik S, Ananthakrishnan AN, Garber JJ, Higuchi LM, Joshi A, Peloquin J, Richter JM, Stewart KO, Curhan GC, Awasthi A. **Identification and characterization of a novel association between dietary potassium and risk of Crohn's disease and ulcerative colitis.** Frontiers in immunology. 2016 Dec 7;7:554.

Knight-Sepulveda K, Kais S, Santaolalla R, Abreu MT. **Diet and inflammatory bowel disease.** Gastroenterology & hepatology. 2015 Aug;11(8):511.

Liu RH. **Health benefits of fruit and vegetables are from additive and synergistic combinations of phytochemicals.** The American journal of clinical nutrition. 2003 Sep 1;78(3):517S-20S.

Liu G, Yu L, Fang J, Hu CA, Yin J, Ni H, Ren W, Duraipandiyan V, Chen S, Al-Dhabi NA, Yin Y. **Methionine restriction on oxidative stress and immune response in dss-induced colitis mice.** Oncotarget. 2017 Jul 4;8(27):44511.

Min B, Fairchild RL. **Over-salting ruins the balance of the immune menu.** The Journal of clinical investigation. 2015 Nov 2;125(11):4002-4.

Poe KL **Plant-Based Diets and Phytonutrients: Potential Health Benefits and Disease Prevention.** ARCHIVES OF MEDICINE ISSN 1989-5216; Vol.9 No.6:7 2017; iMedPub Journals http://www.imedpub.com/; DOI: 10.21767/1989-5216.1000249, © Under License of Creative Commons Attribution 3.0 License; This article is available from: http://www.archivesofmedicine.com/ 1

Ramalingam A, Wang X, Gabello M, Valenzano MC, Soler AP, Ko A, Morin PJ, Mullin JM. **Dietary methionine restriction improves colon tight junction barrier function and alters claudin expression pattern.** American Journal of Physiology-Cell Physiology. 2010 Aug 18;299(5):C1028-35.

Schepens MA, Vink C, Schonewille AJ, Dijkstra G, van der Meer R, Bovee-Oudenhoven IM. **Dietary heme adversely affects experimental colitis in rats, despite heat-shock protein induction.** Nutrition. 2011 May 1;27(5):590-7.

Seril DN, Liao J, West AB, Yang G-Y 2006 **High-Iron Diet: Foe of Feat in Ulcerative Colitis and Ulcerative Colitis-Associated Carcinogenesis.** J Clin Gastroenterol; May/June; 40(5):391–397.

Statovci D, Aguilera M, MacSharry J, Melgar S. **The impact of Western diet and nutrients on the microbiota and immune response at mucosal interfaces.** Frontiers in immunology. 2017 Jul 28;8:838.

Willebrand R, Kleinewietfeld M. **The role of salt for immune cell function and disease.** Immunology. 2018 Feb 21.

Yang Y, Owyang C, Wu GD. **East Meets West: the increasing incidence of inflammatory bowel disease in Asia as a paradigm for environmental effects** on the pathogenesis of immune-mediated disease. Gastroenterology. 2016 Dec 1;151(6):e1-5.

Zhang M, Yang XJ. Effects of a high fat diet on intestinal microbiota and gastrointestinal diseases. World journal of gastroenterology. 2016 Oct 28;22(40):8905.

Chapter 13

The Mediterranean Diet

The Mediterranean dietary pattern was identified in the 1950's and 1960's along the coastal regions of southern European countries, including Italy and Greece, and was associated with a lower mortality rate from coronary heart disease. **~Guilleminault et al., 2017**

The Mediterranean diet is mostly composed of vegetables, whole grains, and fruit, with increased intake of legumes, raw unsalted nuts, and oily fish. **~Hsu et al., 2017**

The traditional Mediterranean diet is characterized by a high intake of olive oil, which is rich in monounsaturated-fat [MUFA], nuts, fruits and legumes, vegetables, and fish and a low intake of red meat, processed meats, and sweets (wine in moderation). In contrast to the low fat diet, which contains up-to 30% fat, 40% of the calories in the Mediterranean diet are derived from fats, mostly MUFA and omega-3 PUFA. MUFA has a favorable effect on lipid profile. **~Romero-Gómez et al., 2017**

T he traditional Mediterranean diet is a dandy, low in animal products, high in plant foods, and great in reward. This makes for a diet that we can learn a lot from in our quest to find a diet that can make all the difference in the battle against ulcerative colitis. It makes for a diet that may even possess the power to protect against IBD.

The Mediterranean diet pattern may have a protective effect on IBD, as the incidence of IBD in the south of Europe is lower than in northern Europe. The Mediterranean diet pattern is a diet that is high in fiber-rich plant-based foods (e.g., cereals, fruits, vegetables, legumes, nuts, seeds and olives), with olive oil as the principle source of added fat, along with high to moderate intakes of fish and seafood, moderate consumption of eggs, poultry, dairy products (cheese and yogurt), wine and low consumption of red meat. A growing body of scientific evidence indicates that the Mediterranean diet pattern has been associated with significant improvements in health status and decreases in inflammatory markers. The protective effect is hypothesized to be derived from the balance in the omega-6/omega-3 ratio of the Mediterranean diet pattern (35% total fat: 15% MUFA (mainly from olive oil), 13% SFA, and 6% PUFA. The mechanisms of how MUFA might be beneficial in colitis are unknown, although adherence to the Mediterranean diet pattern has been shown to beneficially affect the gut microbiome and gut metabolites (metabolome). (Haskey and Gibson, 2017)

Are you beginning to see the Mediterranean diet has a lot to offer the ulcerative colitis patient? So many things found in this diet are found in The Semi-Vegetarian Diet, including a low consumption of red meat (Haskey and Gibson, 2017). I'll bet the Mediterranean diet can easily be transformed (weaponized) into an effective therapy for ulcerative colitis. And like The Semi-Vegetarian Diet, the Mediterranean diet comes with a pyramid, so it has legit written all over it, and obviously should be taken very seriously. I'll describe the pyramid now. We'll start at the bottom, the location where most of the eating occurs. I'll use the Mediterranean diet pyramid according to Guilleminault et al., 2017. The pyramid summarizes the foods allowed, the foods to be consumed day in and day out.

At the bottom of the pyramid are the fruits, vegetables, the cereals (*"wholegrain preferably"*), and olive oil, the preferred oil for cooking. The middle portion of the pyramid, the area where less is consumed, includes white meat, seafood and fish, legumes, eggs, dairy (*"low fat preferably"*), nuts, seeds, and olives. And now we've reached the top. The top of the pyramid is smaller than all the other compartments, allowing limited amounts of sweets, potatoes, processed meats, and red meat. The following quotation summarizes well the characteristics of the Mediterranean diet:

> *The MD [Mediterranean diet] is rich in plant foods (cereals, fruits, vegetables, legumes, tree nuts, seeds and olives), with olive oil as the principal source of added fat, along with high to moderate intakes of fish and seafood, moderate consumption of eggs, poultry and dairy products (cheese and yogurt), low consumption of red meat, and a moderate intake of alcohol (mainly wine during meals).* (Duff et al., 2018)

One thing to keep in mind, the Mediterranean diet is not intentionally designed to induce remission in ulcerative colitis. That would be The Semi-Vegetarian Diet. What is absent in the Mediterranean diet is strict controls on amounts of animal fats and proteins, as well as a limitation on fish consumption. Add stricter controls, in addition to greatly restricting commercially prepared foods (high in sodium, LPS, and harmful food additives), and your chances of turning the Mediterranean diet into weapon in the battle against ulcerative colitis is increased. But even without a makeover, the Mediterranean diet has "success" written all over it.

The success of the Mediterranean diet in decreasing the incidence of Western-style diseases (stroke, heart disease, diabetes, obesity, etc.) is the preponderance of fruits and vegetables, making it a diet high in healthy fiber, high in a wide variety of beneficial nutrients, and high in healthy fats (omega-3 and monounsaturated fatty acids). But the success of the Mediterranean diet is also about what is avoided.

In the spirit of the Mediterranean diet, factory-prepared and fast food are avoided or at least substantially limited. The same is true for the pro-inflammatory omega-6 fatty acids. The diet restricts red meat, which is a plus for the ulcerative colitis patient. So, this feature alone may offer benefit to the patient with ulcerative colitis, for the reasons previously discussed.

As far as I can tell, there are no published studies to date that demonstrate the effectiveness of the Mediterranean diet in the battle against ulcerative colitis. But that is about to change. Currently there is a clinical trial underway to assess the efficacy of the Mediterranean diet as a treatment for ulcerative colitis, to be completed in 2020. The ClinicalTrials.gov Trial identifier is: NCT03053713. I look forward to reading the results of this study.

Since a short chapter is long overdue, I will end our discussion on the Mediterranean diet with this: If you are serious about the use of diet in the battle against ulcerative colitis, learn what you can from the Mediterranean diet—the variety of foods permitted, and the recipes that make eating a plant-based diet a delight—and place controls on your food choices to mimic, within reason, The Semi-Vegetarian Diet. The more plants the better, the less animal products the better. Words to live by.

Putting it all together

There are numerous sites on the web that offer Mediterranean diet recipes free of charge. These will get you started:

–50 Easy Mediterranean Diet Recipes and Meal Ideas by Shape
Magazine
> https://www.shape.com/healthy-eating/healthy-recipes/
> mediterranean-diet-recipes-meal-ideas

–Mediterranean Diet Recipes by Mayo Clinic staff
> https://www.mayoclinic.org/healthy-lifestyle/nutrition-and-
> healthy-eating/in-depth/mediterranean-diet-recipes/art-
> 20046682

Making it Better

The above reference offers these guidelines:

"The Mediterranean diet emphasizes plant-based foods, such as fruits and vegetables, whole grains, legumes and nuts. It replaces butter with healthy fats, such as olive oil and canola oil, and uses herbs and spices instead of salt to flavor foods. **Red meat is limited to no more than a few times a month,** *while fish should be on the menu twice a week."* (Mayo Clinic Staff, emphasis added)

I offer additional recommendations: **1)** Keep things low in fat, overall, with a preference for high-quality olive oil (canola oil as a healthy cooking oil is debatable and may not be acceptable). **2)** When you do eat meat, red meat or otherwise, eat it as a minor part of an entrée. This reduces your intake of animal products—a control measure I believe will make this diet more successful and in line with The Semi-Vegetarian Diet. **3)** Limit prepared, manufactured foods as a measure to reduce the consumption of food additives.

I can't go Paleo

If you were to look at the basic Paleo pyramid, you would notice this: The bottom of the pyramid where most the eating occurs, is largely lean meats. Lean meats are preferred, but the problem of excess exposure to heme and iron are, to me, big red flags. Compared to The Semi-Vegetarian Diet, this pyramid is built upside down! I like to see all the vegetables included in this diet, but they should be on the bottom of the pyramid where most of the eating occurs. However, you can learn a lot from this diet—recipes, and choices of healthy meats and healthy fats—but best not stray from the principles of The Semi-Vegetarian Diet if you want the best chance to achieve remission by diet.

There are ulcerative colitis success stories with the Paleo diet, to be sure. After all, a diet that is not the Western diet typically has features that favor remission in this disease.

What about AIP?

There is a Paleo spinoff diet worth noting, called the Autoimmune Protocol (AIP). This diet is a lot stricter than the parent, Paleo diet—and overall, a lot stricter than The Semi-Vegetarian Diet. Less happiness can be found following this diet.

> *The AIP diet focuses on an initial elimination phase of food groups including grains, legumes [beans], nightshades [white potatoes, tomatoes, bell peppers, and eggplant], dairy, eggs, coffee, alcohol, nuts and seeds, refined/processed sugars, oils and food additives.* (Konijeti et al., 2017)

The rest of the AIP is along the lines of the Paleo diet, with the same positive and negative features. I mention the AIP here because I think we can learn from it. It may be of value to follow the elimination phase recommendations of this diet at the beginning of whatever diet you are following. A little more on the diet before we move on:

> *The premise of the AIP diet, as a whole, involves a staged elimination of food groups that may be associated with immune stimulation and intolerance, maintenance of the eliminated foods, followed by staged reintroduction of certain foods or food groups over time. The purpose of our study was to examine the potential efficacy of the AIP diet for IBD, and as such we focused on the elimination phase and a minimum 1-month maintenance phase. Our study design was adapted from our health coach's online program, which focuses on the 6-week elimination phase. The maintenance phase, in practice, can occur for participants anywhere from 30 to 90 days, although some continue it even longer, before*

starting to reintroduce food groups. The protocol emphasizes
healthy food behaviors aimed at increasing the nutrient density of
the diet, incorporating fresh fruits and vegetables, healthy sources
of fats, lean proteins, fermented foods, and, for our study, modifying
intake according to IBD phenotype (e.g., strictures). (Konijeti et al.,
2017)

The AIP is not the Western diet, so expect the positive features of this diet to produce results. In one study, ulcerative colitis patients who followed this diet showed significant improvement on their disease activity score and experienced *"significantly reduced"* rectal bleeding (Konijeti et al., 2017).

~*References*~

Duff W, Haskey N, Potter G, Alcorn J, Hunter P, Fowler S. **Non-pharmacological therapies for inflammatory bowel disease: Recommendations for self-care and physician guidance.** World journal of gastroenterology. 2018 Jul 28;24(28):3055.

Guilleminault L, Williams E, Scott H, Berthon B, Jensen M, Wood L. **Diet and asthma: is it time to adapt our message?.** Nutrients. 2017 Nov 8;9(11):1227.

Haskey N, Gibson DL. **An examination of diet for the maintenance of remission in inflammatory bowel disease.** Nutrients. 2017 Mar 10;9(3):259.

Hsu CC, Ness E, Kowdley KV. **Nutritional Approaches to Achieve Weight Loss in Nonalcoholic Fatty Liver Disease.** Advances in Nutrition. 2017 Mar 10;8(2):253-65.

Konijeti GG, Kim N, Lewis JD, Groven S, Chandrasekaran A, Grandhe S, Diamant C, Singh E, Oliveira G, Wang X, Molparia B. **Efficacy of the Autoimmune Protocol Diet for inflammatory bowel disease.** Inflammatory bowel diseases. 2017 Sep 29;23(11):2054-60.

Mayo Clinic staff **Mediterranean Diet Recipes** https://www.mayoclinic.org/healthy-lifestyle/nutrition-and-healthy-eating/in-depth/mediterranean-diet-recipes/art-20046682

Romero-Gómez M, Zelber-Sagi S, Trenell M. **Treatment of NAFLD with diet, physical activity and exercise.** Journal of hepatology. 2017 Oct 1;67(4):829-46.

Chapter 14

The DASH diet

Dash is a sodium-restricted (<2400 mg/d) diet rich in vegetables, fruits, whole grains, and low-fat dairy, and low in saturated fats, cholesterol, refined grains, and sweets. ~Hsu et al., **2017**

Given the above quotation, and in context to what we have previously discussed about sodium restriction, it would appear that the DASH diet would be an ideal diet to treat ulcerative colitis. With respect to sodium, previously we have learned that sodium restriction may benefit the ulcerative colitis patient as it reduces Th17 activity and increases both Treg numbers and Treg activity. Let's take a look at what the DASH diet is all about.

DASH is short for Dietary Approaches to Stop Hypertension. Medicine is very proud of this diet because it effectively addresses the problem of sodium excess in those who adhere. In our society, dietary sodium excess *is* a big problem. Restricting sodium has its rewards. It has been estimated *"that reducing the average to 2,300 mg/day could have a striking impact on hypertension, reducing cases by 11 million, saving $18 billion in health care costs, and resulting in 312,000 quality-adjusted live years gained."* (Provenzano et al., 2014) So, to limit the damage and save lives, there is a lot of interest in the DASH diet by the medical community. But is DASH right for ulcerative colitis? Maybe! The pyramid should offer us clues.

Depending upon the source, the DASH pyramid looks something like this: At the bottom portion of the pyramid (where most of the eating occurs), you find the breads, the grains, the pasta, and the potatoes. The next section of the pyramid where a good share of the eating occurs is where you find the fruits and the vegetables. The next section of the pyramid is a smaller section of the pyramid, recommending a somewhat limited consumption of dairy products, meat, fish, legumes, and nuts. Now, we've reached the top of the pyramid. The top portion of the pyramid, where the least of the eating occurs, is where we find the snacks and sweets—foods particularly high in salt, refined sugar, and proinflammatory fats. Be aware, others build the DASH pyramid a little differently than herein described.

However, regardless of the various pyramids put forth, a careful look at the DASH diet reveals a diet less than ideal (let's just say, "unsatisfactory") for the ulcerative colitis patient. Why? The DASH diet allows more animal protein, including red meat, than should probably be consumed by the ulcerative colitis patient. But there is something about this diet that does please me.

What pleases me about the DASH diet is its sodium-restriction recommendations. In as much as a diet high in sodium is harmful—intensifying the Th17 immune response and decreasing Treg numbers and the ability of this cell to suppress and resolve inflammation—the sodium-related recommendations of this diet make it something we can learn from. Recall, *"Within the gastrointestinal tract, increased exposure to dietary salt causes an increased inflammatory milieu [environment]."* (Hernandez et al., 2015)

We previously reviewed the **Cleveland Clinic recommendations** in the gray box at the end of *Chapter 10* (please review . . . daily). Next, let's review at the National Institute of Health recommendations.

TIPS FOR LOWERING SODIUM WHEN SHOPPING, COOKING, AND EATING OUT

Shopping

–Read food labels, choose items that are lower in sodium and salt, particularly convenience foods and condiments.*

–Choose fresh poultry, fish, and lean meats instead of cured food such as bacon and ham.

–Choose fresh or frozen versus canned fruits and vegetables.

–Avoid food with added salt, such as pickles, pickled vegetables, olives, and sauerkraut.

–Avoid instant or flavored rice and pasta.

Cooking

–Don't add salt when cooking rice, pasta, and hot cereals.

–Flavor your foods with salt-free seasoning blends, fresh or dried herbs and spices, or fresh lemon or lime juice.

–Rinse canned foods or foods soaked in brine before using to remove the sodium.

–Use less table salt to flavor food.

Eating out

–Ask that foods be prepared without added salt or MSG, commonly used in Asian foods.

–Avoid choosing menu items that have salty ingredients such as bacon, pickles, olives, and cheese.

–Avoid choosing menu items that include foods that are pickled, cured, smoked, or made with soy sauce or broth.

–Choose fruit or vegetables as a side dish, instead of chips or fries.

Source: National Institute of Health**

*Examples of convenience foods are frozen dinners, prepackaged foods, and soups; examples of condiments are mustard, ketchup, soy sauce, barbecue sauce, and salad dressings.

**https://www.nhlbi.nih.gov/health-topics/dash-eating-plan

Add the Cleveland Clinic recommendations to the National Institute of Health recommendations outlined above, and you are well on your way to a healthier life, perhaps on your way to a kinder and gentler ulcerative colitis, as well. Few seem aware that sodium excess intensifies the inflammatory response pattern associated with ulcerative colitis. Why ignore this driver of inflammation in ulcerative colitis? And why ignore the major sources of dietary sodium?

*Most of the sodium Americans eat comes from **processed and prepared foods**, such as **breads, cold cuts, pizza, poultry, soups, sandwiches** and **burgers, cheese, pasta and meat dishes**, and **salty snacks**. Therefore, healthier choices when shopping and eating out are particularly important.* (National Institute of Health, date not specified, emphasis added)

Have you noticed the chapters are getting shorter and shorter? (That's so not like me.) I'll be sure not to let you down in the next chapter. Since the forthcoming chapter covers a diet that is quite popular in the lay press, I'll need to spend a little more time covering it. And there is a bonus! We get to meet another physician with ulcerative colitis, an individual who went into remission by following the diet we will discuss.

Do you MIND?

Leave it to someone to take the best of both worlds and come up with a new diet and give it a nifty little name. Someone did this and named the diet The MIND diet. The MIND diet is a combination of the Mediterranean diet and the DASH diet. The goal of this diet is, for all intents and purposes, to protect the brain against the evils of Western diet. And following this diet has the potential to reduce the risk of cognitive decline and the risk of neurodegenerative diseases such as Alzheimer's. The diet is simple. The rules are simple. *"Simply eat more of the 10 foods the diet encourages, and eat less of the five foods the diet recommends you limit."* (Pearson, 2005–2018) And guess what's on the list of five things to limit or avoid? Answer: Red meat and the processed meats. It's true! Meat has danger written all over it.

The ten foods to eat are: green leafy vegetables, typical vegetables including sweet potatoes and tomatoes, nuts, berries, beans/legumes, whole grains, fish, poultry, and extra virgin olive oil.

The five foods to limit/avoid are: red meat and processed meat, butter and stick margarine, regular cheese, pastries and sweets in general, and fried foods and fast foods.

The MIND diet emphasizes berries instead of fruits, which is a departure from both the Mediterranean and DASH diets. The reason? Berries are believed to be more beneficial to the brain than fruit.

There are two excellent guides on the MIND diet you should read:

–The MIND Diet: A Detailed Guide for Beginners by Keith Pearson, PhD, RD
https://www.healthline.com/nutrition/mind-diet

–Mind Diet PDF
https://kaiserhealthnews.files.wordpress.com/2017/04/mind_ph_module-1_mind-diet_v2.pdf

If you were to follow the MIND diet in your quest for recovery from ulcerative colitis or to maintain remission, please don't forget the sodium restrictions associated with the DASH diet. Doing so would likely not be wise.

~References~

Hernandez AL, Kitz A, Wu C, Lowther DE, Rodriguez DM, Vudattu N, Deng S, Herold KC, Kuchroo VK, Kleinewietfeld M, Hafler DA. **Sodium chloride inhibits the suppressive function of FOXP3+ regulatory T cells.** The Journal of clinical investigation. 2015 Nov 2;125(11):4212-22.

Hsu CC, Ness E, Kowdley KV. **Nutritional Approaches to Achieve Weight Loss in Nonalcoholic Fatty Liver Disease.** Advances in Nutrition. 2017 Mar 10;8(2):253-65.

National Institute of Health. **DASH Eating Plan.** Date not specified. https://www.nhlbi.nih.gov/health-topics/dash-eating-plan

Provenzano LF, Stark S, Steenkiste A, Piraino B, Sevick MA. **Dietary sodium intake in type 2 diabetes.** Clinical Diabetes. 2014 Jul 1;32(3):106-12. LF, Stark S, Steenkiste A, Piraino B, Sevick MA. Dietary sodium intake in type 2 diabetes. Clinical Diabetes. 2014 Jul 1;32(3):106-12.

Chapter 15

The Specific Carbohydrate Diet

> *The specific carbohydrate diet (SCD) is a nutritional regimen that has been promoted for treating a variety of chronic and auto-immune disorders including IBD, coeliac disease and others. **The SCD strictly limits complex carbohydrates (disaccharides and polysaccharides) and eliminates refined sugar to correct for the imbalance caused by restricting the carbohydrates available to intestinal bacteria and yeasts.*** ~Yamamoto et al., 2009, emphasis added

B oy, does this diet sound restrictive! *And do I know restrictive!* But if restricting specific carbohydrates helps the ulcerative colitis patient achieve or maintain remission, I'm all in. The theory of the diet sounds like a good one, and the goal of this diet is one most noble.

> *This diet is based on the **theory** that disaccharides and polysaccharides pass undigested into the colon, resulting in bacterial and yeast overgrowth, which causes overproduction of mucus. It is further hypothesized that **this malabsorption may cause intestinal injury.** Therefore, strict adherence is recommended to prevent additional mucosal damage. **The SCD permits consumption of only monosaccharides [glucose, fructose, and galactose] and restricts intake of simple carbohydrates.*** (Knight-Sepulveda et al., 2015, emphasis added)

It all seems a little complex—what to include, what to avoid. Perhaps the following table of dos and don'ts will help simplify things a little.

The Specific Carbohydrate Diet Characteristics

Foods allowed

–Vegetables (except canned)

–Unprocessed meats, poultry, fish, eggs

–Legumes including lentils, split peas

–Lactose-free milk/dairy, homemade yogurt fermented at least 24 hours

–Natural cheese (except excluded cheeses)

–Fruit and fruit juices without additives

–Nuts, peanuts in shell, natural peanut butter

–Olive, coconut, soybean, and corn oil; butter

–Wine, weak coffee and tea

–Saccharin, honey

–Mustard, mayonnaise, ketchup

Foods excluded

–All grains

–All canned vegetables

–Canned or processed meats

–Sugars including lactose, sucrose, high-fructose corn syrup, fructose molasses, maltose, isomaltose, fructooligosaccharides

–Ricotta, mozzarella, cottage cheese, cream cheese, fetta, processed cheeses

–Starchy vegetables, including potato, yam, parsnips, corn

–Most legumes including chickpea (garbanzo beans), soybeans, mung beans, bean sprouts, fava beans

–Agar, carrageenan, seaweed

–Milk, instant tea, instant coffee, soymilk, beer

–Canola oil, margarine

–Candy, chocolate, carob

Adapted from: Knight-Sepulveda et al., 2015 and *Web*MD, 2011

So, as you can see, the SCD is quite restrictive. I guess it has its reasons. And its effectiveness is difficult to ignore. Because of its success, the diet is very popular in the lay literature (Haskey and Gibson, 2017); and more interest in the SCD seems to be developing among healthcare professionals. But *"Unfortunately, there is a lack of evidence-based published data on this diet. To date, the evidence for this diet is based on retrospective surveys and case reports."* (Haskey and Gibson, 2017) And with that, I have a case report to share.

Case report: Mako

We'll call her Mako. Mako is an Asian woman with a long-term history of ulcerative colitis. Not that it matters, but our patient is a practicing physician even at the age of 72. And as is so often the case, the course of her disease went fairly well until it didn't. *"In spite of a variety of standard treatments, her condition continued to decline with a significant impact on normal life and functioning."* (Khandalavala and Nirmalraj, 2015) Enter the Specific Carbohydrate Diet.

Formerly, she, like so many other ulcerative colitis patients, was no stranger to the Western diet. And it was only after her condition deteriorated and standard therapy failed, that diet, something other than the Western diet, became of interest. Her condition was indeed serious, based on symptoms and endoscopic documentation of pancolitis. So, something certainly needed to be done. And may I ask? Why do we wait so long before we consider diet as a weapon in the battle against ulcerative colitis? It makes no sense.

Why the SCD was chosen by Mako was not revealed in the report, only that the diet was recommended—presumably by her physician or perhaps by an acquaintance who was aware of its history of success. And after the choice was made to follow this diet, there was no fooling around.

She proceeded to completely exclude wheat, soy, barley, corn and limited rice. No other dairy products other than daily yoghurt were included. Sugar was limited to honey. No starchy vegetables were eaten and potatoes were eliminated. She ate mostly fish, lean meat, certain fruit and restricted nonstarchy vegetables.
(Khandalavala and Nirmalraj, 2015)

The results were pleasing, indeed.

Following this highly restricted diet, within a period of 3-6 months, the patient started noticing improvement with decreased frequency as well as firmer consistency of the stools, blood in the stools was absent and abdominal pain resolved. Within 6 months, she was able to return to her normal activities and career as a physician. Weakness and fatigue dissipated, while weight remained stable, without any regain. Anemia was found to have resolved, and hemoglobin was in the normal range. She continued with strict adherence to the diet due to the remarkable recovery, with dissipation of all of her symptoms over the next 18 months.
(Khandalavala and Nirmalraj, 2015)

There is more to the story.

Subsequent colonoscopy done 2 years after starting the diet was conducted in December 2012, and findings on endoscopy showed a remarkable absence of any inflammation. Biopsies obtained simultaneously confirmed the complete remission of UC with no inflammatory activity present. Since this time, she has noted that accidental consumption of wheat, peppers and other nonapproved SCD foods caused acute flare-ups, and the prompt elimination of these foods resulted in improvement of symptoms within a few days. She has not required hospitalization or additional therapy for UC since the institution of the diet and continues to be essentially in remission from the IBD. A few episodes of self-limited diverticulitis have been noted since. (Khandalavala and Nirmalraj, 2015)

You can find Mako's story in its entirety by searching online for: *Resolution of Severe Ulcerative Colitis with the Specific Carbohydrate Diet*, by Khandalavala BN and Nirmalraj MC, 2015. The authors of the paper believe it to be the first case report in the medical literature of successful remission from ulcerative colitis with SCD. But now Mako has company.

Case report: Sarah

There is another case report in the medical literature, just out, reporting on another ulcerative colitis patient who had a satisfactory response to the SCD. We'll call her Sarah.

Sarah was diagnosed with ulcerative colitis at age 14, complicated by primary sclerosing cholangitis, a rare complication involving inflammation and scarring of the bile ducts. This was successfully treated with antibiotics, yet her ulcerative colitis became progressively more difficult to manage.

This case is most interesting on three levels: **First**, *"all UC symptoms were also controlled as early as one week following the start of the diet."* **Second**, Sarah's gut bacteria composition was analyzed before the SCD *"and showed [a] remarkable loss of bacterial diversity."* **Finally**, it was concluded that vancomycin used to address her primary sclerosing cholangitis negatively altered her gut flora. Surprisingly, only after two weeks on the SCD, *"substantial changes in the fecal bacterial composition"* were documented (see Khandalavala and Nirmalraj, 2015).

The effectiveness of the SCD is attributed to its modification of the gut microbiome (Yamamoto et al., 2009; Khandalavala and Nirmalraj, 2015), so Sarah's experience is, indeed, consistent with the ulcerative colitis/dysbiosis hypothesis.

In the future, more SCD success stories, like the above two case reports, are bound to appear in the research literature. And likely, individual case reports will arise from a team of physicians in Seattle, Washington who embrace SCD as a therapy for IBD, ulcerative colitis included (Obih et al., 2016; Suskind et al., 2016). As to the effectiveness of the SCD, this team of investigators make the following observation:

> Given the constructs of the SCD in which high-fat, high-sugar foods and most food additives (i.e., food emulsifiers) are removed, a potential mechanism of action exists for the clinical benefits we have seen." (Obih et al., 2016)

It looks like the time we spent discussing food additives earlier in the book, including emulsifyers, was not time wasted. I hope you were paying close attention.

Now, for my take on the SCD.

SCD, as a diet for ulcerative colitis, is a diet with major problems. There is no attempt to deal with heme exposure, as does The Semi-Vegetarian Diet, so effectively. And there is no concerted effort to reduce iron exposure secondary to meat consumption. Both problems likely contribute to the perpetuation of ulcerative colitis, as we have previously discussed. Personally, I believe The Semi-Vegetarian Diet is the diet that has the most to offer the ulcerative colitis patient and is so much easier to follow than the SCD diet. Besides, the SCD diet may not be effective for everyone.

> Importantly, the SCD is not an effective symptom management regimen for every IBD patient. Some patients do not experience relief no matter the duration of treatment. (Khandalavala and Nirmalraj, 2015)

There are some concerns about nutrient deficiencies arising from following the SCD. I'm not particularly concerned, because there are plenty of nutritious foods to choose from in the list of allowed foods. Some of these concerns are raised by clinicians who don't seem to mind exposing you to drugs which are dangerous and often fail.

I think I have covered the SCD reasonably well, at least well enough we can move on. But before we reach the next chapter, we have another diet to briefly consider.

The IBD-AID

This diet is a spinoff of the SCD diet, which is why I tack it on to this chapter. *"The development of the IBD-AID is based on the theory that dysbiosis is caused by certain carbohydrates acting as substrates to pathogenic bacteria in the lumen of the gut."* (Knight-Sepulveda et al., 2015, emphasis added) Sounds just like the SCD, but there are some differences.

> *The IBD-AID has 5 basic components: (1) the modification of specific carbohydrates (eg, refined or processed complex carbohydrates and lactose); (2) emphasis on restoring the intestinal flora balance through ingestion of prebiotics and probiotics in the form of soluble fiber such as leek, onion, and fermented foods; (3) focus on decreasing total and saturated fats, eliminating hydrogenated oils, and encouraging the increase in food sources rich in omega-3 fatty acids; (4) review of the overall dietary pattern, identification of food triggers and intolerances, and detection of missing nutrients; and (5) food texture modification to enhance absorption and reduce intact fiber.* (Olendzki et al., 2014, emphasis added)

The food-texture component of this diet makes it special and why it stands out from the SCD as well as the other diets reviewed in this book. *"The initial foods recommended (soft, well-cooked foods without seeds) were based on the severity of the patient's symptoms."* (Knight-Sepulveda et al., 2015)

There are 4 phases to this diet. In **Phase I**, the starting point in the diet, we find the softest of the soft foods (well-cooked, cooked than pureed, no seeds or stems) and a variety of prohibited foods. If things go well, the patient advances to **Phase II**, which allows more food choices than allowed in Phase 1, but still requires foods to be of soft texture, well-cooked pureed or of a tender texture. **Phase III** liberalizes textures, increases food choices, allows soft greens with stems as tolerated. **Phase IV** is the final stage. It means that you have arrived. The food choices are basically SCD food choices. This stage is suitable for an individual who is in remission and without intestinal strictures. The above description of the 4 phases of the IBD-AID is based on the interpretation of this diet by Knight-Sepulveda et al., 2015. This reference is an <u>excellent</u> resource on this and other IBD diets. It's a must have, and available free on the web. The charts and tables of this paper are exceptional. *Exceptional!* Search for:

> Knight-Sepulveda K, Kais S, Santaolalla R, Abreu MT. **Diet and inflammatory bowel disease.** Gastroenterology & hepatology. 2015 Aug;11(8):511.

Making life a little easier

The SCD diet is, indeed, very complex and difficult to follow. Perhaps a kinder and gentler SCD diet is in order. *". . . today significant variations of a carbohydrate-free (reduced) diet exists. For example, a less strict version is a gluten-free diet."* (Ruemmle et al., 2016) Gluten-free dieting is an excellent idea, at least as part of an elimination-diet strategy to see if eliminating gluten for a few weeks helps and reintroducing gluten reverses any gains.

~*References*~

Dubrovsky A, Kitts CL. **Effect of the Specific Carbohydrate Diet on the Microbiome of a Primary Sclerosing Cholangitis and Ulcerative Colitis Patient.** Cureus. 2018 Feb;10(2).

Haskey N, Gibson DL. **An examination of diet for the maintenance of remission in inflammatory bowel disease.** Nutrients. 2017 Mar 10;9(3):259.

Khandalavala BN, Nirmalraj MC. **Resolution of severe ulcerative colitis with the specific carbohydrate diet.** Case reports in gastroenterology. 2015;9(2):291-5.

Knight-Sepulveda K, Kais S, Santaolalla R, Abreu MT. **Diet and inflammatory bowel disease.** Gastroenterology & hepatology. 2015 Aug;11(8):511.

Lewis JD, Abreu MT. **Diet as a trigger or therapy for inflammatory bowel diseases.** Gastroenterology. 2017 Jan 1;152(2):398-414.

Obih C, Wahbeh G, Lee D, Braly K, Giefer M, Shaffer ML, Nielson H, Suskind DL. **Specific carbohydrate diet for pediatric inflammatory bowel disease in clinical practice within an academic IBD center.** Nutrition. 2016 Apr 1;32(4):418-25.

Olendzki BC, Silverstein TD, Persuitte GM, Ma Y, Baldwin KR, Cave D. **An anti-inflammatory diet as treatment for inflammatory bowel disease: a case series report.** Nutrition journal. 2014 Dec;13(1):5.

Ruemmle FM. **Role of diet in inflammatory bowel disease.** Annals of Nutrition and Metabolism. 2016;68(Suppl. 1):32-41.

Suskind DL, Wahbeh G, Cohen SA, Damman CJ, Klein J, Braly K, Shaffer M, Lee D. **Patients perceive clinical benefit with the specific carbohydrate diet for inflammatory bowel disease.** Digestive diseases and sciences. 2016 Nov 1;61(11):3255-60.

*Web*MD, **Specific Carbohydrate Diet: Diet Review.** 2011 Written by Kathleen Zelman, MPH, RD
https://www.webmd.com/digestive-disorders/features/specific-carbohydrate-diet-review#1

Yamamoto T, Nakahigashi M, Saniabadi AR. **Diet and inflammatory bowel disease–epidemiology and treatment.** Alimentary pharmacology & therapeutics. 2009 Jul;30(2):99-112.

Chapter 16
The FODMAP diet

In conclusion, we have shown that an HFM [high FODMAP] diet causes an increase in fecal LPS [lipopolysaccharide, a Gram-negative cell wall component], likely from gut dysbiosis. **This induces mucosal inflammation, impairs permeability,** *and contributes to the development of visceral hypersensitivity. In contrast, an LFM [low FODMAP] diet reduces fecal LPS by modulating gut microbial composition. This decreases mucosal inflammation, improves gut barrier function, and prevents stress-induced visceral hyperalgesia.* **~Zhou et al., 2018, emphasis added**

We discussed FODMAPs earlier, in *Chapter 8*. In this chapter we will look a little deeper to help you see if a low FODMAP diet is the diet right for you. "So, once again, what are FODMAPs?" you ask. "And why should I pay attention to them?" you ask. "Are they evil?" you ask. Let's find out.

FODMAP is an acronym for Fermentable, Oligo-, Di-, Mono-saccharides And Polyols—all easily fermentable carbohydrates that may spell trouble. Bacteria can ferment them, and you get the privilege of experiencing diarrhea in addition to other symptoms. The following explains things a little more scientifically:

Malabsorption of rapidly fermented and osmotically active carbohydrates is not restricted to lactose and fructose. A family of poorly absorbed short-chain carbohydrates is now identified and is collectively termed FODMAPs (Fermentable, Oligo-, Di-, Mono-saccharides And Polyols). FODMAPs include (with examples) fructo-

oligosaccharides (wheat, onions, legumes), lactose (milk, ice-cream), fructose (apples, honey), galactans (legumes) and sorbitol (stone fruits, artificial sweetener). In theory, FODMAPs induce gastrointestinal symptoms via rapidity of gas production from their ready fermentation by intestinal bacteria and by increased fluid delivery to the large bowel via their osmotic effect. (Gearry et al., 2009)

FODMAPS are particularly relevant to patients with irritable bowel syndrome (IBS)—a condition complicated with abdominal bloating and discomfort . . . and perhaps a lot of diarrhea, to boot. You can easily see, should the ulcerative colitis patient have an issue with FODMAPS, trouble could ensue. In one study, *"33% of patients with ulcerative colitis experienced IBS-like symptoms of at least moderate severity in the preceding week."* (Gearry et al., 2009). So, with this elimination diet, the FODMAP diet, you can judge for yourself if FODMAPs are adding to all the misery. When you follow this diet, you <u>strictly</u> eliminate FODMAPs for 6 to 8 weeks (Knight-Sepulveda et al., 2015), then you begin to reintroduce FODMAPS, a few at a time, to see if symptoms worsen or reappear. And for the ulcerative colitis patient, a low FODMAP diet may be both helpful and informative.

A low FODMAP intake can help identify triggers, foods that elicit or exacerbate symptoms. On the other hand, a low FODMAP intake may help you feel better by reducing gut leakiness, and reducing gut inflammation, even in the colon (Zhou et al., 2018). Identifying offending FODMAPs would appear helpful to the ulcerative colitis patient. One benefit would be to decrease the degree of dysbiosis that can occur from high FODMAP consumption (Zhou et al., 2018). You have trouble with dysbiosis, remember?

Following this diet should probably be under medical supervision— as situations may arise and questions may need to be answered. Because of nutritional concern, it is recommended that the diet be no longer than 6 to 8 weeks in duration, as previously mentioned. Then the

reintroduction phase of the diet follows and liberalizes restricted foods. Responses are monitored. During this reintroduction phase a list of offending foods should emerge, revealing the items that should probably be avoided. I guess that's how the diet works. The list of allowed foods is rather large, larger than FODMAP foods to avoid, so it is a relatively easy diet to follow.

Should you be advised to follow this diet, before you begin, obtain a list of the food dos and don'ts, along with advice on how to reintroduce foods and how to identify the offenders. A dietitian familiar with the issues would be nice to have on your team. Also, a list of lactose-free foods would be helpful, as lactose-free milk is a "do" and normal milk and dairy are "don'ts."

For the best of the best FODMAP dos and don'ts food list, go to **IBSDiets.org**, click here and there, or follow this URL:

https://www.ibsdiets.org/wp-content/uploads/2016/03/IBSDiets-FODMAP-chart.pdf

IBSDiet.org has an excellent list of lactose-free foods, at the following address:

https://www.ibsdiets.org/ibs/lactose-free-food-list/

Don't let the brevity of this chapter fool you. The FODMAP diet is a big deal. This diet has helped many, many individuals, and should be helping more. It may help you.

Elimination diets

IBD patients are concerned about food and diet and use various dietary strategies in attempt to control or minimize gastrointestinal distress, as well as improve overall health. Up to 71% of patients with IBD believe diet affects their disease symptoms, with 90% of CD patients and 71% of UC patients employing elimination diets while in remission.
~Haskey and Gibson, 2017

Eliminating the foods that offend certainly sounds like a good practice for the ulcerative colitis patient to follow. To examine the effectiveness of an elimination diet, a study was conducted involving 18 ulcerative colitis patients who were divided equally into two groups. One group, the controls, were asked not to alter their food intake for six weeks, but simply eat a normal diet. The experimental group were asked to avoid foods that seemed to provoke symptoms, also for a 6-week period. *"At the end of the trial the diet [restricted] group displayed significantly fewer symptoms."* (Candy et al., 1995) The following observations certainly point out the individual differences encountered when dealing with the issues of offending foods.

> *There were no foods that provoked symptoms in all patients, though spiced and curried foods and fruits, especially grapes, melon and the citruses, commonly caused diarrhea. In only 2 patients were symptoms reproduced consistently on reintroduction of a particular food, pork in 1 case and yellow cheese in another.* (Candy et al., 1995)

I hope you don't find dairy products on the list of offending foods, as there is so much good in dairy. But consider it a possibility. And consider the possibility that a problem with dairy may simply be due to lactose intolerance.

> *Early investigators into the etiology of UC proposed that an allergy to milk proteins might be involved following observations that the removal of milk from the diet in a group of patients led to clinical improvement, whereas reintroduction of milk was followed by an exacerbation of disease. The discovery of raised circulating antibodies to cow's milk proteins in UC patients supported this theory. However, when sera from 51 UC patients were compared to controls, no differences were observed with respect to IgA or IgG, suggesting a nonimmunological reason, e.g., lactose intolerance for the benefits of a milk-free diet.* (Chapman-Kiddell et al., 2010)

Good luck in discovering the foods you should avoid. Taking the time and effort to discover offending foods, and the effort exerted to avoid them, may just pay off. There are a variety of diets that can help you identify the foods that provoke symptoms. Do your homework. Ask for advice.

A problem with milk fat

While the experts encourage the use of dairy, there is a strong case for making the dairy you consume non-fat. Here's the problem with milk fat: Milk fat has been found to be uniquely responsible for the overgrowth of a sneaky little pathogen named *B. wadsworthia* (Devkota and Chang, 2015).

But there may be an antidote to all this. One team of investigators found that the omega-3 PUFAs block the "blooms" of *B. wadsworthia* (Devkota and Chang, 2015).

~References~

Candy S, Borok G, Wright JP, Boniface V, Goodman R. **The value of an elimination diet in the management of patients with ulcerative colitis.** South African Medical Journal. 1995;85(11).

Chapman-Kiddell CA, Davies PS, Gillen L, Radford-Smith GL. **Role of diet in the development of inflammatory bowel disease.** Inflammatory bowel diseases. 2010 Jan;16(1):137-51.

Devkota S, Chang EB. **Interactions between diet, bile acid metabolism, gut microbiota, and inflammatory bowel diseases.** Digestive diseases. 2015;33(3):351-6.

Gearry RB, Irving PM, Barrett JS, Nathan DM, Shepherd SJ, Gibson PR. **Reduction of dietary poorly absorbed short-chain carbohydrates (FODMAPs) improves abdominal symptoms in patients with inflammatory bowel disease—a pilot study.** Journal of Crohn's'and Colitis. 2009 Feb 1;3(1):8-14.

Haskey N, Gibson DL. **An examination of diet for the maintenance of remission in inflammatory bowel disease.** Nutrients. 2017 Mar 10;9(3):259.

Knight-Sepulveda K, Kais S, Santaolalla R, Abreu MT. **Diet and inflammatory bowel disease.** Gastroenterology & hepatology. 2015 Aug;11(8):511.

Zhou SY, Gillilland M, Wu X, Leelasinjaroen P, Zhang G, Zhou H, Ye B, Lu Y, Owyang C. **FODMAP diet modulates visceral nociception by lipopolysaccharide-mediated intestinal inflammation and barrier dysfunction.** The Journal of clinical investigation. 2018 Jan 2;128(1):267-80.

Chapter 17

Polyphenols to the rescue

Polyphenols have antioxidant activity, modulate cell signaling pathways, and have anti-inflammatory properties. ~**Martin and Bolling, 2015**

*Besides their proven antioxidant qualities, polyphenols show health-promoting effects, because of their **marked ability to modulate inflammatory and immune responses**. In particular, most of them mainly target . . . Nf-κB, which controls the cell signaling cascades that are crucial in the development of IBD.* ~**Biasi et al., 2011, emphasis added**

Each type of polyphenol targets and binds to one or more receptors on immune cells *and thus triggers intracellular signaling pathways that ultimately regulate the host immune response.* ~**Ding et al., 2018, emphasis added**

I've mentioned polyphenols previously, but have not gone into detail. Now, we'll take a deep dive into the subject. Polyphenols have the potential to help rescue you from ulcerative colitis, so we need to have this conversation.

"What is a polyphenol?" You ask. *"Polyphenols are well-known, pharmacologically active compounds with immunomodulatory activity."* (Ding et al., 2018) "And, where do they come from?" They come from plants, plants that become foods. Remarkably, there are components hidden in foods that actively influence the immune system and do so on a regular basis, if given the chance. Typically, the effects are favorable. Remarkably, immune cells have receptors made just for polyphenols, allowing the activation of favorable signaling pathways and the initiation of favorable immune responses.

> Polyphenols promote immunity to foreign pathogens via various pathways. Different immune cells express **multiple types of polyphenol receptors that recognize and allow cellular uptake of polyphenols,** which subsequently activate signaling pathways to initiate immune responses. (Ding et al., 2018, emphasis added)

"Polyphenols also are pumped rapidly out of the cell, often back into the gut lumen" (Kaulmann and Bohn, 2016). Apparently, there are sophisticated systems in play that allow a polyphenol to enter a cell, do its thing, then promptly leave to subsequently enter and influence another cell that could use a little help along the way.

Polyphenols come in various forms and under various names, names such as **flavonoids, phenolic acids, tannins, lignans,** and **stilbenes** (Romier et al., 2009). But you don't need to know their names in order to receive their benefits. All you need to do is eat a healthy, plant-based diet to consume an amount of polyphenols that translate into beneficial responses.

> A vegetarian diet is abundant in polyphenols and antioxidants, which are secondary plant metabolites with many important properties such as anti-inflammatory, antimicrobial, antiradical and anticancer activity. (Duda-Chodak et al., 2015)

Indeed, the intake of polyphenols by ". . . humans on a healthful plant-based diet is approximately I G [gram] a day . . .." (Shapiro et al., 2007) Needless to say, if you don't eat your fruits and vegetables, you are at risk of a polyphenol deficiency. The immune system may suffer. Get used to the word suffer.

At the nutritional level, we normally think of food in terms of fats, proteins, carbohydrates, and vitamins and minerals—all necessary for life and for health. But we should also think of other components in food that offer us an advantage in life, components that favorably regulate the inflammatory response, components that favor overall health. Enter polyphenols. These dietary components are recognized as having special powers.

> Thus, **by reducing proinflammatory mediators and increasing anti-inflammatory markers in damaged intestinal tissues, polyphenols contribute to stopping the uncontrolled intestinal inflammation response, resulting in a decrease of colitis severity.** (Romier et al., 2009, emphasis added)

And we're in luck. There are over 8,000 different polyphenols from which to choose (Ding et al., 2018). These bioactive compounds *"can be subclassified into flavonoids, phenolic acids, tannins, and stilbenes."* (Ding et al., 2018) What should be appreciated here is that polyphenols are not generated for the benefit of the human, they are generated for the benefit of the plant, protecting the plant from insects, viruses, bacteria, and damage from solar radiation (Ding et al., 2018). By killing and eating (the fruit or the vegetable), benefit is transferred, receptors are given something to work with, and the human immune system catches a break. Intriguingly, the benefit is transferred not only to the human; the benefit is also transferred to the teeming multitudes of bacteria that live within the human gut.

> *Polyphenols play a vital role in the microbial community, as they have positive effects on the microbes. Simultaneously, these microbes promote the oxidation and degradation of polyphenols. Therefore*, **polyphenols may change the immune capacity of the host by altering the microbiota**. (Ding et al., 2018, emphasis added)

And speaking of the microbiota, it looks like polyphenols can do a number on the pathogens in your life. *"Regarding immune protection, polyphenols not only regulate the host immune system but also directly target the pathogen.*" (Ding et al., 2018)

So, what are the various benefits we can expect to receive from this or that polyphenol:

- Free radical neutralization (Perron and Brumaghim, 2009; Ding et al., 2018) and the upregulation of genes involved in antioxidant defense (Kaulmann and Bohn, 2016)

- Anti-inflammatory activity, including inhibition of NF-κB and "*reducing the production of several proinflammatory mediators*" (Romier et al., 2009; Ding et al., 2018)

- Regulation of intestinal mucosal responses (Ding et al., 2018)

- Selection of good bacterial resulting in suppressing the growth of pathogenic bacteria (Biasi et al., 2011; Duda-Chodak et al., 2015; Ding et al., 2018)

- Promotion of epithelial tight junction integrity (Biasi et al., 2011)

- Enhancement and stabilization of the intestinal mucus layer (of protection) (Kaulmann and Bohn, 2016)

- Antitumor activity (Ding et al., 2018)

- Iron binding—preventing epithelial cell overexposure to iron-associated free radicals and reducing iron acquisition by pathogenic bacteria (Perron and Brumaghim, 2009)

Although abundant in plant-based foods, polyphenols can also be found in beverages such as coffee, tea, wine—but not so much in a meal of burgers and fries. If one wishes to compensate for burgers and fries, one could eat polyphenolic-rich foods with this or with other meals. "*Rich sources of polyphenols include fruits like strawberry, raspberry, blueberry, cherry, black [current?], and grape; vegetables such as cabbage, beans, radishes, and whole grains; and beverages, namely tea and wine."* (Somani et al., 2015) Foods rich in polyphenols are also rich in other beneficial things, so the benefits received may be due to the combination of the polyphenols in concert with other beneficial things hidden within plant foods (Biasi et al., 2011).   Alternatively, an individual can supplement with polyphenols in a concerted effort to compensate for a lack of polyphenols in his or her diet.

There are a wide variety of plant extracts available, rich in polyphenols, that can be taken in powder or pill form to offset the lack of polyphenols in the diet or to address a particular medical concern.

What follows are the supplements that have captured my attention and may show promise in the battle against ulcerative colitis, demonstrated by the positive results achieved in experimental models and/or human studies of colitis. I'll be relatively brief, although much can be said about the health benefits of each of the following polyphenols. For no particular reason, we'll start with grape seed extract.

Grape seed extract

> *Proanthocyanidins from grape seeds are naturally occurring*
> *polyphenolic flavonoids possessing strong anti-inflammatory activity.*
> **~Somani et al., 2015**

The polyphenols in grape seed extract appear to be of great promise in the treatment of colitis.

> *GSE [grape seed extract] is produced as a by-product of the wine*
> *and grape juice industries. It contains high levels of phytochemicals*
> *such as flavonoids, which have been used for centuries to treat a*
> *wide range of ailments (digestive problem) without fully*
> *understanding their mode of action. The procyanidins in GSE are of*
> *particular interest as they have been shown to be potent*

antioxidants and free radical scavengers, further possessing anti-inflammatory, anti-viral, anti-carcinogenic, anti-bacterial, anti-allergic and vasodilatory properties. (Cheah et al., 2013)

In experimental colitis, grape seed extract ". . . *exerted a protective effect on recurrent colitis in rats by modifying the inflammatory response and promoting damaged tissue repair to improve colonic oxidative stress.*" (Wang et al., 2011) In this model of colitis, NF-κB signaling pathways were blocked by grape seed polyphenols (Wang et al., 2011).

In another model of colitis, it was found that grape seed extract beneficially affected the proximal colon and exerted *"no demonstrable effect"* on more distal regions of the colon (Cheah et al., 2013). The authors of this study raised the possibility that intra-rectal (enema-delivered) or micro-encapsulation of grape seed extract to delay its release could be employed to allow it to reach the distal colon, unabsorbed and unmodified, to treat disease in this region. However, grape seed extract may still help the distal colon if it is unable to physically reach this portion of the bowel, as its antioxidants can travel everywhere, via the bloodstream.

On to the next polyphenol.

Quercetin

Quercetin is a flavonol ubiquitously present in apples, onions, citrus fruits, berries, red grapes, broccoli, and tea. ~**Somani et al., 2015**

The dietary administration of QCN [quercetin] to restore intestinal immune hemostasis and enteric commensal flora balance is a potential and promising strategy IBD therapy. ~**Ju et al., 2018**

This compound, and its metabolites, are among the most studied of the polyphenols (Romier et al., 2009). Notably, quercetin and its metabolites can inhibit the activity of NF-κB (Romier et al., 2009). Recall, NF-κB acts like a master switch for proinflammatory responses. And by inhibiting NF-κB, polyphenols, quercetin included, can reduce the production of proinflammatory cytokines.

Besides placing limits on NF-κB expression, quercetin exhibits *"potent antioxidant activity"* which could come in handy in a disease dominated by oxidative stress (Somani et al., 2015; Serra et al., 2018). In addition, **rutin**, a derivative of quercetin, has been shown to improve experimental colitis by inhibiting TNF-α production and NF-κB signaling (Somani et al., 2015). As with many other polyphenols, rutin is available as a dietary supplement.

Unfortunately, quercetin and its derivatives may not reach the colon in sufficient quantities to make a substantial, <u>direct</u> impact on tissues of the inflamed colon.

> *The inability of quercetin to ameliorate colon inflammation in animal models could be related to the fact that <u>quercetin was rapidly absorbed in the upper intestinal portion and disseminated through the blood stream</u> without being able to reach pharmacological effective concentrations at the required site, i.e. the inflamed colon.* (Comalada et al., 2005, emphasis added)

But even if quercetin does not physically make it to the colon to effect change, not to worry. It may not have to reach the colon to influence the colon.

In one study, *". . . we found that QCN [quercetin] enhanced the bacterial clearance and anti-inflammatory macrophages in the mouse model . . .."* (Ju et al., 2018) This team of investigators found quercetin physically transformes the macrophage, converting it from a pro-inflammatory type (M1) into an anti-inflammatory (M2) type. The M2 macrophage phenotype acts to reduce inflammation and promote wound healing (Ju et al., 2018). As an ulcerative colitis patient, you need all the M2 macrophages you can get your hands on. Perhaps quercetin can come to the rescue in this regard. But there is a catch.

Realistically, high concentrations of quercetin *"cannot be achieved with a normal diet"* (Martin and Bolling, 2015), making supplementation likely necessary in order to achieve results like those achieved in experimental colitis, but caution should be observed (more later).

I think there is a lesson in all this. Even if a polyphenol doesn't make it to the colon, it may still be of value to the inflamed colon by indirect means. However, most polyphenols, perhaps at least some quercetin, reach the colon and exert direct, beneficial effects.

> *Ingested polyphenols are poorly absorbed; most remains in the intestinal lumen, mainly in the colon, where [they] may be particularly concentrated, thus being able to act as direct antioxidants, scavenging oxidant species or preventing their formation.* (Serra et al., 2018)

Pomegranate polyphenols

> *Different preparations of pomegranate, including extracts from peels, flowers, seeds, and juice, show a <u>significant</u> anti-inflammatory activity in the gut.* ~Colombo et al., 2013, emphasis added

From a polyphenol standpoint, pomegranate (PG) packs a punch. Surprisingly, *". . . pomegranate represents one of the most concentrated natural sources of quercetin known to man."* (Harrison and Cooper, 2008) Besides containing quercetin, pomegranate contains *"over 100 different phytochemicals"* (Colombo et al., 2013). (Phytochemicals are the family of plant-derived bioactive compounds that include the polyphenols.) Pomegranate must be something special as, *"Anti-inflammatory properties of PG and its major components have been widely described in the literature."* (Colombo et al., 2013) Given the considerable amount of attention paid to pomegranate, perhaps we should pay at least a little attention to the possibilities when it comes to the treatment of ulcerative colitis.

One advantage pomegranate offers, mentioned above, is its anti-inflammatory properties. In several models of IBD, a wide range of beneficial actions of various pomegranate extracts or other forms have been described (Danesi and Ferguson, 2017). These include decreases in the expression of TNF-α, decreases in colon tissue damage, and decreases in a variety of pro-inflammatory factors (Danesi and Ferguson, 2017).

Another advantage of pomegranate is its effect on the microbiota. Its polyphenols tend to decrease the numbers of pathogenic bacteria, while at the same time encouraging the growth of beneficial bacteria, like bifidobacteria and lactobacilli (Colombo et al., 2013).

It seems likely, the receptors made for polyphenols, mentioned earlier, could use a dose of pomegranate right about now, and perhaps on a regular basis, to lessen the chaos occurring in your colon.

I can't take the time to go into detail on the many health benefits of pomegranate, but you can! You can easily do the study necessary to determine if pomegranate, or any of its different extracts, are worthy of discussing with your physician. And while you're at it, bring up the word cancer.

> *The anti-inflammatory properties of pomegranate may protect against intestinal inflammation and decrease the risk of colon cancer.* (Kim et al., 2017)

Green- and black-tea polyphenols

> *Green-tea polyphenols and their aromatic compounds promote the intestinal growth of commensal Bifidobacterium and Lactobacillus, while repress growth of the pathogenic Clostridium perfringens and C. difficile, and that of Enterobacteriaceae, including the pathogenic Escherichia coli and Salmonella.* **~Biasi et al., 2011**

The most potent inhibitors of microorganism growth are probably the polyphenolic compounds from green and black tea. **~Duda-Chodak et al., 2015**

If you were to isolate a group of intestinal cells and expose them to the polyphenols found in tea, antioxidant effects as well as anti-inflammatory effects would be observed (Oz et al., 2013). If you were to chemically induce colitis in a mouse, you can make the mouse better with green tea polyphenols, and save the day (Oz, 2017). With green tea polyphenols, certain laboratory markers indicating the presence of significant inflammation were *"drastically decreased"* (Oz, 2017). The results were similar to the effects of sulfasalazine on the same markers of inflammation (Oz, 2017).

One of the principal polyphenols in tea is called EGCG, and *"accounts for about 40% of the total polyphenols in tea."* (Oz et al., 2013) Conveniently, EGCG can be taken as a supplement. And to give us a glimpse into its potential in the treatment of ulcerative colitis:

> *Another pilot study investigated the activity of . . . EGCG (400 mg or 800 mg) that was supplied to 15 individuals with mild to moderate UC, whereas another 4 were assigned to a placebo control. The response rate to the treatment after 56 d [day] of therapy was 66.7% and the active treatment remission rate was 53.3%; on the contrary, none of the control subjects showed signs of improvement.* (Salaritabar et al., 2017)

But wouldn't you know, there is a problem or two with EGCG. In animal studies, EGCG can induce macronutrient malabsorption (Salaritabar et al., 2017). This can be worked around to some extent by the coadministration of piperine to allow a lower dose of EGCG to achieve the desired effect (Salaritabar et al., 2017). Piperine enhances the bioavailability of EGCG, and in combination, results in significantly higher anti-inflammatory effects, and at a lower dose (Salaritabar et al., 2017).

Another problem to be aware of is the <u>potential</u> for kidney toxicity when high doses of EGCG are consumed, as observed in studies in mice (Baliga et al., 2014).

As with just about everything in this life, you can get too much of a good thing. Say, you read a study that describes the use of a high dose of EGCG (or a high dose of another polyphenol) required to make a positive impact on experimental colitis. This does not mean that an equivalent dose would be practical or appropriate in you, the human. Hence, the following warning:

> *The evidence indicates that EGCG at high doses exacerbates colitis in rodents, but at lower doses it is protective. It may be prudent for individuals with IBD to avoid excessive doses of supplemental EGCG for colitis management until further evidence of its safety and efficacy in human intervention studies.* (Martin and Bolling, 2015)

In view of the above, before embarking on a course of polyphenol supplementation be sure to seek the advice and approval from your physician. Caution is warranted, particularly with respect to high-dose EGCG.

Olive polyphenols

> *Epidemiological studies about consumption of functional foods, particularly extra virgin olive oil (EVOO) in Mediterranean countries, have showed important beneficial effects as antioxidant, anti-inflammatory, chemopreventive and anticancer.* **~Sánchez-Fidalgo et al., 2013**

"Olive oil is one of the cornerstones of the Mediterranean diet" (Larussa et al., 2019), comprising 40% of the calories consumed by those who follow this traditional dietary practice (Romero-Gómez et al., 2017), and providing *"the majority of the antioxidant activity attributed to the Mediterranean diet."* (Larussa et al., 2019)

Olive oil is rich in monounsaturated fatty acids, fats universally regarded as healthy (Romero-Gómez et al., 2017). If the olive oil under consideration is extra virgin olive oil (EVOO), it was manufactured in a manner that preserves its impressive antioxidant and anti-inflammatory properties (Sánchez-Fidalgo et al., 2013). To be sure, the ulcerative colitis patient can always use impressive antioxidant and anti-inflammatory properties and can certainly benefit from a healthier microbiome and improved gut health.

> It has been widely documented that EVOO is capable of exerting a targeted modulation on gut microbiota in comparison to other fats, and the consequent multiple benefits of this positive impact on intestinal microbiota have been described in mice. In humans, it has been demonstrated that a Mediterranean diet promotes healthy intestinal microbiota and protects from bowel alterations. (Larussa et al., 2019)

And not only is the oil of the olive loaded with polyphenols, so is the leaf of the olive tree.

> Olive leaves are considered to be a mixture of leaves and branches, derived from the pruning of the trees and the cleaning and harvesting process of the fruit. As well as the fruit, olive leaves contain an abundance of biophenols [polyphenols], which can be extracted using special processing techniques. This means that consumers can have access to one of the most beneficial components of olive oil without the necessity of consuming excessive amounts of it, therefore limiting the caloric intake which is still contained in the oil. (Larussa et al., 2019)

It would appear that EVOO, combined with olive leaf polyphenols, would be an impressive polyphenol-based strategy to address the oxidative stress and inflammation taking place in ulcerative colitis.

In one study, EVOO plus additional polyphenols (extracted from olive oil) *"possessed marked protective effects on experimental colitis* (Sánchez-Fidalgo et al., 2013). Alone, EVOO reduced the damage occurring in acute, experimental ulcerative colitis (Saxena et al., 2014).

> *The investigators observed that administering diets enriched with extra virgin olive oil (EVOO) significantly reduced the DSS [a chemical that damages the colon epithelium]-induced mortality by nearly 50 %, attenuated the clinical and histological [tissue] signs of damage, and improved the disease activity index.* (Saxena et al., 2014)

In both olive oil and in the olive leaf, there is a phenolic compound named oleuropenin (OLE). Demonstrated in tissue samples from the colons of ulcerative colitis, *"OLE exerts broad anti-inflammatory actions in inflamed colonic tissue from UC patients."* (Larussa et al., 2017) Furthermore,

> *Interestingly, treatment of biopsy samples with OLE led to an almost complete disappearance of the microscopic features of UC with a prominent decrease in the inflammatory infiltrate, absence of focal cryptitis/crypt abscesses and restoration of mucin-forming goblet cells.* (Larussa et al., 2017)

Clearly, olive oil polyphenols have promise written all over them. Potentially, they are suitable as a complementary therapy for ulcerative colitis.

Apple polyphenols

> *. . . apple ranks second for the total polyphenol concentrations and had the highest portion of free polyphenols when compared with other fruits.* ~**Denis et al., 2016**

Since an apple a day keeps the doctor away, I would be remiss if I didn't bring up the subject of apple polyphenols.

In a study in mice, apple polyphenols in the form of dried apple peel powder (DAPP) was used to see if it could make experimental colitis a bit more tolerable for the mice (Denis et al., 2016). It did (and there was great joy throughout the land). The investigators found the following:

> ". . . DAPP exhibits powerful antioxidant and anti-inflammatory action in the intestine and is associated with the regulation of cellular signaling pathways and changes in microbiota composition." (Denis et al., 2016)

In this study, the dose of apple polyphenols that worked for the mice *"are easily attainable in humans"* (Denis et al., 2016).

Dried apple polyphenols can be purchased online, in both capsule and power form. Hint: The apple peel is particularly high in polyphenols and makes for a great source of dietary fiber, one rounded teaspoon at a time.

Resveratrol and red wine polyphenols

> *Resveratrol, a natural (poly)phenol found in grapes, red wine, grape juice and several species of berries, has been shown to prevent and ameliorate intestinal inflammation.* **~Nunes et al., 2018**

> *Red wine can prevent or delay the progression of IBD by reducing oxidative stress and inflammation through polyphenols acting as free radical scavengers and modulators of inflammation-related genes. Additionally, red wine derived polyphenols can also act as prebiotics and antimicrobial agents. The alcohol within red wine can alter gastrointestinal (GI) pathogens such as Salmonella enterica and E. coli, at low concentrations.* **~Castaneda et al., 2018**

It is the polyphenols in red wine, including resveratrol, that is behind the health benefits and the anti-inflammatory properties of this popular beverage. The alcohol part, not so much. Alternatively, red wine polyphenols can be obtained from red grapes. Furthermore, the most prominent red wine polyphenol, resveratrol, can also be obtained from blueberries, dark chocolate, and peanut butter. But it is the supplement resveratrol that offers us the polyphenol in concentrate form. Let's see if resveratrol, in concentrated form, can influence experimental colitis. There must be some mice around here somewhere with nothing better to do. We'll need some funding.

While waiting for our funding, we might as well see what the other scientists have been up to.

In one study, investigators added a relatively low dose of resveratrol to the food of unsuspecting mice, at a dose equivalent to 58–232 mg in humans *and "which is far below that considered safe in humans"* (Cui et al., 2010). After one week of dietary resveratrol treatment, the chemical agent DSS was given to initiate ulcerative colitis of the mouse, then repeated a couple of times according to an established protocol. Resveratrol was continued at the same dose throughout the experiment until the experiment ended rather abruptly (for the mice), 10 weeks after its start.

And what did the investigators find? *"Significantly"* improved inflammation, downregulated TNF-α production, and a reduction in inflammatory stress (Cui et al., 2010). Furthermore, the investigators found that mice undergoing experimental colitis, and additionally given a cancer-causing agent, had a substantially reduced risk of colon cancer (from 80% down to 20%) if treated with resveratrol. The dose of resveratrol required to achieve such results was a dose equivalent to 300 mg/day in humans. A dose of 300 mg/day is not at all considered to be a high dose of this polyphenol.

That's enough for me! I'm convinced. Resveratrol has potential as a complementary treatment for ulcerative colitis, even at a relatively low dose. I think I'll call off our experiment and refund any research money that comes our way (minus nominal processing and handling fees).

Besides, why complicate the lives of mice when there are plenty of humans around to experiment on.

In a study of humans with ulcerative colitis, 500 mg/day of resveratrol was given for 6 weeks, then the results were evaluated (Samsami-kor et al., 2015; Nunes et al., 2018). In those who received resveratrol, laboratory markers which indicated the presence of inflammation were reduced as well as disease activity scores compared to controls, those who received placebo (fake resveratrol). (Samsami-kor et al., 2015; Nunes et al., 2018) The dose of resveratrol used in the study is well below doses considered safe in humans. And what is considered a safe dose of resveratrol for humans? According to Cui et al, a dose of up to 5,000 mg/day is regarded as safe.

As a treatment for ulcerative colitis, resveratrol is promising, very promising indeed. But so is . . .

Curcumin

Curcumin and resveratrol are two natural products, which have been described as potential anti-inflammatory, anti-tumor, and anti-oxidant molecules. ~**Zhang et al., 2019**

Curcumin is very safe and non-toxic, even when consumed in high doses (e.g. 8g/d). ~**Shapira et al., 2018**

Curcumin had been shown to achieve faster clinical remission and prevents relapse when used as an adjuvant with mesalamine. ~**Iqbal et al., 2018**

Curcumin is derived from the spice tumeric, and appropriately classified as a polyphenol. Curcumin is of great interest to the research community, the subject of a multitude of research studies. Important to the conversation, several studies have demonstrated great promise as a treatment for IBD, ulcerative colitis included. Apparently, people are not waiting for more research to be initiated or completed, they are experiencing the promise now. Curcumin is a very popular over-the-counter supplement for patients with ulcerative colitis. And there are good reasons why.

> *Various studies show that curcumin decreases reactive oxygen species, suppresses activation of nuclear factor kappa, and decreases nitric oxide synthetase expression, all which play an important role in the pathogenesis of UC.* (Iqbal et al., 2018)

Of no surprise (to me), several studies have demonstrated a higher rate of remission or maintenance of remission when curcumin is combined with standard therapy. So, let's take a quick peek at curcumin in action.

In the earlier part of this century, a Japanese team of investigators studied the capacity of curcumin to maintain remission. They gave 43 patients with quiescent ulcerative colitis curcumin, 1 gram orally after breakfast and 1 gram orally after the evening meal, in addition to sulfasalazine or mesalamine (Hanai et al., 2006). The control group of 39 patients, also with quiescent ulcerative colitis, received placebo (fake curcumin) along with sulfasalazine or mesalamine. The treatment period for both groups lasted for 6 months. If given the choice, I'd rather be in the curcumin group. In that group, only 2 of 43 patients relapsed. Whereas in the control group, 8 of the 39 patients experienced relapse. This study demonstrates the potential for curcumin to help maintain remission.

A later study, published in 2015 and performed by Lang and coworkers, curcumin was added to a regime of mesalamine just to see what would happen next (Lang et al., 2015). *"From the 50 patients enrolled and randomized, 26 patients received add-on curcumin, and 24 received add-on placebo."* (Lang et al., 2015) The dose of curcumin was 3 grams/day and the trial lasted for 1 month. And what happened next? *"Clinical improvement after 1 monthly of treatment was achieved in 17 of 26 patients (63.3%) receiving curcumin and in 3 of 24 patients (12.5%)*

receiving placebo . . .." (Lang et al., 2015) Furthermore, *"Endoscopic remission was observed in 8 of 22 patients (36%) in the curcumin arm and in 0 of 16 patients receiving placebo . . .."* (Lang et al., 2015) Endoscopic remission from a 1-month clinical trial is, indeed, quite impressive.

To be fair, other studies investigating curcumin as a treatment for ulcerative colitis have not yielded the same promising results. There are reasons for this, including a curcumin dose that was insufficient.

Hesperidin

> *In our study, colitis induced intestinal inflammation and was significantly improved after hesperidin treatment. These observations may be attributed to intestinal barrier restoration, with enhancement of the Nrf2 antioxidant pathway and regulation of Treg immune response.* **~Guo et al., 2019**

Hesperidin is a flavonoid found in citrus. Flavonoids are polyphenols. Flavonoids are something special.

> *. . . flavonoids are of great nutritional value in inflammatory diseases because they can block many pro-inflammatory proteins and can be considered natural inhibitors of inflammation, ameliorating the intensity of inflammation. In addition to the direct antioxidant activity, flavonoids are capable of activating diverse antioxidant and protective genes via nuclear transcription factors and also of inhibiting inflammatory pathways. Flavonoids influence the composition of the microbial flora, favoring the growth of bifidum and lactobacilli bacteria and stimulating an anti-inflammatory environment.* (Salaritabar et al., 2017)

Could the flavonoid hesperidin come to the rescue as a treatment for ulcerative colitis? Maybe. In a study of experimental colitis in mice by Guo and coworkers, it was discovered

Dietary supplement hesperidin has marked anti-inflammatory properties and restores intestinal barrier damage through regulation of oxidative stress levels involving Nrf2 signaling pathways and increasing the Treg population. (Guo et al., 2019)

Since Nrf2 was mentioned above, I suppose I will need to say more. Nrf2 is a protein within the cell that regulates the expression of specific proteins that protect against oxidative stress. In ulcerative colitis, it must be important, in as much as

Various studies have implied that Nrf-2 pathway is involved in intestinal inflammation and immunity events. Nrf2 pathway as a key anti-inflammatory signal may help with inflammation resolution. It was found that hesperidin had an effective role for anti-inflammation and anti-oxidation, and up-regulated the Nrf2 signaling in vitro and in vivo. (Guo et al., 2019)

Based on their study into the effect of hesperidin on experimental ulcerative colitis, Guo and colleagues concluded this:

Hesperidin can protect against intestinal inflammation via enhanced Nrf2 antioxidant pathway, increases the Treg population, and restores intestinal barrier function. (Guo et al., 2019)

Hesperidin apparently works in a mouse, but will it work in a human? It should be pointed out, the dose of hesperidin used in this mouse study was much higher than is practical for the human. But that doesn't mean that the dose of hesperidin recommended for humans can't help. It doesn't have to pull all the weight. If physician-approved, if you think it could help, you could add hesperidin to all the other flavonoids you will be consuming, once you come to your senses and start eating a plant-based diet.

Naringenin

> . . . *naringenin, which present in high concentrations in citrus fruits, was found to block NF-κB activation resulting in down regulating of the downstream target genes of NF-κB and COX-2 expression.* **~Al-Rejaie et al., 2013**

> *Pre-administration of naringenin significantly reduced the severity of colitis and resulted in down-regulation of pro-inflammatory mediators . . . in the colonic mucosa.* **~Dou et al., 2013**

Another citrus polyphenol worth looking into is naringenin. Like hesperidin, naringenin has demonstrated effectiveness in experimental ulcerative colitis (Saxena et al., 2014). One feature that may set this polyphenol apart from the others is an exceptional ability to dampen the signaling response to pathogenic bacteria (Dou et al., 2013). And why is this important?

> *It is clear that invariably there is dysbiosis in gut inflammatory diseases (e.g. inflammatory bowel disease (IBD)), and along with dysbiosis, there is dysregulation of pattern-recognition receptors that recognize pathogen-associated molecular patterns. Together, these are essential triggers of release of pro-inflammatory cytokines in the gut, which has paved the path towards discovery of pharmacological targets of IBD.* (Dou et al., 2013)

In experimental colitis, naringenin has been found to inhibit the signaling arising from the bacterial sensor TLR-4, and accordingly, acts to suppress NF-κB expression (Dou et al., 2013). Furthermore, *"Naringenin supplementation, significantly and dose dependently increased the colonic mucus content."* (Al-Rejaie et al., 2013) Importantly, suppression of NF-κB, and an increase in mucous production, are needed to achieve remission in ulcerative colitis.

Besides being abundant in citrus, like grapefruit, naringenin is also abundant in tomatoes (Dou et al., 2013). And obviously, it is abundant in a supplement bearing its name. As a supplement, naringenin needs to be regarded as a medication and should be used under physician approval and monitoring. It can interfere with the metabolism of some drugs and risk toxicity by interfering with the enzyme that holds drug levels in check (Mennen et al., 2005).

By no means have I exhausted our search for polyphenols that show promise in the treatment of ulcerative colitis, but I think we can move on. There are, however, a few things that should be considered before the chapter comes to a close.

The downside

*Moreover, a considerable amount of evidence is accumulating which supports the hypothesis that high-dose polyphenols can mechanistically cause adverse effects through pro-oxidative action. Thus, polyphenol-rich dietary supplements can potentially confer additional benefits but **high-doses may elicit toxicity** thereby establishing a <u>double-edge sword</u> in supplement use.* **~Martin and Appel, 2010, emphasis added**

*Nevertheless, administering high doses of polyphenols may also pose a certain risk to subjects already suffering from oxidative stress and inflammation, as **polyphenols could also act as prooxidants**, perhaps **especially when administered in high individual doses.*** **~Kaulmann and Bohn, 2016, emphasis added**

Be wary of high dose anything! Even natural substances can cause problems if taken in excess. For example, high dose quercetin may create more oxidative stress for the IBD patient to deal with, and cause additional harm (Kaulmann and Bohn, 2016). EGCG in high doses may also be problematic.

For example, flavonoids such as epigallocatechin gallate (EGCG), a powerful natural anti-inflammatory substance, inhibited acetic acid-induced colitis in rats at a dose of 50 mg/kg/day, but higher *doses exacerbated inflammation. In that study, the authors concluded: 'It may be prudent for individuals with IBD to avoid excessive doses of supplemental EGCG for colitis management until further evidence of its safety and efficacy in human intervention studies.' Similar to EGCG, green tea polyphenols at doses <0.5% inhibited DSS-induced colitis, whereas doses of 0.5–1% fortified colitis symptoms and mortality.* (Denis et al., 2016)

Although promising, although natural, clearly high-dose polyphenol supplementation is not without risk. In high doses:

- *"They could act as prooxidants, especially when given isolated and in high doses.*

- *"They may perturb absorption of other bioactive compounds, such as drugs or other phytochemicals.*

- *"They may interact and/or saturate pathways related to phase I/II metabolism, likewise increasing the concentration of otherwise more highly metabolized bioactive compounds.*

- *"They may have other negative effects following bacterial metabolism."*
(Kaulmann and Bohn, 2016)

The bottom line: Seek approval from your physician before proceeding with polyphenol supplementation, particularly high-dose polyphenol supplementation. Polyphenols offer great promise in the battle against ulcerative colitis, and certainly should not be ignored in the battle against this disease, but if done they need to be done right. I don't want to discourage you in the use of polyphenol supplementation; I just want to point you in the right direction. The right direction is the use of polyphenol supplementation under the guidance and watchful eye of a physician. This is particularly important, as polyphenols may interfere with the drug therapy your physician is likely to use. And so we read:

. . . caution should be exercised when designing adjuvant polyphenol treatments. Polyphenols can exert pharmacokinetic and pharmacodynamic interactions, leading to enhanced or antagonistic actions. Polyphenols can inhibit or induce Cyp3A4 expression, thus could potentially modulate pharmacokinetics of Cyp3A4-metabolized drugs such as prednisolone, budesonide, clarithromycin, cyclosporine used for IBD. (Martin and Bolling, 2015)

Final thoughts

The risk of consuming high doses of polyphenols from naturally polyphenol-rich foods is low. **~Mennen et al., 2005**

Common polyphenols in the diet are flavanols (cocoa, tea, apples, broad beans), flavanones (hesperidin in citrus fruit), hydroxycinnamates (coffee, many fruits), flavonols (quercetin in onions, apples and tea) and anthocyanins (berries). **~Williamson, 2017**

Rich sources of polyphenols include fruits like strawberry, raspberry, blueberry, cherry, black [current?], and grape; vegetables such as cabbage, beans, radishes, and whole grains; and beverages, namely tea and wine. **~Somani et al., 2015**

To play it safe, consuming a diet rich in a wide variety of polyphenols is perhaps the best approach to take in order to achieve an advantage. Because polyphenols *"originate only from plant-based food"* (Williamson, 2017), a diet that does this best would be a plant-based diet such as The Semi-Vegetarian Diet or the Mediterranean diet. Polyphenols are not stored in the body, as are other dietary components such as vitamins and minerals, so they need to be continually replenished to produce a sustained benefit (see Williamson, 2017). By following the right dietary pattern, and by eating a wide variety of plant foods, you can both supply and continually replenish these invaluable dietary components.

Zinc to the rescue?

> *Zn [Zinc] supplementation can be beneficial to the treatment of ulcerative colitis, because of the anti-inflammatory and antioxidant properties of Zn.* **~Soares et al., 2018**

> *Zn is an <u>indispensable</u> mineral for gut immunity and free-radical protection and both systems are impaired under ZD [zinc deficiency] conditions.* **~Iwaya et al., 2011, emphasis added**

> *Ulcerative colitis patients with zinc deficiency are at higher risk for disease-related complications.* **~Siva et al., 2016**

Zinc to the rescue? Perhaps. Although several studies (Dronfield et al., 1977; Van de Wal et al., 1993; Ananthakrishnan et al., 2015) have failed to find an association between zinc deficiency and the incidence of ulcerative colitis, or its severity, other studies indicate such an association does exist. Indeed, one study found *"a higher intake of zinc has a protective effect on the development of UC."* (Kobayashi et al., 2019) Another study reports *"UC patients who normalized their zinc within 12 months had reduced odds of IBD-related hospitalization and IBD-related complications compared with those who remained deficient."* (Siva et al., 2016)

What does zinc have to offer the ulcerative colitis patient? What does it do? What do you need to know?

- Zinc plays an important role in wound healing (Hwang et al., 2012; Siva et al., 2017)

- Zinc enhances gastrointestinal barrier integrity and function (Skrovanek et al., 2014); whereas zinc deficiency may lead to disruption of the intestinal epithelial barrier (Ananthakrishnan et al., 2015; Kobayashi et al., 2019)

- Zinc possesses anti-inflammatory and antioxidant properties (Soares et al., 2018)

- Zinc deficiency can result from chronic diarrhea (Hwang et al., 2012; Siva et al., 2017)

- Zinc deficiency can impair or completely suppress bacterial clearance by white blood cells (Gîlcă-Blanariu et al., 2018)

- Zinc is involved in the normal life cycle of cells and in DNA repair, with zinc sufficiency potentially protecting against cancers within the GI tract (Skrovanek et al., 2014)

- Low animal-protein diets can lead to zinc deficiency (Skrovanek et al., 2014)

- Diets rich in zinc-binding phylates from whole grains, nuts, and seeds may lead to zinc deficiency (Skrovanek et al., 2014)

- Proton Pump Inhibitors (Prevacid, Prilosec, Aciphex, Protonix, others), drugs used to reduce stomach acid, can lead to zinc deficiency (Skrovanek et al., 2014)

With respect to diets low in animal protein and high in whole grains, nuts, and seeds, such as vegan and vegetarian diets (to include The Semi-Vegetarian Diet), may lead to zinc deficiency, possibly requiring zinc supplementation to correct the problem (see Skrovanek et al., 2014). Should zinc supplementation be advised, attention should also be paid to the copper status of the individual, particularly when zinc doses greater than 50 mg/day are used (Skrovanek et al., 2014).

Certainly, zinc is something you should discuss with your physician.

Normalization of zinc was associated with improvement in these outcomes [hospitalizations, surgeries, disease-related complications] in patients with both CD and UC. (Siva et al., 2017)

And let me add this:

Thus, it is important to note that inflammatory gastrointestinal diseases are associated with changes in zinc metabolism or deficiency. (Paz Matias et al., 2015)

Selenium to the rescue?

Serum Se [selenium] concentrations were significantly influenced by the severity of UC, being higher in those with mild versus severe UC.
~Castro Aguilar-Tablada et al., 2016

Selenium is an *"antioxidant mineral."* (Castro Aguilar-Tablada et al., 2016) Selenium is also an *"essential trace element."* (Kudva et al., 2015) I'm beginning to like selenium already! It must be important.

What does selenium have to offer the ulcerative colitis patient? What does it do? What do you need to know?

- *Selenium deficiency "exacerbates experimental colitis"* (Castro Aguilar-Tablada et al., 2016)

- Selenium supplementation protects against chemically induced, experimental colitis (Barnett et al., 2010)

- Ulcerative colitis patients have low selenium levels (Nettleford and Prabhu, 2018)

- Selenium deficiency is associated with increased disease activity in UC (Gîlcă-Blanariu et al., 2018)

- *"Se concentrations were also positively correlated with the length of time of the disease in UC patients . . .."* (Castro Aguilar-Tablada et al., 2016)

- Selenium has anti-inflammatory and pro-resolving functions (Kudva et al., 2015)

- Selenium can downregulate NF-κB, the master regulator of inflammation (Nettleford and Prabhu, 2018)

- Selenium can upregulate PPAR-γ, a nuclear receptor that can repress proinflammatory signaling pathways associated with NF-κB (Nettleford and Prabhu, 2018)

- Selenium and increase Treg cell numbers (Nettleford and Prabhu, 2018)

- Selenium can influence the character of macrophages, shifting their activity from pro-inflammatory to anti-inflammatory (Castro Aguilar-Tablada et al., 2016)

- Vegetables grown in certain geographical regions known for low soil selenium levels (e.g., New Zealand) may be low in selenium (Barnett et al., 2010)

- Western diets characterized by highly refined foods are thought to be deficient in selenium (Barnett et al., 2010)

- Animal protein foods are good sources of selenium (Castro Aguilar-Tablada et al., 2016)

- Selenium deficiency may negatively alter the gut microbiome, favoring disease susceptibility (Kudva et al., 2015)

For the ulcerative colitis patient, selenium deficiency sounds like a real problem. Get used to the word real. Get used to the word problem. Add selenium to the list of topics to discuss with your physician. Supplementation may be in order.

Se [selenium] deficiency has been recorded in both UC and CD patients, and its deficit was correlated to an increased risk for multiple chronic inflammatory conditions, such as cardiovascular or endocrinological (thyroid) disease. (Gîlcă-Blanariu et al., 2018)

Iron-binding to the rescue

Interestingly, all major types of food polyphenols can strongly inhibit dietary non-haem iron absorption, and a dose-dependent inhibitory effect of polyphenol compounds on iron absorption has been demonstrated.
~Mascitelli and Goldstein, 2011

Furthermore, consumption of polyphenols inhibits nonheme iron absorption and may lead to iron depletion. **~Mennen et al., 2005)**

A high intake of dietary polyphenolic compounds may have important consequences on iron status. For example, tea, red wine and other beverages that are rich in polyphenolic compounds are known to inhibit the absorption on non-heme iron. **~Ma et al., 2011**

I've mentioned the dangers of iron before, particularly in *Chapter 9*, please review (again and again). As you may recall, iron can serve as a growth factor for pathogens, can harm the intestinal epithelia lining, promoting inflammation, and can add fuel to the fire in inflamed tissue. (Erichsen et al., 2005; Kortman et al., 2014) But there is good news.

Polyphenols can reduce the risks imposed by iron in the gut. Polyphenols can bind iron and keep it away from sites of absorption and from pathogen acquisition (Ma et al., 2011; Kortman et al., 2014). This is a win–win for the ulcerative colitis patient, for reasons previously given.

But the win–win can also be a double-edged sword. Notably, EGCG, grape seed extract, and green tea extract does this iron binding thing, perhaps all too well (Ma et al., 2011). Reportedly, polyphenol use can lead to iron depletion, (Mennen et al., 2005), which can lead to iron deficiency anemia. In individuals with an elevated risk for iron deficiency anemia, tea consumption can compound this risk (Mennen et al., 2005).

You to the rescue

By now, it should be obvious that **You** can play a decisive role in achieving and maintaining remission in ulcerative colitis. You can come to the rescue . . . of *you!* Showing up and taking a drug (or two, or three, or more) may work, but it may also not produce the results you desire. Besides, you're in a hurry to get back to normal. But to do things right, run your plans by your physician and receive the cooperation you need to succeed. *You* can learn all you can. *You* can develop a plan. *You* can seek the guidance assistance you need. *You* can succeed.

~References~

Ananthakrishnan AN, Khalili H, Song M, Higuchi LM, Richter JM, Chan AT. **Zinc intake and risk of Crohn's disease and ulcerative colitis: a prospective cohort study.** International journal of epidemiology. 2015 Nov 5;44(6):1995-2005.

Al-Rejaie SS, Abuohashish HM, Al-Enazi MM, Al-Assaf AH, Parmar MY, Ahmed MM. **Protective effect of naringenin on acetic acid-induced ulcerative colitis in rats.** World Journal of Gastroenterology: WJG. 2013 Sep 14;19(34):5633.

Baliga MS, Saxena A, Kaur K, Kalekhan F, Chacko A, Venkatesh P, Fayad R. **Polyphenols in the Prevention of Ulcerative Colitis: Past, Present and Future.** InPolyphenols in Human Health and Disease 2014 Jan 1 (pp. 655-663). Academic Press.

Barnett M, Bermingham E, McNabb W, Bassett S, Armstrong K, Rounce J, Roy N. **Investigating micronutrients and epigenetic mechanisms in relation to inflammatory bowel disease.** Mutation Research/Fundamental and Molecular Mechanisms of Mutagenesis. 2010 Aug 7;690(1-2):71-80.

Biasi F, Astegiano M, Maina M, Leonarduzzi G, Poli G. **Polyphenol supplementation as a complementary medicinal approach to treating inflammatory bowel disease.** Current Medicinal Chemistry. 2011 Nov 1;18(31):4851-65.

Castaneda L, Singharaj B, Martirosyan D. **Functional foods, conventional treatment and bioactive compounds, assist in management of inflammatory bowel disease.** Bioactive Compounds in Health and Disease. 2018 Sep 1;1(4):40-59.

Castro Aguilar-Tablada T, Navarro-Alarcón M, Quesada Granados J, Samaniego Sánchez C, Rufián-Henares J, Nogueras-Lopez F. **Ulcerative colitis and Crohn's disease are associated with decreased serum selenium concentrations and increased cardiovascular risk.** Nutrients. 2016;8(12):780.

Cheah KY, Bastian SE, Acott TM, Abimosleh SM, Lymn KA, Howarth GS. **Grape seed extract reduces the severity of selected disease markers in the proximal colon of dextran sulphate sodium-induced colitis in rats.** Digestive diseases and sciences. 2013 Apr 1;58(4):970-7.

Colombo E, Sangiovanni E, Dell'A'li M. **A review on the anti-inflammatory activity of pomegranate in the gastrointestinal tract.** Evidence-Based Complementary and Alternative Medicine. 2013;2013.

Comalada M, Camuesco D, Sierra S, Ballester I, Xaus J, Gálvez J, Zarzuelo A. **In vivo quercitrin anti-inflammatory effect involves release of quercetin, which inhibits inflammation through down-regulation of the NF-κB pathway.** European journal of immunology. 2005 Feb;35(2):584-92.

Cui X, Jin Y, Hofseth AB, Pena E, Habiger J, Chumanevich A, Poudyal D, Nagarkatti M, Nagarkatti PS, Singh UP, Hofseth LJ. **Resveratrol suppresses colitis and colon cancer associated with colitis.** Cancer prevention research. 2010 Apr 1;3(4):549-59.

Daglia M. **Polyphenols as antimicrobial agents.** Current opinion in biotechnology. 2012 Apr 1;23(2):174-81.

Danesi F, Ferguson L. **Could pomegranate juice help in the control of inflammatory diseases?.** Nutrients. 2017;9(9):958.

Denis MC, Roy D, Yeganeh PR, Desjardins Y, Varin T, Haddad N, Amre D, Sané AT, Garofalo C, Furtos A, Patey N. **Apple peel polyphenols: a key player in the prevention and treatment of experimental inflammatory bowel disease.** Clinical Science. 2016 Dec 1;130(23):2217-37.

Ding S, Jiang H, Fang J. **Regulation of Immune Function by Polyphenols.** Journal of immunology research. 2018;2018.

Dou W, Zhang J, Sun A, Zhang E, Ding L, Mukherjee S, Wei X, Chou G, Wang ZT, Mani S. **Protective effect of naringenin against experimental colitis via suppression of Toll-like receptor 4/NF-κB signaling.** British Journal of Nutrition. 2013 Aug;110(4):599-608.

Dronfield MW, Malone JD, Langman MJ. **Zinc in ulcerative colitis: a therapeutic trial and report on plasma levels.** Gut. 1977 Jan 1;18(1):33-6.

Duda-Chodak A, Tarko T, Satora P, Sroka P. **Interaction of dietary compounds, especially polyphenols, with the intestinal microbiota: A Review** Eur J Nutr. 2015; 54: 325-41. doi: 10.1007/s00394-015-0852-y.

Erichsen K, Ulvik RJ, Grimstad T, Berstad A, Berge RK, Hausken T. **Effects of ferrous sulphate and non-ionic iron–polymaltose complex on markers of** oxidative tissue damage in patients with inflammatory bowel disease. Alimentary pharmacology & therapeutics. 2005 Nov 1;22(9):831-8.

Gîlcă-Blanariu GE, Diaconescu S, Ciocoiu M, Ştefănescu G. **New Insights into the Role of Trace Elements in IBD. BioMed research international. 2018;2018.**

Guo K, Ren J, Gu G, Wang G, Gong W, Wu X, Ren H, Hong Z, Li J. **Hesperidin Protects Against Intestinal Inflammation By Restoring Intestinal Barrier Function and Up Regulating Treg Cells.** Molecular nutrition & food research. 2019 Feb 28:1800975.

Hanai H, Iida T, Takeuchi K, Watanabe F, Maruyama Y, Andoh A, Tsujikawa T, Fujiyama Y, Mitsuyama K, Sata M, Yamada M. **Curcumin maintenance therapy for ulcerative colitis: randomized, multicenter, double-blind, placebo-controlled trial.** Clinical Gastroenterology and Hepatology. 2006 Dec 1;4(12):1502-6.

Harrison AP, Cooper RG. **Quercetin: health benefits with relevance to TNF-alpha-linked inflammatory diseases.** Journal of Pre-Clinical and Clinical Research. 2008;2(2).

Hwang C, Ross V, Mahadevan U. **Micronutrient deficiencies in inflammatory bowel disease: from A to zinc.** Inflammatory bowel diseases. 2012 Apr 5;18(10):1961-81.

Iqbal U, Anwar H, Quadri AA. **Use of curcumin in achieving clinical and endoscopic remission in ulcerative colitis: a systematic review and meta-analysis.** The American journal of the medical sciences. 2018 Oct 1;356(4):350-6.

Iwaya H, Kashiwaya M, Shinoki A, Lee JS, Hayashi K, Hara H, Ishizuka S. **Marginal zinc deficiency exacerbates experimental colitis induced by dextran sulfate sodium in rats.** The Journal of nutrition. 2011 Apr 27;141(6):1077-82.

Ju S, Ge Y, Li P, Tian X, Wang H, Zheng X, Ju S. **Dietary quercetin ameliorates experimental colitis in mouse by remodeling the function of colonic macrophages via a heme oxygenase-1-dependent pathway.** Cell Cycle. 2018 Jan 2;17(1):53-63.

Kaulmann A, Bohn T. **Bioactivity of polyphenols: Preventive and adjuvant strategies toward reducing inflammatory bowel diseases—promises,**

perspectives, and pitfalls. Oxidative medicine and cellular longevity. 2016;2016.

Kim H, Banerjee N, Sirven MA, Minamoto Y, Markel ME, Suchodolski JS, Talcott ST, Mertens-Talcott SU. **Pomegranate polyphenolics reduce inflammation and ulceration in intestinal colitis—involvement of the miR-145/p70S6K1/HIF1α axis in vivo and in vitro.** The Journal of nutritional biochemistry. 2017 May 1;43:107-15.

Kobayashi Y, Ohfuji S, Kondo K, Fukushima W, Sasaki S, Kamata N, Yamagami H, Fujiwara Y, Suzuki Y, Hirota Y, Japanese Case-Control Study Group for Ulcerative Colitis. **Association between dietary iron and zinc intake and development of ulcerative colitis: A case-control study in Japan.** Journal of gastroenterology and hepatology. 2019 Mar 1.

Kortman GA, Raffatellu M, Swinkels DW, Tjalsma H. **Nutritional iron turned inside out: intestinal stress from a gut microbial perspective.** FEMS microbiology reviews. 2014 Nov 1;38(6):1202-34.

Kudva AK, Shay AE, Prabhu KS. **Selenium and inflammatory bowel disease.** American Journal of Physiology-Gastrointestinal and Liver Physiology. 2015 Jun 4;309(2):G71-7.

Lang A, Salomon N, Wu JC, Kopylov U, Lahat A, Har-Noy O, Ching JY, Cheong PK, Avidan B, Gamus D, Kaimakliotis I. **Curcumin in combination with mesalamine induces remission in patients with mild-to-moderate ulcerative colitis in a randomized controlled trial.** Clinical Gastroenterology and Hepatology. 2015 Aug 1;13(8):1444-9.

Larussa T, Imeneo M, Luzza F. **Olive Tree Biophenols in Inflammatory Bowel Disease: When Bitter is Better.** International journal of molecular sciences. 2019 Jan;20(6):1390.

Larussa T, Oliverio M, Suraci E, Greco M, Placida R, Gervasi S, Marasco R, Imeneo M, Paolino D, Tucci L, Gulletta E. **Oleuropein decreases cyclooxygenase-2 and interleukin-17 expression and attenuates inflammatory damage in colonic samples from ulcerative colitis patients.** Nutrients. 2017;9(4):391.

Ma Q, Kim EY, Lindsay EA, Han O. **Bioactive dietary polyphenols inhibit heme iron absorption in a dose-dependent manner in human intestinal Caco-2 cells.** Journal of food science. 2011 Jun;76(5):H143-50.

Martin KR, Appel CL. **Polyphenols as dietary supplements: a double-edged sword.** Nutr Diet Suppl. 2010;2(1):12.

Martin DA, Bolling BW. **A review of the efficacy of dietary polyphenols in experimental models of inflammatory bowel diseases.** Food & function. 2015;6(6):1773-86.

Mascitelli L, Goldstein MR. **Inhibition of iron absorption by polyphenols as an anti-cancer mechanism.** QJ Med. 2011;104:459-61.

Mennen LI, Walker R, Bennetau-Pelissero C, Scalbert A. **Risks and safety of polyphenol consumption.** The American journal of clinical nutrition. 2005 Jan 1;81(1):326S-9S.

Nettleford S, Prabhu K. **Selenium and selenoproteins in gut inflammation—A review.** Antioxidants. 2018 Mar;7(3):36.

Nunes S, Danesi F, Del Rio D, Silva P. **Resveratrol and inflammatory bowel disease: the evidence so far.** Nutrition research reviews. 2018 Jun;31(1):85-97.

Oz H. **Chronic inflammatory diseases and green tea polyphenols.** Nutrients. 2017;9(6):561.

Oz HS, Chen T, de Villiers WJ. **Green tea polyphenols and sulfasalazine have parallel anti-inflammatory properties in colitis models.** Frontiers in immunology. 2013 Jun 5;4:132.

Paz Matias J, Costa e Silva DM, Clímaco Cruz KJ, Gomesda Silva K, Monte Feitosa M, Oliveira Medeiros LG, do Nascimento Marreiro D, do Nascimento Nogueira N. **Effect of zinc supplementation on superoxide dismutase activity in patients with ulcerative rectocolitis.** Nutricion hospitalaria. 2015;31(3).

Perron NR, Brumaghim JL. **A review of the antioxidant mechanisms of polyphenol compounds related to iron binding.** Cell biochemistry and biophysics. 2009 Mar 1;53(2):75-100.

Romero-Gómez M, Zelber-Sagi S, Trenell M. **Treatment of NAFLD with diet, physical activity and exercise.** Journal of hepatology. 2017 Oct 1;67(4):829-46.

Romier B, Schneider YJ, Larondelle Y, During A. **Dietary polyphenols can modulate the intestinal inflammatory response.** Nutrition reviews. 2009 Jul 1;67(7):363-78.

Salaritabar A, Darvishi B, Hadjiakhoondi F, Manayi A, Sureda A, Nabavi SF, Fitzpatrick LR, Nabavi SM, Bishayee A. **Therapeutic potential of flavonoids in inflammatory bowel disease: A comprehensive review.** World journal of gastroenterology. 2017 Jul 28;23(28):5097.

Samsami-kor M, Daryani NE, Asl PR, Hekmatdoost A. **Anti-inflammatory effects of resveratrol in patients with ulcerative colitis: a randomized, double-blind, placebo-controlled pilot study.** Archives of medical research. 2015 May 1;46(4):280-5.

Sánchez-Fidalgo S, Cárdeno A, Sánchez-Hidalgo M, Aparicio-Soto M, de la Lastra CA. **Dietary extra virgin olive oil polyphenols supplementation modulates DSS-induced chronic colitis in mice.** The Journal of nutritional biochemistry. 2013 Jul 1;24(7):1401-13.

Saxena A, Kaur K, Hegde S, Kalekhan FM, Baliga MS, Fayad R. **Dietary agents and phytochemicals in the prevention and treatment of experimental ulcerative colitis.** Journal of traditional and complementary medicine. 2014 Oct 1;4(4):203-17.

Serra G, Incani A, Serreli G, Porru L, Melis MP, Tuberoso CI, Rossin D, Biasi F, Deiana M. **Olive oil polyphenols reduce oxysterols-induced redox imbalance and pro-inflammatory response in intestinal cells.** Redox biology. 2018 Jul 1;17:348-54.

Shapira S, Leshno A, Katz D, Maharshak N, Hevroni G, Jean-David M, Kraus S, Galazan L, Aroch I, Kazanov D, Hallack A. **Of mice and men: a novel dietary supplement for the treatment of ulcerative colitis.** Therapeutic advances in gastroenterology. 2018 Jan 3;11:1756283X17741864.

Shapiro H, Singer P, Halpern Z, Bruck R. **Polyphenols in the treatment of inflammatory bowel disease and acute pancreatitis.** Gut. 2007 Mar 1;56(3):426-36.

Siva SS, Rubin DT, Gulotta G, Wroblewski K, Pekow J. P151 **Ulcerative colitis patients with zinc deficiency are at higher risk for disease-related complications.** Journal of Crohn's and Colitis, Volume 10, Issue suppl_1, 1 March 2016, Pages S166–S167.

Siva S, Rubin DT, Gulotta G, Wroblewski K, Pekow J. **Zinc deficiency is associated with poor clinical outcomes in patients with inflammatory bowel disease.** Inflammatory bowel diseases. 2017 Jan 1;23(1):152-7.

Skrovanek S, DiGuilio K, Bailey R, Huntington W, Urbas R, Mayilvaganan B, Mercogliano G, Mullin JM. **Zinc and gastrointestinal disease.** World journal of gastrointestinal pathophysiology. 2014 Nov 15;5(4):496.

Soares NR, de Moura MS, de Pinho FA, Silva TM, de Lima Barros SÉ, de Castro Amorim A, Vieira EC, Neto JM, Parente JM, e Cruz MD, do Nascimento Marreiro D. **Zinc supplementation reduces inflammation in ulcerative colitis patients by downregulating gene expression of Zn metalloproteins.** PharmaNutrition. 2018 Sep 1;6(3):119-24.

Somani SJ, Modi KP, Majumdar AS, Sadarani BN. **Phytochemicals and their potential usefulness in inflammatory bowel disease.** Phytotherapy research. 2015 Mar;29(3):339-50.

Van de Wal Y, Veer AV, Verspaget HW, Mulder TP, Griffioen G, Van Tol EA, Peña AS, Lamers CB. **Effect of zinc therapy on natural killer cell activity in inflammatory bowel disease.** Alimentary pharmacology & therapeutics. 1993 Jun;7(3):281-6.

Wang YH, Ge B, Yang XL, Zhai J, Yang LN, Wang XX, Liu X, Shi JC, Wu YJ. **Proanthocyanidins from grape seeds modulates the nuclear factor-kappa B signal transduction pathways in rats with TNBS-induced recurrent ulcerative colitis.** International immunopharmacology. 2011 Oct 1;11(10):1620-7.

Williamson G. **The role of polyphenols in modern nutrition.** Nutrition bulletin. 2017 Sep;42(3):226-35.

Zhang L, Xue H, Zhao G, Qiao C, Sun X, Pang C, Zhang D. **Curcumin and resveratrol suppress dextran sulfate sodium-induced colitis in mice.** Molecular medicine reports. 2019 Apr 1;19(4):3053-60.

Chapter 18
Bile acid advantage

*Dietary fat affects bile acid metabolism, because the absorption of fat requires an increase in bile flow. Consequently, **a high-fat diet elevates the fecal concentration of bile acids**. ~Stenman et al., 2012, emphasis added*

Bile acid levels are specific to an individual due to individual gut microbiome compositions. ~Heinken et al., 2017

Altered BA [bile acid] transformation in the gut lumen can erase the anti-inflammatory effects of some BA species on gut epithelial cells and could participate in the chronic inflammation loop of IBD. ~Duboc et al., 2013, emphasis added

It is likely bile acids play some kind of role in ulcerative colitis, but I doubt if the subject has come up during any one of your many doctor appointments. Not sure why. Perhaps it is thought that there is not much the patient can do about what his or her bile acids are up to. In this chapter, let's see if there is a thing or two we can do that may give you a bile acid advantage in your battle against ulcerative colitis.

Let's begin with this:

Notably, in colonic biopsies from UC patients with active disease, there has been shown to be . . . a reduction in the enzymes responsible for detoxification process from BAs [bile acids] in the epithelial cells. (Tiratterra et al., 2018)

This is significant, given the fact that if not properly handled, bile acids can harm the very individual who created them. Keep this in mind as we continue.

There are other problems associated with bile acids the ulcerative colitis patient is likely dealing with, silently, and all alone. We will explore all this shortly. But first, let's get the basics out of the way. And to keep things streamlined, I will cover the basics referring only to a few references, as most of what follows is well established.

Bile acid basics

Bile acids are a peculiar family of steroidal molecules generated by the coordinated cooperation between host and its intestinal microbiota. **~Fiorucci et al., 2018**

*. . . the past two decades have seen a renaissance in research activity that has firmly placed **bile acids** as being <u>central</u> to maintenance of our overall health.* **~Hegyi et al., 2018, emphasis added**

Bile acids (also called bile salts) are a family of molecules synthesized in the liver and sent forth to serve. They are formed from cholesterol, discharged to collect within the gall bladder, and subsequently expelled from the gall bladder into the upper small intestine (duodenum) when required to break dietary fat into tiny little pieces to aid in its uptake. But I'm getting a little ahead of the story. It's not yet dinner time.

In the liver, newly synthesized bile acids, called **primary bile acids**, are ultimately formed (joined/conjugated) to include a molecule of glycine or a molecule of taurine, both of which are amino acids. **Significantly, <u>unless acted upon by bacteria in a special way, a primary bile acid remains a primary bile acid</u> as it travels unchanged through the small intestine, assisting in the breakdown of fat for uptake by this**

portion of the bowel. However, should the primary bile acid meet up with a bacterium equipped with the skills to "deconjugate," the magic happens. Off comes the glycine or the taurine and the primary bile acid is subsequently exposed to other bacterial actions that can further modify the primary bile acid molecule and turn it into one of a variety of what are called **secondary bile acids.** The change from a primary to a secondary bile acid alters the biological activity of the bile acid, determines how it will relate to the intestinal epithelial cell, and determines how it will interact with what are called **bile acid receptors.** But let's back up a little.

Typically, the primary bile acid cannot leave the small intestine unless it is first deconjugated by a bacterium. In its conjugated state, it exists in a form that prevents its passage through the epithelium, and simply cannot leave unless it passes into the colon (Laukens et al., 2014). However, once it is deconjugated by a bacterium, at any location within the small intestine, it is then able to easily transfer, *"passively,"* through the epithelium and return to the liver for reprocessing (Hofmann, 1999; Asgharpour et al., 2015; Dawson and Karpen, 2015). But let's assume for a moment that none of this has occurred and the primary bile acid reaches the terminal ileum (end portion of the small intestine), wholly intact. Then what?

Having escaped deconjugation, upon arriving in the terminal ileum the primary bile acid is given the opportunity to establish contact with specialized transporters built into the ileal epithelial cell. These transporters, in association with intracellular transport proteins, can *"actively"* transport the primary bile acid, as is, in and through the cell, and direct it back to the liver via the portal vein. The liver will subsequently take the steps necessary to return it back to the upper small intestine, via the gallbladder, to once again assist in the digestion of dietary fat or do the other things that bile acids do. The circulation of bile acids from the liver to the intestine then back to the liver then back to the intestine then back to the liver and so on is called the **enterohepatic**

circulation. A particular bile acid may serve with dignity and distinction within the intestine then return to the liver, then back to the intestine, up to 10 times a day (Stamp and Jenkins, 2008).

How are you doing so far? I know, all this can be a little difficult to wrap one's mind around. Just hang on for a few more moments and we'll have the basics under our belt. Do your best. That's all I ask.

Both active and passive transport of bile acids out of the small intestine—be it a primary bile acid or a secondary bile acid—is quite efficient, allowing only approximately 5% of all bile acids created to transfer from the terminal ileum into the colon and give the bacteria in the colon something important to do. Ordinarily, colonic bacteria deconjugate all the primary bile acids they can get their hands on and further transform them into secondary bile acids. These actions will allow the bile acid to easily leave the colon, by passive diffusion through the colonocyte, and will allow it to return to the liver for further processing, for reconjugation, and for recirculation (Hegyi et al., 2018). That being said, apart from passive diffusion, there is at least some chance the primary bile acid will recirculate from the colon and back to the liver, intact, via specialized transporters build into the colonocyte (Nguyen et al., 2018). However, the cells of the colon are not generally recognized for receptor-mediated uptake of primary bile acids, probably indicating a minor role for receptor-mediated uptake at the level of the colonocyte. So, in order to get back to the liver, the primary bile acid will need to rely upon first being transformed into a secondary bile acid.

Before the secondary bile acid diffuses into the colonocyte and returns to the liver, the secondary bile acid has something important to do. It has an opportunity to meet up with a cell-surface receptor (more later) and initiate a variety of biological effects, some of which favorably influence the immune system and some of which promote the integrity of the intestinal barrier (Baars et al., 2015; Fiorucci et al., 2018; Hegyi et al., 2018).

If the uptake of either primary or secondary bile acids by the colonocyte, either passively or actively, fails to occur, the bile acid will be lost in the feces, never to return, gone for good, totally forgotten. Ordinarily, only a small amount of bile acids are lost each day in this manner.

This ends the bile acid basics. You made it through! (Your certificate of achievement is in the mail.) With the basics now out of the way, we can get down to business.

Problems worth mentioning

A high concentration of bile acids in the intestine may have a significant role in the pathophysiology of ulcerative colitis at active phase. ~Tanida et al., 1986, emphasis added

Dysregulation of microbial/bile acid interactions can negatively impact mucosal function, contributing to the onset of intestinal and metabolic disorders. ~Hegyi et al., 2018

Altered BA [bile acid] transformation in the gut lumen can erase the anti-inflammatory effects of some BA species on gut epithelial cells and could participate in the chronic inflammation loop of IBD. ~Duboc et al., 2013

. . . BAs [bile acids] act as strong stimulators of colorectal cancer (CRC) initiation by damaging colonic epithelial cells, genomic destabilization, apoptosis [programed cell death] resistance, and cancer stem cells-like formation. ~Nguyen et al., 2018

If you paid close attention to the above references, you learned a number of important things: **1)** high levels of bile acids may play a role in active ulcerative colitis; **2)** some bile acids have anti-inflammatory effects—but this can all be erased by altered bile acid transformation, such as occurs in IBD; **3)** bile acids can initiate and perpetuate intestinal inflammation; and, **4)** bile acids are strong stimulators of colorectal cancer.

And if you place the above in context with the finding that the ulcerative colitis patient has *"a reduction in the enzymes responsible for detoxification process from BAs in the epithelial cells"* (Tiratterra et al., 2018), you can easily see why bile acid dysregulation is a real threat to the patient with ulcerative colitis. So, perhaps you can easily see why bile acids are worthy of discussion.

At this point in the conversation you may be wondering what is behind all the bile acid dysfunction in ulcerative colitis? That would be dysbiosis.

> *We demonstrated that IBD-associated <u>dysbiosis leads to impaired BA metabolism</u> characterised by <u>defective deconjugation,</u> transformation and desulphation. Moreover, we demonstrated that IBD-associated BA dysmetabolism within the gut lumen might enhance the intestinal epithelial inflammatory response, and thus, worsen IBD.* (Duboc et al., 2013, emphasis added)

> *In IBD patients, <u>fecal conjugated bile acid levels are higher while secondary bile acid levels are lower,</u> and **<u>the deconjugation and transformation abilities of IBD-associated microbiomes are impaired</u>**.* (Heinken et al., 2017, emphasis added)

Looking a little closer, it has been determined that the bacterial species that convert primary to secondary bile acids are *"depleted"* in ulcerative colitis (Heinken   et al., 2017).   This is important, in that *"<u>Complementary</u> microbe-microbe interactions are required for secondary bile acid biosynthesis in individual communities."* (Heinken et al., 2017, emphasis added)

So, here's the deal: **In the context of dysbiosis, IBD patients have reduced microbial diversity leading to impaired <u>bacterial</u> conversion of primary to secondary bile acids** (Heinken et al., 2017; Van den Bossche et al., 2017), **leading to *"reduced production of secondary bile acids and*** *decreased levels of sulfated bile acids"* (Joyce and Gahan 2017, emphasis added). However, in one respect, this might come in handy as secondary bile acids—particularly the one called lithocholic acid (LCA)—have been singled out as particularly toxic (Ajouz et al., 2014). In fact, **LCA is *"the most toxic substance produced in the body* and a known carcinogen."** (Stamp and Jenkins, 2008, emphasis added) Additionally, another secondary bile acid, **DCA**, also has carcinogenic potential (Ajouz et al., 2014; Martínez-Augustin and de Medina, 2008). So less of these things hanging around the better, particularly so if one is serious about decreasing the elevated risk of colon cancer associated with ulcerative colitis.

> *The secondary bile acids, such as deoxycholic acid [DCA] and lithocholic acid [LCA], have been considered to be cytotoxic for normal colonic crypt cells, resulting in an increased compensatory proliferation of colonic epithelium cells, which is associated with an increased risk of colon cancer.* (Han et al., 2009)

But the cancer risk is not just related to the secondary bile acid. Primary bile acids also pose a risk for colon cancer.

> *. . . **primary bile acids retain carcinogenic action**, and a high concentration of primary bile acids together with the similar concentration of lithocholic acid [LCA] in colitis patients should be taken into consideration.* (Tanida et al., 1986, emphasis added)

Apart from cancer risk, an excess of either primary or secondary bile acids can have a negative effect on intestinal barrier function.

> *. . . if levels of luminal conjugated [AKA, primary] bile acids increase sufficiently, loss of tight junction integrity occurs . . ..* (Hegyi et al., 2018)

Elevations in the levels of secondary bile acids . . . are believed to increase epithelial permeability, leading to enhanced bacterial translocation and prolonged low-grade mucosal inflammation, ultimately contributing to cancer development. (Hegyi et al., 2018)

Besides cancer risk and impaired integrity of the intestinal epithelial barrier, there are other bile acid-associated problems facing the ulcerative colitis patient, to be sure. But you get the idea. I could go on and on, but your eyes are noticeably glazed over, strongly suggesting that I am pushing the limit and we need to move on. I hope the message got through to you, loud and clear: **You have a problem with bile acids, and your bile acid issues should be addressed.** (My opinion.)

*Bile acid levels are specific to an individual due to individual gut microbiome compositions. Consequently, alterations in bile acid human-microbiome co-metabolism in disease states are also **individual-specific and interventions should be targeted.*** (Heinken et al., 2017, emphasis added)

So, what can be done?

*. . . the **Western diet**, which is **rich in fat** and **low in fiber**, leads to alterations in the enterohepatic circulation <u>leading to increased synthesis and colonic delivery of bile acids</u>.* **~Hegyi et al., 2018, emphasis added**

And just like that, we have a couple of things to do, related to diet, related to the Western diet, related to dietary fat, related to fiber, related to you. Let's start with dietary fat. This one is easy!

Low-fat dieting

The Western high-fat/high-sugar/low-fiber diet, which is associated with the development of many diseases, including CRC [colorectal cancer],

*IBD, IBS, obesity, and diabetes, is also **associated with a significantly altered bile acid signature.** These changes occur, at least partly, as a consequence of __increased hepatic bile acid biosynthesis in response to the high intake of fat__ and partly to their altered metabolism due to the presence of a "Westernized" microbiota in the colon . . ..*

. . . avoidance of a Western diet in favor of one containing less fat and more fiber appears to be __the simplest approach__ to modulate the intestinal bile acid signature for prevention of intestinal diseases.
~Hegyi et al., 2018, emphasis added

Can you see why I previously expended a great deal of time and effort discussing diet, particularly low-fat dieting? I wanted you to gain a bile acid advantage. And now, does my promotion of The Semi-Vegetarian Diet make complete and total sense? (You're nodding "Yes," aren't you?) This diet makes sense because, among other things, it reduces the production of bile acids in excess, an excess that can reach the colon, an excess known to provoke a variety of negative effects (in excess).

__Dietary fat affects bile acid metabolism__*, because the absorption of fat requires an increase in bile flow. Consequently, **a high-fat diet elevates the fecal concentration of bile acids.*** (Stenman et al., 2012, emphasis added)

A diet high in meat has been shown to significantly increase both the levels of taurine conjugation to bile acids and the production of hydrogen sulfide in the colon. A relationship exists between the generation of hydrogen sulfide in the colon and chronic GI illness, such as inflammatory bowel disease and colon cancer. (Ridlon et al., 2006)

And in this context, let's not forget about dietary fiber.

In addition, diets rich in fat and poor in fiber can increase more than 10-fold the amount of taurine conjugated BAs [bile acids] reaching the colon, due to higher conjugation and production (higher conjugation reduces ileal absorption). (Martínez-Augustin and de Medina, 2008)

With The Semi-Vegetarian Diet, all bases are covered here, low in fat, high in fiber, replete with advantage—a diet that reduces bile acid production and colonic bile acid exposure, while at the same time provides the dietary fiber fire power needed to deal with the bile acids that reach the colon in excess. And how does dietary fiber help deal with the dangers of colonic bile acid excess? Dietary fiber can bind bile acids and keep them from interacting with the colonic epithelium. It also assists in their elimination.

Dietary fiber (prebiotics)

The consequences of consuming a diet low in fiber cannot be ignored. Low-fiber diets have been associated with heart disease, type 2 diabetes, inflammatory bowel disease (IBD), and certain types of cancer. **~Rose et al., 2007**

Dietary fibers (from vegetables and fruits) can bind LCA and aid in its excretion in stool; as such, fibers can protect against colon cancer. **~Ajouz et al., 2014**

This one is easy, too!

Recognized is the ability of dietary fibers and fiber supplements to bind bile acids to prevent their physical contact with colonic tissues. But binding is not the final step, they also need to be ushered out and sent on their way to the local sewage treatment plant. The dietary fiber that escapes digestion is headed there anyway, so why not take a bunch of bile acids with it?

The Western diet is correctly characterized as a low-fiber diet, so forsaking this diet and adopting a plant-based diet, rich in fiber, offers the individual the advantage of increased bile acid binding capacity. One clear advantage offered by a plant-based diet is a reduction in cancer risk.

Binding bile acids and preventing their circulation results in reduced fat absorption, excretion of cancer-causing toxic metabolites and cholesterol utilization to synthesize more bile acids. This is believed to be the mechanism by which food fractions lower cholesterol and prevent cancer. (Kahlon et al., 2007)

It stands to reason that binding bile acids with dietary fiber has other benefits, too, other than reducing the risk of colon cancer. A strong case could be made that binding bile acids can reduce colonic inflammation as well as decrease the risk of colitis—given the toxicity of bile acids, both primary and secondary, coupled with the impaired detoxification of bile acids that occurs in ulcerative colitis.

The bile acid binding capacity of various vegetables can depend on methods of preparation. *"Steaming resulted in highest bile acid binding values, whereas boiling the lowest."* (Kahlon and Chui, 2018) But let's not worry too much over methods of preparation, as raw vegetables, even microwaved vegetables, provide plenty of dietary fibers to bind plenty of bile acids (Kahlon and Chui, 2018).

Although most dietary fibers can bind bile acids, the insoluble fibers from cereal grains appear to do it best (Rose et al., 2007).

In general, it is estimated that an intake of 30 g [grams] of dietary fiber per day is associated with a 50% reduction in risk of colon cancer, and insoluble cereal fibers seem to be more effective than soluble fibers. (Rose et al., 2007)

One class of dietary fiber we should discuss at this point in the conversation is cellulose. Sorry! No usefulness here with regard to bile acid binding. Other fibers do this, but apparently *"cellulose does not"* (Kahlon et al., 2018). You don't have to avoid cellulose—actually, you can't—there's a ton of it found in vegetables. It is beneficial in that it helps bulk-up the stool, and thereby helps prevent constipation, but that's about it. Cellulose is incapable of binding bile acids. Unfortunately, processed foods may have added cellulose (from trees) as a fiber component. Not good from a bile acid binding standpoint, and probably is another dumb idea. Get used to dumb ideas.

We can move on.

Probiotics

> Plausible mechanisms for the protective properties of **L. reuteri** could involve a precipitation of the deconjugated bile salts and **a physical binding of bile salts by the bacterium, thereby making harmful bile acids less bioavailable.** ~De Boever et al., 2000, emphasis added

This is where things get a little crazy. Secondary bile acids, particularly LCA and DCA, although cytotoxic, *"exert anti-inflammatory effects in human colonic epithelial cells"* (Duboc et al., 2013).

> Indeed, **BAs have been repeatedly shown to be anti-inflammatory molecules** able to decrease the synthesis of proinflammatory cytokines, like TNF-α in monocytes and macrophages, through NF-κB inhibition. (Duboc et al., 2013)

Things are so confusing and contradictory here, no wonder no one wants to talk about these issues, or so it seems. On the one hand, bile acids certainly pose a danger. Yet, on the other hand, they can be beneficial. I suppose it has something to do with excess and something to do with balance. And with respect to ulcerative colitis,

> Fecal bile acid profiles in colitis patients differed distinctly from those in healthy subjects and from those with colonic tumors. It was **characterized by increased concentration, and <u>high proportion</u> of primary bile acids** and their amino acid conjugates. (Tanda et al., 1986, emphasis added)

Given the fact that the ulcerative colitis patient is having trouble with converting primary to secondary bile acids (Heinken et al., 2017), perhaps there is a role for primary to secondary converting probiotics to come to the rescue. The bacterial enzyme responsible for this action is called **BSH**, for short. Therefore, the probiotic needed here is one containing bacteria that express BSH activity.

Of course, you will need your physician on board to sort things out, to determine the best course of action to take—and particularly so should you wish to take a BSH-active probiotic to achieve a bile acid advantage.

Some probiotics excel in primary-to-secondary bile acid conversion, like *L. reuteri* mentioned above, like the common probiotics found in yogurt and kefir, the bacterial strains in VSL#3, and in probiotic supplements readily available on the market. However, some common probiotic species or strains do not possess this ability (Baars et al., 2015). So, if your physician believes you might benefit from a probiotic that excels in converting primary to secondary acids, which is notably impaired in ulcerative colitis, be sure to ask for help in choosing the right probiotic for this purpose. And what is the goal, here? The goal is to achieve a bile acid advantage (and reduce inflammation). And there are at least a couple ways a probiotic can do this.

First, before a bacterium converts a primary to a secondary bile acid, it needs to internalize the primary bile acid (Urdaneta and Casadesús, 2017). If the bacterium is lost (think BM), with a primary bile acid tucked away inside, there goes the bile acid, never to return and never allowed an opportunity to harm. Similarly, it may be that a BSH-active probiotic bacterium will **deconjugate, then bind and hang on tightly, leading to reduced availability** (see De Boever et al., 2000; Ridlon et al., 2006).

Second, an alternative way to remove a primary bile acid from the scene is to simply convert it into a secondary bile acid, which will then allow it to passively transfer out of the colon, to be sent on its way to the liver for reprocessing. This is a normal event, even in health. However, we don't want too much of this going on due to the cancer risk from excess exposure to secondary bile acids. Hence, a low-fat diet is likely the best measure to take to reduce the production of all bile acids, both primary and secondary. Yet, it appears that the ulcerative colitis patient needs more secondary bile acids than he or she is producing. So, **the answer does not appear to be more bile acid delivery to the colon (as per the high-fat, Western diet), but rather to have less primary bile acids to deal with, combined with the increased deconjugation of a limited amount of primary bile acids, converting them into secondary bile acids.**

And there is a good reason to have more secondary bile acids available (within reason). There are cellular receptors for secondary bile acids in need of activation. One such receptor is called TGR5.

TGR5, also known as GPBAR1, is a cell-surface receptor capable of triggering a variety of beneficial cellular events—a receptor *"activated by both conjugated as well as unconjugated BAs"* (Baars et al., 2015), yet ***"mostly activated"* by secondary bile acids LCA and DCA** (Duboc et al., 2013). TGR5 is located on the surface of the average intestinal epithelial cell (Bunnett, 2014; Hegyi et al., 2018). It resides on the surface of a variety of immune cells, as well (Baars et al., 2015). Importantly, TGR5 can be activated by bile acids in the intestinal lumen as well as bile acids that reach the intestinal epithelial cell from the inside via the circulation (Bunnett, 2014).

When activated by whichever bile acid gets there first, TGR5 performs a variety of beneficial actions, such as holding in check pro-inflammatory cytokine production by macrophages and other closely-related immune cells, and regulating the tight junctions positioned between intestinal epithelial cells (Baars et al., 2015; Hegyi et al., 2018). TGR5 also helps regulate *"the synthesis, uptake, transportation, and detoxification of bile acids"* (Martin et al., 2018, emphasis added). Recall in ulcerative colitis, there is a problem with the detoxification of bile acids (Tiratterra et al., 2018). TGR5 activation could come in handy in this regard.

There is another bile acid receptor to add to the discussion, a nuclear receptor called **FXR**. This receptor is found deep within a variety of cells, including the cells that line the colon, and is capable of triggering a variety of genetically driven events (Stojancevic et al., 2012). Two such events, potentially offering a benefit to the ulcerative colitis patient, are a downregulation of inflammation and a reduction in epithelial permeability.

> Activation of FXR in the intestinal tract decreases the production of proinflammatory cytokines such as interleukin (IL) 1-beta, IL-2, IL-6, tumor necrosis factor-alpha and interferon-gamma, thus contributing to a reduction in inflammation and epithelial permeability. (Stojancevic et al., 2012)

Furthermore,

> At the intestinal level, FXR activity alleviates inflammation and preserves the integrity of the intestinal epithelial barrier in many ways by regulating the extent of the inflammatory response, maintaining the integrity and function of the intestinal barrier, and preventing bacterial translocation into the intestinal tract. (Stojancevic et al., 2012)

Importantly, FXR is expressed in the colonocyte (Hegyi et al., 2018). However, the colonocyte is not particularly capable of the uptake of conjugated bile acids. Therefore, **deconjugation and passive transport is most necessary before a bile acid can readily enter this cell and activate the FXR** (Hegyi et al., 2018). Why this is important is because <u>**the ulcerative colitis patient basically has a secondary bile acid deficiency,**</u> **one that is not solved by adding more primary bile acids to the mix, a deficiency that does not address the needs of the colonic FXR.** This deficiency in secondary bile acids (and reduced FXR expression) leads to increased inflammation and compromise of the intestinal barrier, which can lead to increased bacterial translocation. However, you don't want too many secondary bile acids in play, as this, too, may contribute to increased epithelial permeability, may enhance bacterial translocation, and may increase colon cancer risk (Hegyi et al., 2018).

To close out this section: It seems likely that there is a place for primary-to-secondary bile acid converting probiotics in the management of ulcerative colitis. Your physician will advise (unless he or she does not want to talk about it).

Hang on! Only one more topic to discuss before this chapter comes to a merciful end. Next, we will discuss a bile acid that can be safely taken to deal with a secondary bile acid deficiency, and to deal with a few other problems as well.

TUDCA

> *Bile salts are important regulators of cell viability* in the gastro-intestinal lumen. Recently, *decreased concentrations of secondary bile salts have been found in fecal samples of patients with IBD*. **~Laukins et al., 2014, emphasis added**

> *Because* **secondary bile acids exhibit immunomodulatory functions, increasing secondary bile acid levels in the intestinal lumen could be an efficient therapeutic approach for IBD.** **~Van den Bossche et al., 2017, emphasis added**

> *Recent studies have also shown that the protective effects of the taurine conjugate of UDCA (TUDCA) in experimental colitis in vivo [in the organism] are also associated with increased colonic mucus secretion.* **~Hegyi et al., 2018**

Briefly, TUDCA is a rather unique secondary bile acid created when the liver adds (conjugates) taurine to another secondary bile acid known as UDCA. The parent <u>primary</u> bile acid of both UDCA and TUDCA is called chenodexeoxycholate acid, or CDCA for short. (Can you see why I prefer using abbreviations whenever possible?) Continuing . . .

Once TUDCA enters the small intestine, a bacterium can internalize it, remove the taurine, and release it back into the small intestine lumen to send it on its way. Deconjugation by the bacterium returns the TUDCA back into UDCA. And, so we see, **a <u>secondary</u> bile acid becomes a**

secondary bile acid. (If I were to venture a guess, your eyes are beginning to glaze over again. So, I will hurry things along.)

Since you, the ulcerative colitis patient, have a secondary bile acid deficiency, perhaps taking a secondary bile acid supplement makes perfect sense. And you're in luck! TUDCA is available as a dietary supplement, no prescription required. But you should have your physician's approval first, as there are likely contraindications and caveats that should be placed under consideration. Besides, an effective dose will need to be determined. But if approved, and you follow through, you will be supplementing with a bile acid that appears to have a lot to offer you, the ulcerative colitis patient.

Keep in mind, supplementing with TUDCA is basically the same as supplementing with UDCA, as both *"TUDCA and UDCA are essentially identical molecules"* (Vang et al., 2014). Of note, UDCA is a prescription drug your physician is likely familiar with. And both bile acids seem to have a place in the treatment of ulcerative colitis. With respect to UDCA,

> *The naturally occurring secondary bile acid, ursodeoxycholic acid (UDCA), has well-established anti-inflammatory and cytoprotective actions and may be effective in treating IBD.* (Ward et al., 2017)

Studies in mice have shown that both UDCA and TUDCA can offer a protective effect in experimental colitis and can prevent or correct the type of dysbiosis associated with experimental colitis (Van den Bossche et al., 2017). In one mouse study, UDCA *"attenuated the release proinflammatory cytokines from colonic epithelial cells in vitro [in the lab] and was protective against the development of colonic inflammation of in vivo [in the organism]."* (Ward et al., 2017) Now, remember, a mouse is not a human, but studies in mice often correctly predict a certain therapy will offer a benefit to the human.

There are several things about TUDCA that make it a tempting therapy for ulcerative colitis. For instance, as a secondary bile acid, TUDCA can activate TGR5 (Yanguas-Casás et al., 2017). And if it can hold on to its taurine, it is an even more potent TGR5 activator (Hegyi et al., 2018). But if it can't hold on, it is still a secondary bile acid (transformed into UDCA), and as such, can activate TGR5 then diffuse easily into the colonocyte and offer another benefit or two as it passes through (Berger and Haller, 2011). Importantly, TUDCA is a cell- and tissue-friendly bile acid, considered to be *"cytoprotective"* (Hatipoğlu et al., 2013). Simply put, ***"TUDCA is not toxic to colonocytes"*** (Laukins et al., 2014, emphasis added). From the sound of things, TUDCA has safety written all over it.

Besides activating TGR5, TUDCA helps prevent an accelerated or early death of the intestinal epithelial cell, thereby acting to prevent gaps from forming in the intestinal epithelial barrier, gaps that weaken the barrier and invite bacterial translocation (Laukins et al., 2014).

Another advantage offered by TUDCA is a reduction in **endoplasmic reticulum stress** (Berger and Haller, 2011). The endoplasmic reticulum is a cell structure that assembles and sorts proteins—and performs other useful tasks. Cells under duress, including intestinal epithelial cells, develop what is called endoplasmic reticulum stress (Berger and Haller, 2011). This leads to problems with protein synthesis and proper protein formation which can contribute to the persistence of ulcerative colitis.

Substantial evidence has accumulated that unresolved endoplasmic reticulum stress owing to a variety of environmental factors might also be a prevalent secondary cause of intestinal inflammation or important factors in the perpetuation of intestinal inflammation once induced by other causes. (Kaser et al., 2010)

In addition, ER stress in intestinal epithelial cells is associated with activation of host immune response and intestinal dysbiosis, which are critical factors implicated in the pathogenesis of intestinal diseases including IBD and mucosal disease. (Ma et al., 2017)

It certainly looks like endoplasmic reticulum stress should be targeted in the management of ulcerative colitis, and it is. Anti-inflammatory medications do this, but so does TUDCA. So why not use it for this purpose and to gain an advantage?

> A _remarkable_ secondary bile salt that has long been studied for its cytoprotective actions is TUDCA, which is only found in trace amounts in human bile. **The use of TUDCA has been proposed as a new therapeutic option for UC because of its ability to inhibit endoplasmic reticulum stress induced by inflammatory stimuli.** (Laukens et al., 2014, emphasis added)

> We conclude that TUDCA and UDCA are potent anti-aggregants for the resolution of ER [endoplasmic reticulum] stress in intestinal epithelial cells and **should be considered as a potential drug target to resolve ER stress mechanisms underlying the pathology of IBD.** (Berger and Haller, 2011, emphasis added)

As promising as TUDCA is, let's not forget about the promise of UDCA. _". . . UDCA has the capacity to prevent the elevated cytokine levels and the increased epithelial permeability associated with intestinal inflammation."_ (Ward et al., 2017) And regarding ER stress, UDCA _"is 10 times more effective in alleviating ER stress than TUDCA"_ in intestinal epithelial cells (Ma et al., 2017).

Given the weight of the evidence, personally, I would find some way to weave TUDCA and UDCA into an upcoming discussion with my physician.

Conclusion

> **In IBD patients, fecal conjugated bile acid levels are higher while secondary bile acid levels are lower, and the deconjugation and transformation abilities of IBD-associated microbiomes are impaired.**
> ~Heinken et al., 2017, emphasis added

> *Because secondary bile acids exhibit immunomodulatory functions, increasing secondary bile acid levels in the intestinal lumen could be an efficient therapeutic approach for IBD.* ~Van den Bossche et al., 2017, emphasis added

Let me sum things up this way: Bile acids influence the cells that line the intestine, both in a positive and in a negative way. **In ulcerative colitis, bile acids are in excess, <u>and</u> there is a dysbiosis-driven excess of primary bile acids as well as a dysdiosis-driven deficiency of secondary bile acids.** Bile acid excess can be addressed by a plant-based, low-fat diet. The deficiency of secondary bile acids can be addressed by correcting dysbiosis, BSH-active probiotics, and supplementation with TUDCA. That's it in a nutshell.

Can't wait for the results of this study

There is a study being currently conducted using TUDCA as a therapy for ulcerative colitis. It is scheduled to be completed at the end of 2020. A paper should follow, a few months later. The official title of the study: *A Phase 1 Open Label Study of the Efficacy and Safety of TUDCA in Ulcerative Colitis.* Trial identifier: NCT04114292.

You might want to look this study up to see if it is available. If not, try later. I'm hopeful the study will show encouraging results.

Remission, so unexpectedly

This is by far the most unusual case of remission in ulcerative colitis that has crossed my path. And I know the guy! You won't believe his story, but I'll tell it to you anyway. To protect his privacy, I'll call him Brian.

I met Brian almost 20 years ago in the hospital where I worked for more than 35 years until retirement. He was there to visit his son who was recovering from an ulcerative colitis-related surgery. Not that it matters, his son is a physician. I established a friendship with his son approximately a year prior to meeting Brian. Of interest, before the day of his surgery, I had no idea my physician friend had a long history of ulcerative colitis.

On my initial trip to visit my physician friend, on the day of his surgery, I met Brian and was invited by him to sit down in the waiting room to visit. One of the first things he said to me was "I wish my son would have had the same experience that I had"—then preceded to tell me the story of how he himself went into remission in ulcerative colitis, now some 40-plus years ago. And how it occurred is most unusual.

Brian was in his early thirties at the time of his remission, following more than a decade of battling ulcerative colitis. And it was, indeed, a battle. Ongoing therapy, and at times aggressive therapy, eventually failed to halt the progression of this disease, and the disease process became so severe that Brian was faced with what seemed to be an inevitable colectomy to remove his diseased colon. But there was one hope left. A new drug, one showing great promise in the battle against ulcerative colitis, became available and was offered to Brian as a therapy of last resort. The drug was an immunosuppressant called azathioprine (Imuran).

At the start of therapy, I'm certain that Brian felt at least some sense of optimism, or not—as this disease brings out a sense of defeat even in the best of us. Whatever the case, Brian was started on Imuran. And the result? For Brian, ***the drug was a disaster!*** (But led to a most unusual case of remission.) To be fair, Imuran has been a success story for many individuals with ulcerative colitis (Neurath and Travis, 2012; Sood et al., 2015).

Shortly after Imuran was started, Brian developed acute pancreatitis. This happens to be one of the dangers of taking this drug. Acute pancreatitis is serious business. Those who contract this disease are often extremely ill and have a 20% mortality rate (Fu et al., 2007).

Brian's new disease produced severe symptoms, so much so that he was promptly hospitalized. Not to worry! (OK, worry if you want to.) Surprisingly, only two weeks after admission, Brian walked out of the hospital, recovering from acute pancreatitis and completely free of the symptoms of ulcerative colitis. And the symptoms of ulcerative colitis never returned. Forty-plus years later, Brian is still in remission. No medications were required, ever, to treat his ulcerative colitis following his hospitalization. It's as if he left it all behind the day he left the hospital and headed for home. As recently as last year (2018), a routine colonoscopy to screen for colon cancer showed no evidence of active ulcerative colitis and, astonishingly, no evidence the disease was ever present.

The clues

So, how did it all happen? How did Brian promptly go into remission? To find answers these questions, let's go back in time to see what occurred during his hospitalization. Details are a little sketchy, as memories fade, but what Brian relayed to me may give us a clue or two we can follow up on to get a sense of what may have occurred. There are some instances found in the medical literature where the onset of a new disease healed a preexisting one or prevented another disease from emerging, but I have found nothing like what Brian experienced.

Acute pancreatitis can be so severe that admission to the intensive care unit (ICU) is necessary. Such was the case for Brian. Furthermore, acute pancreatitis can lead to a condition called **ileus**. An ileus is basically a loss of effective movement of the intestine and can be quite painful. It usually requires the patient to be NPO (nothing by mouth) and the placement of a nasogastric (NG) tube, connected to suction to remove any bile that collects in the stomach. And collect it does! Bile acid production and flow does not stop during an ileus. In my days as a critical care nurse, I regularly emptied hundreds of cc's of bile each shift from the suction canisters of my ileus patients. In Brian's situation, he was made NPO and a nasogastric tube was indeed placed to remove the bile that had only one way to go—up, into the stomach and out through the NG tube. To me, **Clue #1 is ileus with bile acid removal/depletion**. As Brian recalls, he had an NG tube most, if not all, of his ICU stay. Did Brian achieve some kind of bile acid advantage? We'll explore this shortly.

Brian relayed to me that, to the best of his knowledge, he was not placed on any new medication, be it anti-inflammatory or immuno-suppressant, during his hospitalization. Furthermore, he believes his ulcerative colitis medications were promptly held once he was admitted to the hospital.

Before identifying the next clue, I need to mention that while Brian was NPO (nothing by mouth) with the NG tube in place, he was maintained on a clear IV solution to meet his fluid needs. All this occurred before the days of TPN, a yellow IV solution that supplies calories and nutrients. During his hospitalization, Brian "fasted" (no oral caloric intake) for the better part of two weeks. Fasting for a period of time translates into "bowel rest." Fasting/bowel rest is known to exert beneficial effects in IBD (see Wild et al., 2007). So, **Clue #2 is fasting/bowel rest.**

The next clue has something to do with something that customarily occurs in acute pancreatitis. Acute pancreatitis provokes a large increase in circulating IL-10 levels within the bloodstream (Van Laethem et al., 1998; Chen et al., 1999). IL-10 is a powerful anti-inflammatory cytokine that impedes the production of proinflammatory cytokines like TNF-α. Attempts have been made to use IV IL-10 as a therapy for IBD in the past, but without notable success (Herfarth and Schölmerich, 2002). But that doesn't mean elevating circulatory IL-10 levels can't give someone an edge. The immune system uses IL-10 to limit inflammation and bring the inflammatory process to an end. So, **Clue #3 is**

systemically elevated IL-10 levels. One last clue, then we'll wrap things up.

For Brian, acute pancreatitis, along with the nature of his hospital course, created a period of time that allowed several generations of new, healthy intestinal epithelial cells to replace the older, disease-challenged and impaired/dysfunctional epithelial cells. Recall, epithelial cell turnover occurs every 3-5 days. So perhaps Brian's intestinal epithelial cells simply outgrew the disease process, not having to deal with the normal, everyday challenges like the detoxification of a continual supply of bile acids—and doing so at a time when pro-inflammatory forces (cytokines) were held in check by several mechanisms, possibly by increased IL-10 exposure. Epithelial cell turn-over is a force for good, helping to rebuild and create a more formidable barrier of protection. So, **Clue #4 is a tincture of time, allowing several new generations of intestinal epithelial cells to come into being, remodeling and strengthening the intestinal epithelial barrier.** I guess this is a big clue, as it took a lot of words to describe it.

Clearly, the following is speculation on my part. But hear me out. I believe it was acute pancreatitis that set the stage for Brian's remission. His unfortunate reaction to Imuran, serendipitously lead to events that, together, halted the inflammatory response and allowed healing programs to be unleased and proceed. And the rest is history.

Per Clue #1, Brian may have benefited from bile acid withholding. By removing the bile that collected in his stomach, day after day, a lot of bile acids were removed, never to return, never to reach the colon, never to complicate, gone for good. The removal of bile acids in great numbers, some most toxic—and without continuous exposure to bile acids that normally occurs from the consumption of 3 meals a day (plus snacks)—may have given Brian's colon a much-needed break from dealing with a never-ending supply of bile acids, some quite toxic.

Per Clue #2, fasting/bowel rest may have reduced the negative impact certain dietary components have on the cells that form the intestinal barrier. For example: Fasting certainly reduces the intake of dietary iron, a dietary component that poses daily challenges to the intestinal epithelium. And so we read,

> *Besides the effects of iron on the gut microbiota, which may cause a shift towards a more pathogenic profile and an increase in virulence of enteric pathogens, iron may also directly exert unfavorable effects on the gut epithelium most likely by the promotion of redox stress.* (Kortman et al., 2014, emphasis added)

Per Clue #3, the elevated circulating IL-10 levels that occur with acute pancreatitis, and presumably experienced by Brian, may have restrained gastrointestinal intestinal inflammation just enough (or perhaps more than enough) to turn things around and head Brian in the right direction and promote healing. And finally:

Per Clue #4, the rapid rate of intestinal epithelial cell turnover, and under unusual yet favorable circumstances, may have given Brian a cellular-turnover advantage. Epithelial cell turnover rebuilds and renews the intestinal barrier, and each new intestinal epithelial cell is likely to be healthier than the one it replaced. A healthier epithelial cell, one living in a renewed defensive barrier, is likely better able to defend and likely better able to serve. It is also less likely to succumb to disease.

~References~

Ajouz, H., Mukherji, D. and Shamseddine, A., 2014. **Secondary bile acids: an underrecognized cause of colon cancer.** *World journal of surgical oncology,* *12*(1), p.164.

Asgharpour A, Kumar D, Sanyal A. **Bile acids: emerging role in management of liver diseases.** Hepatology international. 2015 Oct 1;9(4):527-33.

Baars A, Oosting A, Knol J, Garssen J, van Bergenhenegouwen J. **The gut microbiota as a therapeutic target in IBD and metabolic disease: a role for the bile acid receptors FXR and TGR5.** Microorganisms. 2015 Dec;3(4):641-66.

Berger E, Haller D. **Structure–function analysis of the tertiary bile acid TUDCA for the resolution of endoplasmic reticulum stress in intestinal epithelial cells.** Biochemical and biophysical research communications. 2011 Jun 17;409(4):610-5.

Bunnett NW. **Neuro-humoral signaling by bile acids and the TGR5 receptor in the gastrointestinal tract.** The Journal of physiology. 2014 Jul 15;592(14):2943-50.

Chen CC, Wang SS, Lu RH, Chang FY, Lee SD. **Serum interleukin 10 and interleukin 11 in patients with acute pancreatitis.** Gut. 1999 Dec 1;45(6):895-9.

Dawson PA, Karpen SJ. **Intestinal transport and metabolism of bile acids. Journal of lipid research.** 2015 Jun 1;56(6):1085-99.

De Boever P, Wouters R, Verschaeve L, Berckmans P, Schoeters G, Verstraete W. **Protective effect of the bile salt hydrolase-active Lactobacillus reuteri against bile salt cytotoxicity.** Applied microbiology and biotechnology. 2000 Jun 1;53(6):709-14.

Duboc H, Rajca S, Rainteau D, Benarous D, Maubert MA, Quervain E, Thomas G, Barbu V, Humbert L, Despras G, Bridonneau C. **Connecting dysbiosis, bile-acid dysmetabolism and gut inflammation in inflammatory bowel diseases.** Gut. 2013 Apr 1;62(4):531-9.

Fiorucci S, Biagioli M, Zampella A, Distrutti E. **Bile acids activated receptors regulate innate immunity.** Frontiers in immunology. 2018;9.

Fu CY, Yeh CN, Hsu JT, Jan YY, Hwang TL. **Timing of mortality in severe acute pancreatitis: experience from 643 patients.** World journal of gastroenterology: WJG. 2007 Apr 7;13(13):1966.

Guo C, Chen WD, Wang YD. **TGR5, not only a metabolic regulator.** Frontiers in physiology. 2016 Dec 26;7:646.

Han Y, Haraguchi T, Iwanaga S, Tomotake H, Okazaki Y, Mineo S, Moriyama A, Inoue J, Kato N. **Consumption of some polyphenols reduces fecal deoxycholic acid and lithocholic acid, the secondary bile acids of risk factors of colon cancer.** Journal of agricultural and food chemistry. 2009 Aug 27;57(18):8587-90.

Hatipoğlu AR, Oğuz S, Gürcan Ş, Yalta T, Albayrak D, Erenoğlu C, Sağıroğlu T, Sezer YA. **Combined effects of tauroursodeoxycholic acid and glutamine on bacterial translocation in obstructive jaundiced rats.** Balkan medical journal. 2013 Dec;30(4):362.

Hegyi P, Maléth J, Walters JR, Hofmann AF, Keely SJ. **Guts and gall: bile acids in regulation of intestinal epithelial function in health and disease.** Physiological reviews. 2018 Aug 1;98(4):1983-2023.

Heinken A, Ravcheev DA, Baldini F, Heirendt L, Fleming RM, Thiele I. **Personalized modeling of the human gut microbiome reveals distinct bile acid deconjugation and biotransformation potential in healthy and IBD individuals.** BioRxiv. 2017 Jan 1:229138.

Herfarth H, Schölmerich J. **IL-10 therapy in Crohn's'disease: at the crossroads.** Gut. 2002 Feb 1;50(2):146-7.

Hofmann AF. **The continuing importance of bile acids in liver and intestinal disease.** Archives of internal medicine. 1999 Dec 13;159(22):2647-58.

Joyce SA, Gahan CG. **Disease-associated changes in bile acid profiles and links to altered gut microbiota.** Digestive Diseases. 2017;35(3):169-77.

Kahlon TS, Chapman MH, Smith GE. **In vitro binding of bile acids by okra, beets, asparagus, eggplant, turnips, green beans, carrots, and cauliflower.** Food chemistry. 2007 Jan 1;103(2):676-80.

Kahlon T, Chui MC. **A Review—In Vitro Bile Acid Binding of Various Vegetables.** Medical Research Archives. 2018 Feb 15;6(2).

Kaser A, Martínez-Naves E, Blumberg RS. **Endoplasmic reticulum stress: implications for inflammatory bowel disease pathogenesis.** Current opinion in gastroenterology. 2010 Jul;26(4):318.

Kortman GA, Raffatellu M, Swinkels DW, Tjalsma H. **Nutritional iron turned inside out: intestinal stress from a gut microbial perspective.** FEMS microbiology reviews. 2014 Nov 1;38(6):1202-34.

Laukens D, Devisscher L, Van den Bossche L, Hindryckx P, Vandenbroucke RE, Vandewynckel YP, Cuvelier C, Brinkman BM, Libert C, Vandenabeele P, De Vos M. **Tauroursodeoxycholic acid inhibits experimental colitis by preventing early intestinal epithelial cell death.** Laboratory investigation. 2014 Dec;94(12):1419.

Ma X, Dai Z, Sun K, Zhang Y, Chen J, Yang Y, Tso P, Wu G, Wu Z. **Intestinal epithelial cell endoplasmic reticulum stress and inflammatory bowel disease pathogenesis: an update review.** Frontiers in immunology. 2017 Oct 25;8:1271.

Martin G, Kolida S, Marchesi J, Want E, Sidaway J, Swann JR. **In vitro modeling of bile acid processing by the human fecal microbiota.** Frontiers in microbiology. 2018;9:1153.

Martínez-Augustin O, de Medina FS. **Intestinal bile acid physiology and pathophysiology.** World journal of gastroenterology: WJG. 2008 Oct 7;14(37):5630.

Neurath MF, Travis SP. **Mucosal healing in inflammatory bowel diseases: a systematic review.** Gut. 2012 Jan 1:gutjnl-2012.

Nguyen TT, Ung TT, Kim NH, Do Jung Y. **Role of bile acids in colon carcinogenesis.** World journal of clinical cases. 2018 Nov 6;6(13):577.

Ridlon JM, Kang DJ, Hylemon PB. **Bile salt biotransformations by human intestinal bacteria.** Journal of lipid research. 2006 Feb 1;47(2):241-59.

Rose DJ, DeMeo MT, Keshavarzian A, Hamaker BR. **Influence of dietary fiber on inflammatory bowel disease and colon cancer: importance of fermentation pattern.** Nutrition reviews. 2007 Feb 1;65(2):51-62.

Sood R, Ansari S, Clark T, Hamlin PJ, Ford AC. **Long-term Efficacy and Safety of Azathioprine in Ulcerative Colitis.** Journal of Crohn's'and Colitis. 2015;191:197.

Stamp D, Jenkins G. **An overview of bile-acid synthesis, chemistry and function. Bile acids: toxicology and bioactivity.** Cambridge, UK: Royal Society of Chemistry. 2008 Jul 24:1-3.

Stenman LK, Holma R, Korpela R. **High-fat-induced intestinal permeability dysfunction associated with altered fecal bile acids.** World journal of gastroenterology: WJG. 2012 Mar 7;18(9):923.

Stojancevic M, Stankov K, Mikov M. **The impact of farnesoid X receptor activation on intestinal permeability in inflammatory bowel disease.** Canadian Journal of Gastroenterology and Hepatology. 2012;26(9):631-7.

Tanida N, Hikasa Y, Dodo M, Sawada K, Kawaura A, Shimoyama T. **High concentration and retained amidation of fecal bile acids in patients with active ulcerative colitis.** Gastroenterologia Japonica. 1986 Jun 1;21(3):245-54.

Tiratterra E, Franco P, Porru E, Katsanos KH, Christodoulou DK, Roda G. **Role of bile acids in inflammatory bowel disease.** Annals of gastroenterology. 2018 May;31(3):266.

Urdaneta V, Casadesús J. **Interactions between bacteria and bile salts in the gastrointestinal and hepatobiliary tracts.** Frontiers in medicine. 2017 Oct 3;4:163.

Van den Bossche L, Hindryckx P, Devisscher L, Devriese S, Van Welden S, Holvoet T, Vilchez-Vargas R, Vital M, Pieper DH, Bussche JV, Vanhaecke L. **Ursodeoxycholic acid and its taurine/glycine conjugated species reduce colitogenic dysbiosis and equally suppress experimental colitis in mice.** Applied and environmental microbiology. 2017 Jan 23:AEM-02766.

Vang S, Longley K, Steer CJ, Low WC. **The unexpected uses of urso-and tauroursodeoxycholic acid in the treatment of non-liver diseases.** Global advances in health and medicine. 2014 May;3(3):58-69.

Van Laethem JL, Eskinazi R, Louis H, Rickaert F, Robberecht P, Devière J. **Multisystemic production of interleukin 10 limits the severity of acute pancreatitis in mice.** Gut. 1998 Sep 1;43(3):408-13.

Ward JB, Lajczak NK, Kelly OB, O'D'yer AM, Giddam AK, Gabhainn JN, Franco P, Tambuwala MM, Jefferies CA, Keely S, Roda A. **Ursodeoxycholic acid and lithocholic acid exert anti-inflammatory actions in the colon.** American Journal of Physiology-Heart and Circulatory Physiology. 2017 Mar 30.

Wild GE, Drozdowski L, Tartaglia C, Clandinin MT, Thomson AB. **Nutritional modulation of the inflammatory response in inflammatory bowel disease-from the molecular to the integrative to the clinical.** World journal of gastroenterology: WJG. 2007 Jan 7;13(1):1.

Yanguas-Casás N, Barreda-Manso MA, Nieto-Sampedro M, Romero-Ramírez L. **TUDCA: An agonist of the bile acid receptor GPBAR1/TGR5 with anti-inflammatory effects in microglial cells.** Journal of cellular physiology. 2017 Aug;232(8):2231-45.

Chapter 19

Berberine

The potential benefit of berberine in IBD therapy could arise from its widely known antibacterial effects including activity against E. coli.
~Habtemariam, 2016

Notably, in our study [in mice] 30-day treatment with berberine significantly reduced colonic mucosal inflammation as demonstrated by macroscopic and histological [tissue] examination. **~Li et al., 2016**

When I first heard of berberine, a proposed therapy for ulcerative colitis, I decided to take a closer look and share with you what I found. It didn't take long for me to recognize that berberine is something special.

Berberine, a simple herb with a centuries-long, time-honored history of combating gastrointestinal disease (Chen et al., 2014), has properties the ulcerative colitis patient is desperately in need of. Indeed, somewhere on earth (China, to be exact) berberine *"has been widely used in the treatment of ulcerative colitis."* (Cui et al., 2018)

So, what's so special about berberine? Berberine

- Blocks proinflammatory cytokines and pathways

- Stimulates anti-inflammatory pathways

- Kills bacteria known to be problematic in ulcerative colitis, such as *E. coli*

- Supports the growth of friendly bacteria

- Shifts the gut microbiome to a less pathogenic profile

- Reinforces the integrity of the junctions that keep the intestinal epithelial cells close together, reducing epithelial permeability and blocking unwanted passage of noxious molecules and bacteria

- Impairs the ability of bacteria to adhere to mucosal and epithelial cell surfaces

- Possesses potent anti-diarrheal effects

- Decreases discomfort associated with gastrointestinal disturbances

- Promotes antitumor activity in the colon

The above list is taken from Chen et al., 2014. But this team of investigators are not the only ones who are telling the berberine story. Numerous authors report similar and additional properties exhibited by this herb, an herb believed to have *"low acute toxicity"* and is generally well tolerated at doses of *"0.2–1.0 g/day"* (Chen et al., 2014). Berberine seems to be designed just for the disordered gastrointestinal system.

One property of berberine is its ability to bind a receptor called PPARγ (Chen et al., 2014, Wang et al., 2018). Binding PPARγ reduces colonic inflammation (Lewis et al., 2008). Remarkably, people with mild to moderate ulcerative colitis have clinically improved or have gone into remission by targeting this important anti-inflammatory pathway (Lewis et al., 2008). In fact, mesalamine targets PPARγ, and is one of the reasons for its effectiveness. But that's not all.

Berberine can reduce your exposure to LPS. *"Alteration in the gut microbiota induced by berberine resulted in a significant reduction in bacterial lipopolysaccharide [LPS] levels in portal [major vein leading to the liver] plasma."* (Xu et al., 2017) Furthermore, berberine is capable of *"direct interaction"* with the bacterial component LPS, augmenting berberine's antibacterial effect (Habtemariam, 2016). And this could come in handy:

> *. . . berberine supplementation alleviated metabolic endotoxemia and subsequent systemic inflammation, via restoring the integrity of the gut barrier through increasing the expression and restoring the distribution of tight junction proteins.* (Xu et al., 2017)

And let me add this (as if you have any choice in the matter): Berberine acts as an antioxidant (Habtemariam, 2016). Furthermore, it can enhance antioxidant defenses and reduce the formation of free radicals (Habtemariam, 2016). All this sounds great, particularly in a disease (UC) where free radicals are everywhere and inflicting damage. And the following could certainly come in handy:

Berberine is a killer! *"While killing harmful gut bacteria, berberine is generally known to have little effect on beneficial bacteria such as Bifidobacterium adolescentis and Lactobacillius acidophillus."* (Habtemariam, 2016) So, with berberine, we have an opportunity to spare the lives of good bacteria while destroying the lives of bacteria that can cause us harm (Habtemariam, 2016).

Finally, another property of berberine is its promotion of a favorable Treg/Th17 balance (Cui et al., 2018, Li et al., 2016). In *Chapter 9* we learned of the importance of a favorable balance between the Treg's and the Th17 cells, and an excess in Th17 cell numbers and activity leads to increased disease activity in ulcerative colitis. Enter berberine. Berberine exerts a *"suppressive effect"* on Th17 cells; and does so *"without affecting Treg cells"* (Habtemariam, 2016). Indeed, *"A number of studies including in humans have shown a direct inhibitory effect on the Th17 [cell]."* (Habtemariam, 2016) Surprisingly, you can give berberine to a mouse undergoing experimental ulcerative colitis, improve the mouse's Treg/Th17 balance by this means, then transplant the poop from this mouse into a recipient mouse, one suffering from experimental ulcerative colitis, and the recipient mouse gets better, exhibits an improved Treg/Th17 balance, and lives a healthier, happier life. (see Cui et al., 2018).

I guess someone should ask this question: "Why is berberine not customarily used in the treatment of ulcerative colitis?" To me, it sounds like the perfect therapy for the disease. And it has safety (*"low toxicity"*) written all over it! (Wang et al., 2018)

Now if you live in China, it would probably be easy to receive permission from your gastroenterologist to give berberine a try. China appears to be the center of gravity for both berberine research and its clinical use. This makes sense as the Chinese have been using berberine for centuries for various GI ailments, including what would now be recognized as ulcerative colitis (Li et al., 2016). But no need to move to China to take advantage of the benefits of berberine. You can easily purchase berberine online or at your favorite supplement store. Before purchase and use, however, get permission from your gastroenterologist. Some individuals have run into trouble. *"There are only a few reports on the side-effects of berberine in the GI tract, including mildly upset stomach after oral administration."* (Chen et al., 2014) Furthermore, constipation could occur (Chen et al., 2014).

An additional consideration: One physician who takes berberine herself offers the following recommendation:

> *It's recommended that you take berberine for only 8 weeks at a time and then take a holiday owing to the effect of the herb on cytochromes P450 (CYPs) in the liver.*

When you see an effect of berberine on cytochromes P450, it may lead to drug-drug interactions, which should be reviewed with a knowledgeable clinician and/or pharmacist. Many supplements should be used in this way—pulsed in an 8-week cycle, and then off for some length of time such as two to four weeks, then restarted if symptoms aren't resolved. (Gottfried, 2015)

Like so many promising therapies, berberine has a problem or two that may come into play. I'll discuss one problem momentarily, before we end our discussion on berberine.

Currently, there are at least two clinical trials evaluating the use of berberine for ulcerative colitis, one trial to determine the efficacy of berberine to maintain remission (Trial identifier: NCT02962245), the other trial to determine the efficacy of berberine to prevent colorectal cancer in patients with ulcerative colitis (Trial identifier: NCT02365480). No results are available yet, but later, perhaps in a year or two, you should be able to go online and read the results of these two clinical trials.

Before we move on, please do your best with the following quotation. I place it here primarily for the physician (lots of doctor talk along with a few translation issues), but by now I'm sure you can get the gist of what is being said.

*The anti-inflammatory effect of berberine has been acknowledged for long history. Current investigations have revealed that berberine exerts the anti-inflammatory activities in the intestinal lumen by regulating their transcription and therefore ameliorating proinflammatory cytokine-induced intestinal epithelial damage, which is mediated mainly through activation of AMPK and inhibition of transcription factor activator protein 1 (AP1) and NF-kB. For example, berberine inhibits mucosal generation of interleukin-8 (IL-8), which is responsible for polymorphonuclear neutrophils infiltration in intestinal lesions of intestine bowel disease (IBD) and ulcerative colitis. **Similar effects were observed in metformin**.* (Wang et al., 2018, emphasis added)

Metformin! Hmm. Could metformin be used as a therapy for ulcerative colitis? We'll take a look. But first . . .

Bile acid <u>dis</u>advantage

Various doses of BBR increased primary BAs, whereas it decreased secondary BAs, and has effects on BA metabolism and related genes as well as intestinal flora, which provides insight into many pathways of BBR effects. ~Guo et al., 2016

There seems always a tradeoff when it comes to therapy for IBD, and that would include ulcerative colitis. Berberine is no exception. You may benefit from the positive effects of berberine, outlined near the beginning of this chapter. However, you may not benefit from the negative influence berberine has on bile acid metabolism.

Apparently, berberine increases bile acid production (Guo et al., 2016). You likely do not need this, as fecal bile acids are already elevated in IBD (Heinken et al., 2017). Importantly, elevated bile acid production contributes to the risk of colorectal cancer in ulcerative colitis. So this effect of berberine is a big negative.

Berberine does one more thing that you likely do not need. **Berberine impairs the ability of BSH-active bacteria to convert primary bile acids into secondary bile acids** (Sun et al., 2017).

Recall from *Chapter 18*, the ulcerative colitis patient typically has a secondary bile deficiency, brought on by reduced BSH activity. This unfortunate situation increases intestinal inflammation and impairs the integrity of the intestinal epithelial barrier. So, indeed, berberine may not be helpful from a bile acid standpoint. However, many other therapies do not address bile acid dysmetabolism and may actually contribute to it, yet they offer an advantage. Similarly, berberine may be helpful, perhaps very helpful, apart from its negative effects on bile acid metabolism.

Berberine is yet another example of why you should not go out on your own in treating your ulcerative colitis. You need guidance every step of the way to keep you out of more trouble than you are already in. But remember, every therapy for ulcerative colitis seems to have its share of negative side effects. Likewise, the positive effects of berberine may outweigh the negative effects.

Me, too

"Metformin is the subject of clinical trials for various diseases as it has a potent antioxidant, anti-inflammatory and anti-carcinogenic properties." (Samman et al., 2018) Which, of course, makes metformin a promising agent for use in the battle against ulcerative colitis.

Under experimental conditions (involving a mouse), metformin can inhibit the induction of colon inflammation, when given rectally (Lee et al., 2015). (Try explaining *this* to a mouse!) Moreover, giving oral metformin to a mouse can *"significantly attenuate the severity of colitis"* as well as significantly reduce the development of colon cancer (Koh et al., 2014).

In view of the above, perhaps in the future we will see more interest in the use of metformin as a therapy for ulcerative colitis.

Trouble ahead?

As with everything that is useful in medicine, berberine has a problem or two that should be placed under consideration.

Likely, it should not be taken during pregnancy or while nursing, or given to the baby (Gottfried, 2015). Additionally, caution should be taken when adding berberine to the mix while one is also taking medications that are metabolized by the same CYP enzyme (Rad et al., 2017). Your physician can sort this all out for you. The issue of drug interactions is yet another reason why you should not go out on your own but have a physician guide you each and every step of the way. Berberine use in no exception.

~References~

Chen C, Yu Z, Li Y, Fichna J, Storr M. **Effects of berberine in the gastrointestinal tract—a review of actions and therapeutic implications.** The American journal of Chinese medicine. 2014;42(05):1053-70.

Cui H, Cai Y, Wang L, Jia B, Li J, Zhao S, Chu X, Lin J, Zhang X, Bian Y, Zhuang P. **Berberine regulates Treg/Th17 balance to treat ulcerative colitis through modulating the gut microbiota in the colon.** Frontiers in pharmacology. 2018;9.

Gottfried S. **For the Love of Berberine: What It Is and Why I Take It to Lower Blood Sugar, Bad Cholesterol, and Weight (plus 5 FAQs).** Oct 2015. https://www.saragottfriedmd.com/for-the-love-of-berberine-what-it-is-and-why-i-take-it-to-lower-blood-sugar-bad-cholesterol-and-weight-plus-5-faqs/

Guo Y, Zhang Y, Huang W, Selwyn FP, Klaassen CD. **Dose-response effect of berberine on bile acid profile and gut microbiota in mice.** BMC complementary and alternative medicine. 2016 Dec;16(1):394.

Habtemariam S. **Berberine and inflammatory bowel disease: A concise review.** Pharmacological research. 2016 Nov 1;113:592-9.

Heinken A, Ravcheev DA, Baldini F, Heirendt L, Fleming RM, Thiele I. **Personalized modeling of the human gut microbiome reveals distinct bile acid deconjugation and biotransformation potential in healthy and IBD individuals.** BioRxiv. 2017 Jan 1:229138.

Koh SJ, Kim JM, Kim IK, Ko SH, Kim JS. **Anti-inflammatory mechanism of metformin and its effects in intestinal inflammation and colitis-associated colon cancer.** Journal of gastroenterology and hepatology. 2014 Mar;29(3):502-10.

Lee SY, Lee SH, Yang EJ, Kim EK, Kim JK, Shin DY, Cho ML. **Metformin ameliorates inflammatory bowel disease by suppression of the STAT3 signaling pathway and regulation of the between Th17/Treg balance.** PloS one. 2015 Sep 11;10(9):e0135858.

Lewis JD, Lichtenstein GR, Deren JJ, Sands BE, Hanauer SB, Katz JA, Lashner B, Present DH, Chuai S, Ellenberg JH, Nessel L. **Rosiglitazone for active ulcerative** colitis: a randomized placebo-controlled trial. Gastroenterology. 2008 Mar 1;134(3):688-95.

Li YH, Xiao HT, Hu DD, Fatima S, Lin CY, Mu HX, Lee NP, Bian ZX. **Berberine ameliorates chronic relapsing dextran sulfate sodium-induced colitis in C57BL/6 mice by suppressing Th17 responses.** Pharmacological research. 2016 Aug 1;110:227-39.

Rad SZ, Rameshrad M, Hosseinzadeh H. **Toxicology effects of Berberis vulgaris (barberry) and its active constituent, berberine: a review.** Iranian journal of basic medical sciences. 2017 May;20(5):516.

Samman FS, Elaidy SM, Essawy SS, Hassan MS. **New insights on the modulatory roles of metformin or alpha-lipoic acid versus their combination in dextran sulfate sodium-induced chronic colitis in rats.** Pharmacological Reports. 2018 Jun 1;70(3):488-96.

Sun R, Yang N, Kong B, Cao B, Feng D, Yu X, Ge C, Huang J, Shen J, Wang P, Feng S. **Orally administered berberine modulates hepatic lipid metabolism by altering microbial bile acid metabolism and the intestinal FXR signaling pathway.** Molecular pharmacology. 2017 Feb 1;91(2):110-22.

Wang H, Zhu C, Ying Y, Luo L, Huang D, Luo Z. **Metformin and berberine, two versatile drugs in treatment of common metabolic diseases.** Oncotarget. 2018 Feb 9;9(11):10135.

Xu JH, Liu XZ, Pan W, Zou DJ. **Berberine protects against diet-induced obesity through regulating metabolic endotoxemia and gut hormone levels.** Molecular medicine reports. 2017 May 1;15(5):2765-87.

Chapter 20

Fat chance

Mechanistically, we have shown that CLA ameliorates . . . colitis by enhancing PPARγ activity and thereby suppressing immune cell infiltration, inflammation, and epithelial erosion in the gut mucosa. **~Evans et al., 2010**

*PPARγ is a member in the superfamily of nuclear receptors implicated in the regulation of intestinal inflammation. There are studies demonstrating that **its activation could potentially reduce the severity of IBD by inhibiting excessive immunoinflammatory responses.*** ~Sánchez-Fidalgo **et al., 2013, emphasis added**

The fact that PPARγ is highly expressed in the colonic epithelium makes it an attractive target for IBD therapy. **~Borniquel et al., 2012**

Inadequate expression of PPARγ leads to activation of inflammatory cascade leading to IBD. **~Ray, 2008**

T his chapter is about fat, but not just any fat. This chapter is also about a receptor, but not just any receptor. The receptor in question is activated by fat, but not just any fat.

The fat I have in mind is called conjugated linoleic acid (CLA). The receptor activated by CLA is called PPARγ. You can find this receptor prepositioned in the nucleus of a variety of cells including the macrophage and the T cell (Evans et al., 2010). *"PPARγ is also abundant in the gastrointestinal track, where it is **highly expressed in epithelial cells**."* (Necela and Thompson, 2008, emphasis added) Importantly, PPARγ is *"implicated in the regulation of intestinal inflammation"* (Sánchez-Fidalgo et al., 2013) and when activated has the power to decrease mucosal inflammation (Hontecillas et al., 2002). And you can see it all in action.

Take a mouse, one that you are not particularly fond of, and give the mouse an agent that reliably creates colitis. Then, once the mouse develops colitis (and the suffering begins), add CLA to the mouse's diet and he or she will experience less colonic inflammation and will be protected from developing colon cancer (Evans et al., 2010). You will come across as some kind of hero. But it is CLA, not you, that should receive all the glory, as **CLA is** *"a polyunsaturated fat with <u>potent</u> anti-inflammatory effects."* (Bassaganya-Riera et al., 2012, emphasis added)

CLA is found in varying amounts in dairy and beef, and obviously, in CLA supplements. You can also find impressive amounts of CLA in mutton and in kangaroos. But likely you are not into mutton. And most likely not into kangaroo. Besides dairy, beef, mutton, and kangaroo, there is another place where CLA can be found. It can be made, on site, in the colon—created by bacteria with the skills required to perform this task (Dubuquoy et al., 2006; Bassaganya-Riera et al., 2012). Furthermore, *"CLA seems to be endogenously formed [created within] in humans from trans vaccenic acid found in dairy fat."* (Risérus et al., 2004)

CLA is not the only compound that activates PPARγ. One compound that does this you are likely familiar with. The time-honored, first-line ulcerative colitis medication, **5-ASA** (Asacol; Pentasa; sulfasalazine), activates PPARγ (Bassaganya-Riera et al., 2010; Byndloss et al., 2019). And that's a good thing.

Other fats besides CLA also activate PPARγ. **Butyrate**, a fat produced by colonic bacteria acting on soluble fibers, activates PPARγ, and is one of the reasons for the effectiveness of butyrate as a therapy for ulcerative colitis (Byndloss et al., 2017). **The polyphenols in extra virgin olive oil** also activate PPARγ (Sánchez-Fidalgo et al., 2013). And this should come as a surprise: **Red clover metabolites** can activate this receptor (Martin, 2009; Wang et al., 2014). So, get out there and do some grazing!

Actually, grazing is the reason why cows, their milk, and their butter become rich sources of CLA (Kay et al., 2004). Soon you will learn, grass fed-cows are the cows you should develop a close relationship with.

The reasons for targeting PPARγ, a cellular sensor fundamentally involved in the inflammatory response, and thus involved the pathogenesis of ulcerative colitis (see Martin, 2009; Wada et al., 2001), are many. Here are a few:

- PPARγ downregulates pro-inflammatory pathways, including NF-κB and MAPK (Ray, 2008)

- PPARγ stimulates production of the anti-inflammatory cytokine IL-10 by immune cells (Martin, 2009)

- PPARγ stimulates production of antibiotic-like molecules called defensins (Chamaillard and Dessein, 2011)

- PPARγ expands Treg cell numbers (Housley et al., 2009)

- PPARγ *"regulates a very large cohort of genes that are involved in maintenance of the cellular cytoskeleton, in cell-cell adhesion, and in cellular motility."* (Thompson, 2007)

- PPARγ activates intestinal healing programs (Borniquel et al., 2012)

- PPARγ regulates macrophage polarization, and when activated, PPARγ promotes a shift from a proinflammatory M1 macrophage phenotype to an anti-inflammatory M2 macrophage phenotype, one which calms inflammation and promotes healing (Schuster et al., 2018)

Given these and other actions, is it any wonder, soon after a new drug showed up on the scene that excelled in binding PPARγ, a clinical trial was conducted to see what it would do for ulcerative colitis? The drug was not just any drug. The drug was one of those "wonder" drugs that didn't pan out, named rosiglitazone (Avandia).

Reported in 2001, a clinical trial involving fifteen patients with mild to moderate ulcerative colitis was conducted (Lewis et al., 2001). Each participant in the trial was given rosiglitazone 4 mg twice a day for a period of 12 weeks. *"In this pilot study, 27% of patients achieved a clinical remission, 20% achieved an endoscopic remission, and 53% had a clinical improvement within 12 wk of starting therapy."* (Lewis et al., 2001) Well, that's a start! Rosiglitazone appeared promising, indeed. Perhaps this drug, or other drugs of this class, would be a suitable treatment for ulcerative colitis.

In 2008, two studies reported results similar to the study mentioned above. Both studies (Lewis et al., 2008 and Liang and Ouyang, 2008) combined rosiglitzazone with 5-ASA, and both studies showed beneficial results of combining these two drugs. In an article evaluating the results of all three studies reported here, the following was written:

> *Can rosiglitazone be added to our conventional therapeutic guidelines and recommended in patients with active ulcerative colitis? The ability of rosiglitazone to <u>induce a rapid response</u> in more than 40% of UC patients intolerant or refractory to aminosalicylates (≥ 2 g/day for at least 4 weeks), with a similar efficacy in all subgroups of patients according to varying extent of disease and their ability to respond to steroids or immune-modulators, is attractive.* (Desreumaux and Dubuquoy 2009, emphasis added)

Too bad there is a catch. Rosigitazone (and a related drug, piolitazone, AKA Actose) was found to cause serious side effects. Once it was realized that the development of congestive heart failure will likely do the ulcerative colitis patient no favors, the interest in using this drug and drugs of this class faded and a conclusion was reached.

Most notably, the PPARγ agonist rosiglitazone showed therapeutic efficacy in humans with UC. However, rosiglitazone and other drugs belonging to the thiazolidinedione (TZD) class of anti-diabetic drugs are unlikely to be adopted for the treatment of IBD because of their significant side effects (i.e., fluid retention, hepatotoxicity, weight gain and congestive heart failure) and a U.S. Food and Drug Administration (FDA)-mandated "black box warning" for rosiglitazone [Avanda] and pioglitazone [Actose]. (Mohapatra et al., 2010)

Perhaps these PPARγ agonists, *rosiglitazone and pioglitazone,* are just too good at what they do. It has been suggested that agents that strongly bind PPARγ, may not be as effective as agents that only have a moderate affinity to this receptor (see Martin, 2009). Apparently, a strong binding to PPARγ can lead to unwanted side effects. The cell must need some wiggle room. I suspect the PPARγ agonist CLA has wiggle room written all over it.

9-CLA to the rescue

It is now well established that CLA have antiproliferative [anti-cancer] and anti-inflammatory effects on colonocytes, so provision of CLA in the intestinal lumen could be considered beneficial, particularly for inflammatory bowel diseases, such as ulcerative colitis and Crohn's disease. **~Devillard et al., 2007**

. . . CLA milk fat is considered a natural inflammation fighter as it has the ability to reduce the TNF-α and IL-6 expression. **~Kanwar et al., 2016**

Sounds like targeting PPARγ is something "we" should do. And since CLA targets this receptor, and has anti-inflammatory properties, perhaps we should consider its use in the battle against ulcerative colitis. It works for mice, and it works for pigs.

In a hallmark study (Hontecillas et al., 2002), pigs were used to evaluate the potential for CLA as a therapy for ulcerative colitis. Pigs were chosen because humans and pigs closely resemble each other (some more than others). The study basically found that the administration of CLA, prior to infecting the pig with a bacterium that predictably creates colitis, prevented or lessened the severity of colitis. The investigators state: *"This is the first-time observation demonstrating that dietary CLA supplementation prevents or ameliorates the onset of experimental colitis in pigs."* (Hontecillas et al., 2002)

One may be tempted to go to the supplement store and buy a bottle of CLA, thinking this is the path to take to gain an advantage by targeting PPARγ. This may not be a good idea, as CLA supplementation in this form can lead to oxidative stress and insulin resistance and has not lived up to all the hype (Benjamin et al., 2015). Let's look a little deeper.

The CLA found in CLA supplements is a mixture of CLA forms, 70% of which being a 50:50 mix of *cis-9, trans-11* and *trans-10, cis-12* (Benjamin et al., 2015). As opposed to *trans-10, cis-12*, ***cis-9, trans-11*** **is the** ***"biologically active"*** **and** ***"natural"*** **CLA form** (Benjamin et al., 2015). Importantly, **1)** *"trans-10, cis-12 isoform are* <u>not</u> *normally found in nature,"* **2)** are *"normally rare in the diet,"* and **3)** actually <u>antagonizes</u> PPARγ rather than activates PPARγ (Martin, 2009), making CLA supplements a dubious choice, at least for humans.

It should be noted, however, the "pig" study mentioned above used a mixture of CLA isomers synthesized from sunflower oil, likely similar to the CLA supplements currently on the market. In my view, they should have given the pigs a more natural form of CLA called "rumenic acid," otherwise known as 9-CLA. Last time I looked, you can't buy rumenic acid, but last time I looked, you can eat rumenic acid. That's where the cow comes in.

The "natural" method of obtaining 9-CLA is by diet, not by supplementation. For our benefit, cows make 9-CLA for us—actually, it is the bacteria in cows that make 9-CLA for us by acting on the linoleic acid (a fat) found in various grasses. Similarly, the bacteria in humans can make it for us, too, but that takes a healthy microbiome to pull this off (Wikipedia, 2019).

Since the experts (and me) want you to limit meat consumption, and because you may need to limit dairy consumption due to your ulcerative colitis, what you're left with is butter. And when it comes to 9-CLA, the best butter is the butter from grass-fed cows. And with respect to butter:

> Intake of butter *naturally* enriched with cis-9,trans-11 CLA reduced systemic inflammatory mediators in healthy adults. (Kanwar et al., 2016, emphasis added)

So here's the deal: Butter from grass-fed cows will supply you with several times more 9-CLA than average, store-bought butter (Wikipedia, 2019). This could give you an advantage. This fat, 9-CLA, acts to suppress inflammation. Other fats are recommended for this purpose, so why not promote the use of 9-CLA? And why not promote a food particularly high in this fatty acid? To gain an advantage in this life, I, personally, use a grass-fed butter imported from Ireland called **Kerrygold**™. Call me crazy, but I have no interest contracting cancer, including colorectal cancer. 9-CLA, clearly, has anti-cancer properties written all over it. One study, involving 60,708 women, found

> . . . women who consumed four or more servings of high-fat dairy foods per day (including whole milk, full-fat cultured milk, cheese, cream sour cream and butter) showed half the risk of developing colorectal cancer, compared to women who consumed less than one serving per day. (Benjamin et al., 2015)

9-CLA should probably be added to the list of fats that are healthy fats. And it looks like the best source for 9-CLA is butter from grass-fed cows. This fat, 9-CLA, activates PPARγ (it must "butter" it up). Perhaps activating PPARγ in this manner will help you in your battle against ulcerative colitis.

> As CLA is mainly found in milk and meat products and may also be generated from linoleic acid by human gut microflora, these studies are important, identifying for the first time that PPARγ natural ligands present in food or synthesized by commensal flora may improve colon inflammation. (Dubuquoy et al., 2006)

Other PPARγ agonists

In addition to 9-CLA, there are other substances that bind and activate PPARγ, a substance you are already familiar with. Briefly:

Fish oil

Fish oil is regarded as a "potent" PPARγ agonist (activator) (Su et al., 1999). Its use could be helpful in reducing colon inflammation, but as I pointed out in *Chapter 9*, fish oil supplementation can be problematic (please review). So, as in all things ulcerative colitis, seek the advice of your physician before you proceed with fish oil supplementation, even though PPARγ activation (agonism) is a noble endeavor.

EVOO

We discussed EVOO in *Chapter 17* and briefly mentioned it near the beginning of this chapter. Recall, EVOO stands for extra-virgin olive oil. This oil is rich in polyphenols, reportedly able to bind and activate PPARγ (Sánchez-Fidalgo et al., 2013), and is considered a healthy fat.

Prebiotics

Prebiotics, fiber-rich foods, and resistant starch promote the production of short chain fatty acids (SCFA), which go into the production butyrate, a known PPARγ agonist (Byndloss et al., 2017). In this manner, wise dietary choices impact the PPARγ pathway. In *Chapter 8* I discuss butyrate at length. Please review.

Another benefit of butter besides its CLA content, related to SCFAs, is a component in butter called **tributyrin**, Unlike CLA, which is absorbed in the small intestine (Bassaganya-Riera et al., 2012), tributyrin degrades in the large intestine and boosts butyrate concentrations (Byndloss et al., 2017). You can find tributyrin as a supplement online, often combined with butyrate.

Probiotics

> *While dietary CLA can be absorbed in the small intestinal and enter the plasma pools, CLA produced by the microbiota is not being absorbed in the large intestine but exerts local immune modulatory and protective effects.*
> **~Bassaganya-Riera et al., 2012**

Although indirectly, certain probiotics can activate PPARγ, including the bacterial strains found in VSL#3 (Bassaganya-Riera et al., 2012). They do this by first converting linoleic acid to CLA in the small intestine. Subsequently, the CLA is absorbed into the bloodstream to circulate and to find a PPARγ receptor in waiting, with benefits to follow. But if not absorbed into the bloodstream, the CLA that reaches the colon *"exerts local immune modulatory and protective effects."* (Bassaganya-Riera et al., 2012)

In conclusion

There are other natural PPARγ agonists to consider in the treatment of ulcerative colitis. Among them is **quercetin, naringenin**, and a flavonoid found in red clover called **biochanin A** (Martin, 2009). Although not a direct PPARγ agonist, **curcumin** and the active ingredient in ginger, **zingerone**, upregulate this receptor, thereby contributing to the anti-inflammatory role of PPARγ agonists (Martin, 2009). *"Inadequate expression of PPARγ leads to activation of inflammatory cascade leading to IBD."* (Ray, 2008, emphasis added) So, increasing the expression of PPARγ sounds pretty important to me. Adding PPARγ agonists to the mix sounds pretty important to me.

One last thing. Selenium deficiency can negatively impact PPARγ (Nettleford and Prabhu, 2018). And typically, ulcerative colitis patients are low in selenium (Nettleford and Prabhu, 2018). One laboratory demonstrated *"a critical role"* for selenium in the activation of PPARγ (Nettleford and Prabhu, 2018). And you certainly need this: Activated PPARγ has the ability to downregulate NF-κB (Nettleford and Prabhu, 2018). Have you discussed selenium with your physician lately?

> . . . *Se (selenium) supplementation mitigates inflammation, while increasing pro-resolutory pathways, suggesting that Se may be a potential therapeutic candidate for IBD.* (Nettleford and Prabhu, 2018)

A bit of a myristery

Palm and coconut oil are regarded by many individuals as healthy fats. However, both oils are relatively high in a fatty acid called **myristic acid**. Unfortunately, one study found that in ulcerative colitis patients, maintained in remission by mesalamine, myristic acid consumption was uniquely associated with an increased risk of disease flare (Barnes et al., 2017). Also, unfortunately, dairy also contains a fair amount of this fatty acid.

As we discussed in this chapter, 9-CLA is a good fat, but other fats in dairy may be problematic. So, it just makes sense to limit fat consumption, overall, in the battle against ulcerative colitis, yet make attempts to consume the fats that are the healthiest and most beneficial. Importantly, we do need fat in our diet, so making wise choices here is a wise course of action. As we have previously learned, in ulcerative colitis, limiting saturated fat is favorable, limiting omega-6 fatty acids is desirable, and increasing the consumption of the omega-3s and 9-CLA appears to be warranted. With respect to butter, it stands to reason that choosing grass-fed butter, a butter with a higher proportion of CLA than regular butter, translates into a butter with a lower percentage of myristic acid. Myristic acid is even in breast milk, so it is probably something that is useful and should not be avoided entirely.

~References~

Barnes EL, Nestor M, Onyewadume L, de Silva PS, Korzenik JR, Aguilar H, Bailen L, Berman A, Bhaskar SK, Brown M, Catinis G. **High dietary intake of specific fatty acids increases risk of flares in patients with ulcerative colitis in remission during treatment with aminosalicylates.** Clinical Gastroenterology and Hepatology. 2017 Sep 1;15(9):1390-6.

Bassaganya-Riera J, Hontecillas R. **Dietary CLA and n-3 PUFA in inflammatory bowel disease.** Current opinion in clinical nutrition and metabolic care. 2010 Sep;13(5):569.

Bassaganya-Riera J, Viladomiu M, Pedragosa M, De Simone C, Carbo A, Shaykhutdinov R, Jobin C, Arthur JC, Corl BA, Vogel H, Storr M. **Probiotic bacteria produce conjugated linoleic acid locally in the gut that targets macrophage PPAR γ to suppress colitis.** PloS one. 2012 Feb 21;7(2):e31238.

Benjamin S, Prakasan P, Sreedharan S, Wright AD, Spener F. **Pros and cons of CLA consumption: an insight from clinical evidences.** Nutrition & metabolism. 2015 Dec;12(1):4.

Borniquel S, Jädert C, Lundberg JO. **Dietary conjugated linoleic acid activates PPARγ and the intestinal trefoil factor in SW480 cells and mice with dextran sulfate sodium-induced colitis.** The Journal of nutrition. 2012 Oct 17;142(12):2135-40.

Byndloss MX, Olsan EE, Rivera-Chávez F, Tiffany CR, Cevallos SA, Lokken KL, Torres TP, Byndloss AJ, Faber F, Gao Y, Litvak Y. **Microbiota-activated PPAR-γ signaling inhibits dysbiotic Enterobacteriaceae expansion.** Science. 2017 Aug 11;357(6351):570-5.

Byndloss MX, Litvak Y, Bäumler AJ. **Microbiota-nourishing immunity and its relevance for ulcerative colitis.** Inflammatory bowel diseases. 2019 Jan 30;25(5):811-5.

Chamaillard M, Dessein R. **Defensins couple dysbiosis to primary immunodeficiency in Crohn's disease.** World Journal of Gastroenterology: WJG. 2011 Feb 7;17(5):567.

Desreumaux P, Dubuquoy L. **PPARγ agonists as a new class of effective treatment for ulcerative colitis.** Inflammatory bowel diseases. 2009 Jun;15(6):959-60.

Devillard E, McIntosh FM, Duncan SH, Wallace RJ. **Metabolism of linoleic acid by human gut bacteria: different routes for biosynthesis of conjugated linoleic acid.** Journal of bacteriology. 2007 Mar 15;189(6):2566-70.

Dubuquoy L, Rousseaux C, Thuru X, Peyrin-Biroulet L, Romano O, Chavatte P, Chamaillard M, Desreumaux P. **PPARγ as a new therapeutic target in inflammatory bowel diseases.** Gut. 2006 Sep 1;55(9):1341-9.

Evans NP, Misyak SA, Schmelz EM, Guri AJ, Hontecillas R, Bassaganya-Riera J. **Conjugated linoleic acid ameliorates inflammation-induced colorectal cancer in mice through activation of PPARγ.** The Journal of nutrition. 2010 Jan 20;140(3):515-21.

Hontecillas R, Wannemeulher MJ, Zimmerman DR, Hutto DL, Wilson JH, Ahn DU, Bassaganya-Riera J. **Nutritional regulation of porcine bacterial-induced colitis by conjugated linoleic acid.** The Journal of nutrition. 2002 Jul 1;132(7):2019-27.

Housley WJ, O'C'nor CA, Nichols F, Puddington L, Lingenheld EG, Zhu L, Clark RB. **PPARγ regulates retinoic acid-mediated DC induction of Tregs.** Journal of leukocyte biology. 2009 Aug;86(2):293-301.

Kanwar JR, Kanwar RK, Stathopoulos S, Haggarty NW, MacGibbon AK, Palmano KP, Roy K, Rowan A, Krissansen GW. **Comparative activities of milk components in reversing chronic colitis.** Journal of dairy science. 2016 Apr 1;99(4):2488-501.

Kay JK, Mackle TR, Auldist MJ, Thomson NA, Bauman DE. **Endogenous synthesis of cis-9, trans-11 conjugated linoleic acid in dairy cows fed fresh pasture.** Journal of Dairy Science. 2004 Feb 1;87(2):369-78.

Lewis JD, Lichtenstein GR, Stein RB, Deren JJ, Judge TA, Fogt F, Furth EE, Demissie EJ, Hurd LB, Su CG, Keilbaugh SA. **An open-label trial of the PPARγ ligand rosiglitazone for active ulcerative colitis.** The American journal of gastroenterology. 2001 Dec;96(12):3323.

Lewis JD, Lichtenstein GR, Deren JJ, Sands BE, Hanauer SB, Katz JA, Lashner B, Present DH, Chuai S, Ellenberg JH, Nessel L. **Rosiglitazone for active ulcerative** colitis: a randomized placebo-controlled trial. Gastroenterology. 2008 Mar 1;134(3):688-95.

Liang HL, Ouyang Q. A clinical trial of combined use of rosiglitazone and 5-aminosalicylate for ulcerative colitis. World journal of gastroenterology: WJG. 2008 Jan 7;14(1):114.

Martin H. Role of PPAR-gamma in inflammation. Prospects for therapeutic intervention by food components. Mutation research. 2009 Oct;669(1-2):1-7.

Mohapatra SK, Guri AJ, Climent M, Vives C, Carbo A, Horne WT, Hontecillas R, Bassaganya-Riera J. Immunoregulatory actions of epithelial cell PPAR γ at the colonic mucosa of mice with experimental inflammatory bowel disease. PLos One. 2010 Apr 20;5(4):e10215.

Necela BM, Thompson EA. Pathophysiological Roles of PPARγ in Gastrointestinal Epithelial Cells. PPAR research. 2008;2008.

Nettleford S, Prabhu K. Selenium and selenoproteins in gut inflammation—A review. Antioxidants. 2018 Mar;7(3):36.

Ray G. Advances in the Management of Inflammatory Bowel Disease. Medicine Update 18(Chapter 34) 2008;264–270.

Risérus U, Vessby B, Ärnlöv J, Basu S. Effects of cis-9, trans-11 conjugated linoleic acid supplementation on insulin sensitivity, lipid peroxidation, and proinflammatory markers in obese men. The American journal of clinical nutrition. 2004 Aug 1;80(2):279-83.

Sánchez-Fidalgo S, Cárdeno A, Sánchez-Hidalgo M, Aparicio-Soto M, de la Lastra CA. Dietary extra virgin olive oil polyphenols supplementation modulates DSS-induced chronic colitis in mice. The Journal of nutritional biochemistry. 2013 Jul 1;24(7):1401-13.

Schuster S, Cabrera D, Arrese M, Feldstein AE. Triggering and resolution of inflammation in NASH. Nature Reviews Gastroenterology & Hepatology. 2018 Jun;15(6):349.

Su CG, Wen X, Bailey ST, Jiang W, Rangwala SM, Keilbaugh SA, Flanigan A, Murthy S, Lazar MA, Wu GD. A novel therapy for colitis utilizing PPAR-γ ligands to inhibit the epithelial inflammatory response. The Journal of clinical investigation. 1999 Aug 15;104(4):383-9.

Thompson EA. **PPARγ Physiology and Pathology in Gastrointestinal Epithelial Cells.** Molecules & Cells (Springer Science & Business Media BV). 2007 Oct 1;24(2).

Wada K, Nakajima A, Blumberg RS. **PPARγ and inflammatory bowel disease: a new therapeutic target for ulcerative colitis and Crohn's'disease.** Trends in molecular medicine. 2001 Aug 1;7(8):329-31.

Wang L, Waltenberger B, Pferschy-Wenzig EM, Blunder M, Liu X, Malainer C, Blazevic T, Schwaiger S, Rollinger JM, Heiss EH, Schuster D. **Natural product agonists of peroxisome proliferator-activated receptor gamma (PPARγ): a review.** Biochemical pharmacology. 2014 Nov 1;92(1):73-89.

Wikipedia **Conjugated Linoleic Acid.** 2019
https://en.wikipedia.org/wiki/Conjugated_linoleic_acid

Chapter 21

Of all the nerve!

> *Inflammation is a local, protective response to microbial invasion or injury. It **must be fine-tuned and regulated precisely**, because deficiencies or excesses of the inflammatory response cause morbidity and shorten lifespan. The discovery that cholinergic neurons inhibit acute inflammation has qualitatively expanded our understanding of how the nervous system modulates immune responses. **The nervous system reflexively regulates the inflammatory response <u>in real time</u>**, just as it controls heart rate and other vital functions. The opportunity now exists to apply this insight to the treatment of inflammation through selective and reversible 'hard-wired' neural systems.* ~Tracey, 2002, emphasis added

> *Recent evidence supports the idea that **the central nervous system interacts dynamically via the vagus nerve with the intestinal immune system to modulate inflammation** through humoral and neural pathways, using a mechanism also referred to as the intestinal cholinergic anti-inflammatory pathway.* ~Goverse et al., 2016, emphasis added

> ***Autonomic imbalance plays a <u>pivotal role</u> in the pathophysiology of inflammatory bowel disease (IBD).*** ~Seyedabadi et al., 2018, emphasis added

The nervous system is *so* into control. It's in control of your breathing, your sweating, your digestion, your voluntary and involuntary movements, your just about everything. Surprisingly, the nervous system also exerts control over the immune system, a system that responds to insult and injury and works to keep you safe. I'm so surprised! Who would have thought?

Based on ground-breaking research, we now know that the cells of the immune system communicate with the cells of the nervous system and the cells of the nervous system communicate right back . . . and *"in real time."* Who would have thought?

When I first heard of this, I said to myself *"This . . . changes . . . everything!"* And I still believe this. In this chapter I will share with you what I know about the so-called Cholinergic Anti-inflammatory Pathway, and what it can do for you, the patient with ulcerative colitis. I tell a most interesting story.

> In this sense, the regulation of inflammation seems to be considered in terms of checkpoints. Among these mechanisms, **<u>the nervous system is the main regulator of the immune system</u>**. (Peña et al., 2011, emphasis added)

A most interesting story

> The main task of the immune system is to distinguish and respond accordingly to 'danger' or 'non-danger' signals. **This is of critical importance in the gastrointestinal tract** in which immune cells are constantly in contact with food antigens, symbiotic microflora and potential pathogens. **~Goverse et al., 2016, emphasis added**

> The nervous system integrates the inflammatory response: it gathers information about invasive events from several local sites, mobilizes defenses and creates memory to improve chances for survival. **~Tracey, 2002**

> The vagus nerve not only is essential in the detection of inflammation but also provides an important route through which the central nervous system can respond. **~Van Westerloo et al., 2005**

This most interesting story goes something like this:

Once upon a time—actually, in the year 2000—a team of investigators revealed for the first time a pathway that can inhibit inflammation, involving a major nerve in the body, the vagus nerve (Goverse et al., 2016). This gave way to other, related discoveries. Not only could vagal stimulation (electrical or otherwise) block or reduce inflammation, but there is a unique receptor intimately involved, called the **α7 nicotinic acetylcholine receptor (α7nAChR)**. In fact, *"The anti-inflammatory properties of the vagus nerve depend on activation of α7nAChR."* (Seyedabadi et al., 2018) Importantly, the α7 nicotinic acetylcholine receptor resides notably on the surface of the macrophage and dendritic cell—and is responsive to the vagus nerve via the molecule it releases to get things done, **acetylcholine** (Goverse et al., 2016). Funny thing, this receptor is also responsive to nicotine, hence the inclusion of nicotine in its name. Long known is the anti-inflammatory effect of smoking in preventing or reducing the severity of ulcerative colitis. It is the Cholinergic Anti-inflammatory Pathway that explains it all.

So, let's get this straight. The vagus nerve controls the inflammatory response, and it uses acetylcholine to stimulate a receptor situated on the surface an immune cell to pull this off. But what controls the vagus nerve? That would be the brain. *"As the activity of this pathway is controlled by neural signals, it provides a way for the brain to regulate the cytokine response in a localized, controlled, and organ-specific manner."* (Tracey, 2005) Ironically, this is the same brain that can arrive at the conclusion that smoking is the cool thing to do. Yes, the same brain that allows you to do stupid stuff in life and make decisions that are so unwise, even deadly. (Hint!)

If a pathway can control the inflammatory response, wouldn't it be wise to take advantage of it? Or we could simply ignore it and go on our merry way. I, personally, would not go on my merry way.

The advantages of taking advantage of the Cholinergic Anti-inflammatory Pathway include:

- Reduction in pro-inflammatory cytokine production without affecting the production of anti-inflammatory cytokines (Pavlov and Tracey, 2006; Giebelen et al., 2009)

- Reduction in mucosal inflammation (Ji et al., 2014)

- Reduction in intestinal permeability (Van Der Zanden et al., 2009)

- Protection of involved tissues by inhibiting a local, excessive inflammatory response (Tracey, 2010)

- Enhancing the ability of the macrophage to devour the pathogen (De Winter and De Man, 2010)

- Inhibition of proinflammatory, M1 macrophages (Bonaz et al., 2018)

Clearly, targeting this pathway *is* something worthwhile to do. We'll discuss the ways to do this in a few minutes, but first we need to tuck a few more concepts under our belt.

The vagus nerve is part of what is called the autonomic nervous system, which serves to control a multitude of bodily functions. The autonomic nervous system originates in the brain, the fibers of which extend outward or downward in networks, and is divided into two branches, the sympathetic nervous system and the parasympathetic nervous system. This sets up a dynamic whereby one branch can counteract the other branch, to a degree, as they modulate various bodily functions. Importantly, both have an influence on the immune system. Higher sympathetic activity (tone) can be proinflammatory; whereas, higher parasympathetic activity (tone) can be anti-inflammatory. According to the scheme of things, *"Parasympathetic impairment results in a dominant sympathetic drive, and it is known that this enhances* _colonic inflammation."_ (Ghia et al., 2007) And **this** is why you take advantage of the Cholinergic Anti-inflammatory Pathway!

"What would impair the parasympathetic nervous system and create a dominant sympathetic drive?" You ask. Stress will do it.

The stresses of life (anxiety, worry, ongoing uncomfortable situations, depression, dysfunctional relationships, the rat race, etc.) can increase sympathetic tone and impair parasympathetic tone. Unfortunately, the major nerve of the parasympathetic nervous system, **the vagus nerve, is negatively impacted by stress**—the very nerve at the heart of the Cholinergic Anti-inflammatory Pathway. And with that, I have a story to tell. I've told this story before, in my book **More to Consider in the Battle Against Crohn's**. What follows is an excerpt from the book.

A story within a story

Various sensory and cognitive signals then converge to activate a stress response that triggers several adaptive processes in the body and brain aimed at restoring homeostasis. If stressful situations become chronic and uncontrollable, then an imbalance may occur that can exert deleterious effects on virtually all organs. **~Lucassen et al., 2010**

Stress is an environmental stimulus that flares from a variety of circumstances and has become ingrained in human society. Small bouts of stress are believed to enhance the host's immune response; however, **prolonged periods of stress can be detrimental through excess production of neuroendocrine-derived mediators that dampen immune responses to invasive pathogens.**

Stress-related molecules dampen immune responses . . . bacteria can use these factors to enhance microbial pathogenesis during stress.

Collectively, increased sympathetic stimulation, presumably during periods of stress, may increase the susceptibility to the host to pathogenic *infection by influencing virulence capacity related to adhesion and antimicrobial defenses.* ~**Radek, 2010, emphasis added**

I *never* thought we could *ever* run out of mice to experiment on, but apparently shortly after World War II, a mouse shortage of biblical proportions occurred. But, hey, there are always plenty of college students around to experiment on. So it was off to the headache lab for anyone wanting to make a quick buck.

In this experiment, college students—in this case, medical students (how fun)—were each fitted with a helmet, with not 16, not 17, but 18 screws, all exiting from what could correctly be identified as an implement of torture. But college students are used to doing stupid stuff, so it was easy to prey on the willing.

The study was intended to see if a stressor like pain, like headache pain, would produce a negative effect on the bowel. And so the screws were tightened, one by one—not enough for the eyes to pop out, but just enough to simulate Excedrin Headache #37. They did not tell the students what was up next. A colonoscope was up next! (My skill as a humorist is certainly coming in handy.)

So here we have, in one place, screwed medical students and scientists holding colonoscopies. (Try not to go into great detail in creating a mental image of this scene.) A procedure is about to be performed. Of course, this happened in 1947, or thereabouts, so the procedure is now over, the medical students are all grown up (probably retired or worse), and a report has finally made it to my desk. According to the study . . .

The students were fitted with a metal helmet containing 18 large screws that could be tightened against the head to produce a painful distressing headache lasting 30 min during which time visual colonoscopic evaluation of the sigmoid colon was recorded. In each case the authors visualized severe colonic spasm, which was sufficient to occlude the lumen. Marked mucosal hyperemia and engorgement with intermittent blanching and flushing (perfusion/

reperfusion) was also noted. During periods of maximum engorgement, gentle movement of the proctoscope caused a superficial injury with hemorrhage. Nausea often accompanied visualized episodes of colonic spasm. This study indicates that stress can cause severe alterations in colonic function and predispose to colonic hypoxia and reoxygenation (perfusion/reperfusion) injury (sequential blanching and hyperemia with mucosal engorgement). Thus, local stress-induced colonic spasm is mediated via the enteric nervous system, which results in spastic contraction of colonic smooth muscle leading to transient local tissue hypoxemia with subsequent reoxygenation upon colonic smooth muscle relaxation. (Pravda, 2005)

This study is *so* fascinating (and I still can't shake the mental image that I have created). It demonstrates quite clearly that what happens in the brain does not stay in the brain—and explains why we feel it in our gut when we experience stressful events that come our way as we journey through this life.

Coincidentally, when I was writing this chapter, a friend of mine, whose Crohn's was currently in remission had her symptoms briefly return while she was going through a stressful period in her life, dealing with a serious life-and-death issue involving one of her closest relatives. One can only guess what her bowel was going through, but it must not have been a pretty sight. During this challenging time, I encouraged her to study ways to reduce the level of stress she was experiencing. I even went so far as to tell her funny stories about medical students in compromising situations simply to distract her and to make her laugh. I think it helped! Humor *is* the best medicine. In time, and after the stress had passed, she returned to her previous state of remission and has remained so for several years.

Sure, extreme stress can negatively impact the bowel, but what about ongoing stress, what about psychological stress?

Mammals are under relentless bombardment by environmental stressors, including psychological anxiety, microorganisms, and physical insult. Although humans cannot distinguish between physical and psychological stressors, there exists a dramatic difference in the manner and degree to which stress is perceived and dealt with depending on the tolerance and coping mechanisms of the organism. As early as the 1970s, PS [psychological stress] was implicated in the suppression of immune responses believed to contribute to a higher incidence of infection and cancer. Stress has also been shown to exacerbate epithelial inflammatory diseases such as . . . Crohn's disease. (Radek, 2010)

Perhaps one of the most damaging effects of stress is its negative effect on the integrity of the mucosal barrier of the bowel, a barrier already compromised in Crohn's disease. Of course, a compromised mucosal barrier will require more purposeful inflammation in order to deal with the situation.

The stress-induced barrier defects via neuroendocrine proteins and their respective receptors may permit uptake of immunogenic material into the intestinal mucosa, which initiates or exacerbates intestinal inflammation frequently seen in recurring intestinal inflammatory diseases, such as Crohn's disease. (Radek, 2010)

I've made a great case for limiting stress, stress of any kind, as a strategy of war in our battle against Crohn's, but there is more to the story. There is one more issue to discuss concerning the negative effect of stress on the individual with Crohn's disease.

Previously, I spent a great deal of time on the battle over iron between pathogen and host. The pathogen is winning as long as it can obtain iron. The host is winning if iron is being successfully withheld (or the death of the pathogen can somehow be achieved). Surprisingly, stress makes iron more available to the pathogen! What, pray tell, is *this* all about?

Briefly, stress—major stress producing a negative effect on the host—causes iron to be released from the binding molecules that we use to sequester iron and prevent it from being accessible to bacteria (Radek 2010). This, of course, is good news for the pathogen that needs this iron, not only to survive, but to become more mobile, adherent, menacing, and more difficult to eradicate. It is the catecholamines, the signaling molecules/hormones that are excessively produced by the sympathetic nervous system during stress, that act to release iron from transferrin and lactoferrin and make iron more environmentally available for pathogen acquisition. Stress, to the pathogen, is the gift of iron! And so iron withholding, as an effective strategy of war—host vs. pathogen—should probably include the management of stress, even psychological stress.

Together, PS [psychological stress] acts to disrupt normal iron metabolism in the host via neuroendocrine hormones that result in metabolic disturbances, such as hypoferremia, which can increase the ability of invasive pathogens to proliferate and evade host antimicrobial mechanisms.

Concentrations of catecholamines . . . increase in the intestinal lumen following traumatic stress.

*The correlation among bacterial growth, iron limitation, and virulence has been recognized for over a decade, where **low host iron reserves present as a major impediment to microbial growth.*** (Radek, 2010, emphasis added)

Stress reduction should definitely be a part of your battle plan as you wage war against this disease we call Crohn's, or any disease for that matter. Managing stress may be all that it takes to turn things around and point you in the right direction. I am *very* serious. Stress allows for easier iron acquisition for the ambitious pathogen. *This* must stop!

Many clinicians have observed that emotional conflicts appear to provoke exacerbation of colitis.

In a more rigorous study using a larger sample of 124 IBD patients, Duffy et al. evaluated monthly life events with symptoms of pain, bowel dysfunction and bleeding. At baseline, patients with a history of major life events had a greater risk of active disease and there was a persisting twofold increased risk at 6 months followup. Another study of 10 patients with Crohn's disease found a significant association between acute daily stressors and bowel symptoms. (Bhatia and Tandon, 2005)

And speaking of stressors, I find writing this chapter to be quite stressful. I'd better bring it to a close (before it's too late).

This ends the excerpt from *More to Consider in the Battle Against Crohn's.* And I have good news. There are a few (million) copies left for purchase. Let's continue. There is more to the story.

More to the story

*Hence, this "cholinergic anti-inflammatory pathway" provides the host with **a powerful mechanism** for "sensing" inflammation via sensory pathways that relay information to the brain, as well as for counteracting excessive inflammation in a very fast, discrete, and localized way through acetylcholine release by the efferent vagus nerve.*

The vagus nerve not only is essential in the detection of inflammation but also provides an important route through which the central nervous system can respond. ~Van Westerloo et al., 2005, emphasis added

Clinical evidence indicates that when vagus nerve activity is deficient, inflammation is excessive. ~Huston and Tracey, 2011, **emphasis added**

Taking advantage of the Cholinergic Anti-inflammatory Pathway can be as easy as limiting the stresses of life. As easy as addressing depression with appropriate antidepressants. As easy as giving medications that allow acetylcholine to hang around longer and exert an influence before being metabolically disassembled. As easy as taking substances that activate the α7nAChR receptor. As easy as mechanically or electrically stimulating the vagus nerve. As easy as deep breathing exercises. As easy as saying "No" to fish oil supplementation. As easy as . . .

Let's look at the many ways to take advantage of this anti-inflammatory pathway.

Stress reduction

> *A study of stable IBD patients who were followed for over five years explored the influence of stress on exacerbating the disease. Those patients with high prolonged stressful life events were found to have a 90% recurrence rate of their colitis as compared to only 40% recurrence in low stress patients.* **~Hollander, 2004**

> *Indeed, stress increases intestinal permeability, modifies immunity and stimulates the sympathetic nervous system whilst inhibiting the vagus nerve (VN) thus disturbing the equilibrium of the autonomic nervous system (ANS).* **~Bonaz et al., 2017**

Do you really need to work your butt off just to become employee of the month . . . six months in a row? Do you really need to go for two master's degrees . . . while holding down a full-time job? Do you really need to get up a 4 AM, day after day, to drive your daughter across town before school for harmonica lessons? Do you really need to play video games all the livelong day? There are a lot of things that increase life's stresses that can be scaled back so a person can lead a less stressful life. Besides taking your life out of overdrive, there are other things you can do to reduce stress, increase vagal tone, and take advantage of the Cholinergic Anti-inflammatory Pathway.

Deep breathing exercises are an excellent way to cope with stress and increase vagal tone (Breit et al., 2018). So simple. *". . . slow breathing and long exhalation phase leads to an increase in parasymphetic tone."* (Breit et al., 2018)

Deep breathing actually forces you to meditate at the same time—both activities legendary at reducing stress and increasing vagal tone. Surprisingly, splashing your face with cold water stimulates the vagus nerve. (Try doing this every few minutes, all day long!) It is reported that chewing gum increases vagal tone. (Actually, you can do this all day long.) Also reported, lying on your right side while resting/sleeping increases vagal tone.

Then there is yoga, tai chi, singing, humming, laughing (at the funny things written in this book), listening to soothing music, biofeedback, thoughts of love and kindness—all activities that reduce stress and increase vagal tone.

You get the idea. Activities and situations that increase stress should be limited and activities and situations that relieve stress should be encouraged in order to take advantage of the Cholinergic Anti-inflammatory Pathway in the battle against ulcerative colitis.

A dominate sympathetic drive, which can simultaneously occur with impaired vagus nerve activity, has been associated with enhanced colonic inflammation. (Ji et al., 2014)

Emotional/psychological state and coping skills

Many clinicians have observed that emotional conflicts appear to provoke exacerbation of colitis. **~Bhatia and Tandon, 2005**

Separate investigations of HRV [heart rate variation] in IBD, CD and UC have revealed that during remission, some patients exhibit low vagal tone.

In an initial study, we observed that vagal tone was related to the emotional adjustment of patients (high vs. low negative emotions) and to their way of coping with the disease. A positive coping style had a biological cost, for instance in CD, as it was associated with low vagal tone. In contrast in UC, a positive coping style was associated with high vagal tone. This study revealed the importance of (i) separating populations of patients with IBD within studies and (ii) psychological factors on vagal tone. **~Bonaz et al., 2017**

The tone of the vagus nerve can be assessed clinically. It's complicated, but heart rate variability, evaluated under controlled conditions, can point to a problem with vagal tone (Bonaz et al., 2017; Breit et al., 2018). But let's just assume you do have a vagal tone problem, for you have ulcerative colitis and likely things are not going too well.

Perhaps of no surprise, emotions and an individual's psychological state play a role in the scheme of things. Emotions also imply coping skills. The bottom line here: If you have emotional or psychological issues that negatively impact your life, and you are not able to get control of your life, now is the time to get a handle on things. The Cholinergic Anti-inflammatory Pathway is at stake.

Since, the vagal tone is correlated with capacity to regulate stress responses and can be influenced by breathing, its increase through meditation and yoga likely contribute to resilience and the mitigation of mood and anxiety symptoms.

*It has been shown that self-generated positive emotions via loving-kindness meditation lead to an increase in positive emotions relative to the control group, an effect moderated by baseline vagal tone. In turn, **increased positive emotions produced increases in vagal tone**, which is probably mediated by increased perceptions of social connections. Individuals suffering from depression, anxiety, and chronic pain have benefited from regular mindfulness meditation training, demonstrating a remarkable improvement in symptom severity.* (Breit et al., 2018, emphasis added)

Cholecystokinin (CCK)

Clinical studies have demonstrated that high-fat nutrition could effectively increase vagus nerve activity, reduce the production of inflammatory mediators and improve inflammatory bowel disease, rheumatoid arthritis and cardiovascular disease. **~Wang et al., 2019**

Although it is well known that CCK regulates pancreatic secretion, gallbladder function, intestinal motility, and satiety, recent studies have provided new insights into the effects of CCK in these areas and have introduced a novel role of CCK in intestinal inflammation. **~Chandra and Liddle, 2007**

Most interestingly, dietary fat stimulates the Cholinergic Anti-inflammatory Pathway (Pavlov and Tracey, 2006). It does this by stimulating the release of the gut hormone cholecystokinin (CCK).

Mechanistically, once consumed, dietary fat establishes contact with specialized cells in the duodenum, jejunum, upper ilium, and can eventually reach specialized nerve cells located in the brain, via the bloodstream (Chandra and Liddle, 2007). In response to such contact, the cells in question produce cholecystokinin. Cholecystokinin then promptly goes to work, stimulating gall bladder contraction, stimulating intestinal motility, and stimulating the vagus nerve and activating the alpha7 nicotinic receptor (Luyer et al., 2005, Chandra and Liddle, 2007). A win-win!

Attention please! Although most dietary fat triggers cholecystokinin release, some fats such as saturated fats should probably be limited in a diet that favors remission in ulcerative colitis. We discussed this at length in *Chapter 10*, please review). Don't worry, there are other fats you can choose from that do an excellent job of stimulating cholecystokinin release.

One such fat is called **oleic acid**, *"known to be **a very potent stimulus for the release of the gastrointestinal hormone cholecystokinin."** (Jakob et al., 2001, emphasis added) Fortunately, it is relatively easy to add oleic acid to your diet. Both olive oil and avocados are high in this exceptional fatty acid (Jakob et al., 2001; Lerman-Garber et al., 1994).

I've warned against fish oil supplementation before in *Chapter 9*, again please review. I'm going to say **no** with respect to large amounts of fish oils with respect to the Cholinergic Anti-inflammatory Pathway. According to one study, **fish oils substantially decrease the release of cholecystokinin by 85%** (Riber et al., 1996).

Interestingly, there are cholecystokinin receptors on vagal nerve fibers (Breit et al., 2018). And, as mentioned, there are cholecystokinin receptors in various portions of the brain where cholecystokinin *"functions as a neurotransmitter."* (Breit et al., 2018) I guess, the production of this hormone should not be interfered with, as it plays an important role in the Cholinergic Anti-inflammatory Pathway. Even short-chain fatty acids, like butyrate, often deficient in the ulcerative colitis patient, can stimulate the vagus nerve *"in a CCK-dependent mechanism"* (Breit et al., 2018). This association between short-chain fatty acids and the Cholinergic Anti-inflammatory Pathway reinforces the rationale for following a plant-based diet as a therapy for ulcerative colitis, a diet that generates plenty of short-chain fatty acids.

Antidepressants

> *Depression is associated with abnormalities in innate and adaptive immune function, including increased production of pro-inflammatory cytokines, decreased production of anti-inflammatory cytokines and increased expression of surface markers associated with immune cell activation.* ~**Huston and Tracey, 2011**

> *. . . depressive-like behaviors in mice increased susceptibility to intestinal inflammation by interfering with the tonic vagal inhibition of proinflammatory macrophages and that tricyclic antidepressants restored vagal function and reduced inflammation.* ~**Ghia et al., 2008**

Major depression is characterized by significantly depressed mood and the reduced responsiveness to pleasurable stimuli (anhedonia) coupled with behavior and cognitive changes such as sleep alterations, weight gain or weight loss, and difficulty concentrating and making decisions. This psychological disorder is multifaceted, and it significantly affects an individual's mental and physical health.

Endocrine and autonomic changes associated with depression . . . are not unlike those accompanying exposure to stress. **~Grippo and Johnson, 2002, emphasis added**

Importantly, it has been proven that several antidepressants exert anti-inflammatory effects in the brain as well as in the periphery by different mechanisms. **~Ondicova et al., 2019**

Need I say more? Yes. My guess is, some antidepressants work better than others when it comes to influencing the anti-inflammatory pathway in question.

Prozac (fluoxine), is an antidepressant which *"exerts* **potent** *anti-inflammatory effects,"* and does so, in part, by favorably influencing the vagus nerve (Ondicova et al., 2019, emphasis added). So, with Prozac, we have both an antidepressant and an anti-inflammatory. Could come in handy.

However, not all antidepressants are the same when it comes to modulating vagal nerve activity (Dawood et al., 2009). So, careful choice of antidepressants, and proper dose of the chosen antidepressant, is required, or the opposite effect may occur—and increase in sympathetic activity with a decrease in vagal activity (Dawood et al., 2009). Prozac seems like a good drug choice, should depression be part of the life of the ulcerative colitis patient. If the ulcerative colitis patient does not have depression (or anxiety) and wishes to give it a try to influence the vagus nerve and produce other anti-inflammatory effects, perhaps the "off-label" use of Prozac may be justified. But there are other ways and there are other means.

Clonidine

An overall increase of sympathetic activity characterized active UC. Normalization of the autonomic profile by clonidine was accompanied by an improvement of the disease.

Taken together, these findings indicate the existence of an abnormally enhanced sympathetic activity in subjects suffering from active UC.
~Furlan et al., 2006

This is interesting!   A medicine used to lower blood pressure, clonidine, can influence the nervous system by lowering sympathetic nervous tone, and has the power to improve the lives of the patients with ulcerative colitis. This caught my eye, and I had to share it with you.

On the surface, the clonidine story may be more about dealing with sympathetic overactivity than dealing with parasympathetic underactivity; however, per the scheme of things, a reduced sympathetic drive automatically translates into increased parasympathetic drive, which increases vagal tone.

Amiodarone

*The cardiac anti-arrhythmic drug **amiodarone** has been identified as an inhibitor of TNF syntheses in monocytes in vitro, but it also functions as a **potent stimulator of vagus nerve activity**.* **~Tracey, 2002, emphasis added**

Amiodarone led to a dramatic healing of both oral and colonic ulcers. This effect lasted 7 years for the colon and 9 years for the mouth. **~Maroy, 2009**

It is unlikely your gastroenterologist will jump at the chance to give you this drug. This is understandable, in as much as amiodarone is not in the Gastroenterology playbook and has the potential to cause serious side effects. But you never know—he or she is a specialist in the use of dangerous drugs irrespective of potential side effects, and just may consider a therapeutic trial of amiodarone, particularly after reading the following case report.

From an article written in 2009 by Maroy, the story is told of a 71-year-old gentleman who presented with a complex history that included chronic skin lesions, mouth ulcers *"continuous for 55 years,"* and was repeatedly besieged by other horrible things. (A boil is a horrible thing.) And if all that wasn't enough, here come the tummy troubles, which led to the discovery of a large ulceration in the beginning portion of his colon, some 15 years after receiving the diagnosis of **Behçet's syndrome**.

Curiosity got the best of me, so I went online and reviewed pictures of several patients with this disease. All I can say is, be thankful you have ulcerative colitis! I noticed that the images of the diseased colons of Behçet's syndrome patients look a lot like your hideous looking colon. Continuing with our case report . . .

Some 4 years after the start of tummy troubles, our gentleman's tummy troubles continued, refractory to conventional treatment—and a follow-up colonoscopy showed a progression of his colonic ulceration. Additionally, his oral ulcerations, *"which were almost permanent,"* persisted. Then, here comes cardiac problems . . . fortunately!

For reasons not entirely clear, our patient developed a relatively common abnormal cardiac rhythm called **atrial fibrillation**. And here is the fortunate part: The drug amiodarone was prescribed to control the abnormal heart rhythm. And surprise surprise!

Within a couple of days after the start of amiodarone, the mouth ulcer healed. A colonoscopy one month later revealed the ulceration in the colon to be *"completely healed"* (Maroy, 2009). This must have been *very* exciting! And there was more good news: The original colon ulcerations remained healed; however, a small, newly acquired ulceration in the same region showed up along the way but was short-lived as amiodarone therapy continued. Last look (with a colonoscope), 7 years later, the ulcerations remained healed. In the light of this study, perhaps the gastroenterology community should seriously explore the potential for amiodarone in the battle against ulcerative colitis. Perhaps. Maybe hearing that amiodarone is a *"potent stimulator of vagus nerve activity,"* and has anti-inflammatory effects, will help make the case.

> *Amiodarone decreases TNF alpha and IL 6 secretion and has also anti-inflammatory and anti-oxydative [sic] properties. These properties could explain its benefit for the patient.* (Maroy, 2009)

Acetylcholinesterase inhibition

> *An interesting way to downregulate macrophages is to interfere with the cholinergic anti-inflammatory pathway; for instance, by the use of α7 nicotinic acetylcholine receptors agonists, direct vagal stimulation or the use of acetylcholine esterase inhibitors.* ~**De Winter and De Man, 2010**

There are multiple ways to target the Cholinergic Anti-inflammatory Pathway. One way is to inhibit an enzyme that exists to disassemble acetylcholine moments after it is released. Inhibiting this enzyme, **acetylcholinesterase**, allows acetylcholine to have a little more hangtime and ability to accumulate, and thereby increases vagal stimulation of the target cell (Wang et al., 2018). Don't underestimate this approach to place the brakes on excessive inflammation. And with that, I have a story to tell.

Not sure any sane person would do this, even on a dare, but when it comes to medical research, people do the strangest of things. Punching a hole in the intestine of a mouse is, in my book, not a particularly normal behavior. But if you are a scientist, you can do stuff like this all day long and no one raises an eyebrow. Astonishingly, you can make a good living doing this sort of thing.

In a mouse model of sepsis (bacteria entering the bloodstream), created by creating a hole in the intestine to allow bacteria to escape and invade, the Cholinergic Anti-inflammatory Pathway was put to the test

(Hofer et al., 2008). The purpose of the study was to see if inhibiting acetylcholinesterase would blunt the inflammatory response. In sepsis, the inflammatory response goes into overdrive, and can be intense enough to kill.

During this experiment, it was found that giving a drug that inhibits the breakdown of acetylcholine, <u>significantly increased</u> the survival and *"resolution of sepsis"* of the treated mice, compared with those untreated (Hofer et al., 2008). It should be noted, some mice were given nicotine instead of an acetylcholinesterase inhibitor, which also attenuated the lethal inflammatory response to sepsis and promoted survival. We'll talk about nicotine later.

There are several medications currently available that inhibit acetylcholinesterase. One such is **Aricept** (Donepezil), a drug given to help the brains of Alzheimer's patients work better. Another medication, **Rasadyne** (Galantamine), is used for the same reason, to inhibit acetylcholinesterase and improve neurological function (Ji et al., 2014). There are other medications of this class, all with the risk of side effects that may make their use undesirable. But there is one "medication" that *"appears to have few side effects"* (University of Southern California, 2012). It is a dietary supplement, readily available over the counter, called **huperzine A**.

Huperzine A *is both "a cholinergic nicotinic receptor agonist and a potent and reversable inhibitor of ACh esterase [acetylcholinesterase]."* (Kolgazi et al., 2013) Great! Sounds like huperzine A could be helpful in the battle against ulcerative colitis, due to its ability to favorably influence the Cholinergic Anti-inflammatory Pathway.

Berberine, another over-the-counter supplement, discussed at length in ***Chapter 19***, is also an acetylcholinesterase inhibitor (Wang et al., 2019)—and could certainly be used with that purpose in mind. However, as you will recall, berberine impairs the ability of BSH-active bacteria to turn primary bile acids into secondary bile acids (Sun et al., 2017), could be a problem. Although berberine offers many benefits that the ulcerative colitis is clearly in need of, like the blocking of pro-inflammatory cytokines and pathways and the stimulation of anti-inflammatory pathways (Chen et al., 2014), its use should be under physician approval and supervision. As with berberine, huperzine A use should be under physician approval and supervision, as even over-the-counter medications and supplements can cause harm—hence the warning: *"children, pregnant or nursing women, or those with high blood pressure or severe liver or kidney disease should not take huperzine A except on a doctor's recommendation."* (University of Southern California, 2012)

Choline/Lecithin

In this study, we provide evidence that choline functions as an anti-inflammatory molecule through an α7nAChR-dependent mechanism.

Choline dose-dependently suppressed NF-κB activation in response to endotoxin. ~Parrish et al., 2008

. . . lecithin raises blood choline concentrations far more effectively than equimolar doses of choline chloride, causing elevations that persist for more than 8 hours. ~Magil et al., 1981

In a series of experiments by Parrish et al, once again a hole was made in the intestine of a mouse to allow bacteria to escape and eventually wind up in the bloodstream. This can cause all sorts of problems for the mouse, including the serious problem of death—a death that, in this situation, stems from overwhelming release of proinflammatory cytokines in response to bacterial invasion, leading to what is called sepsis. However, if the mouse is supplemented with choline, its chance of survival will rise from 20% up to 63% (Parrish et al., 2008). This is impressive! And a tribute to the power of the Cholinergic Anti-inflammatory Pathway.

Choline is an essential nutrient, involved in numerous metabolic processes, and just happens to be able to inhibit the release of cytokines from the macrophage (Parrish et al., 2008). Among its many actions, choline activates α7nAChR, the receptor essential to the Cholinergic Anti-inflammatory Pathway. Choline should probably be in adequate supply. Likely, it is not.

Recent analyses indicate that large portions of the population (ie, approximately 90% of Americans), including most pregnant and lactating women, are well below the AI [Adequate Intake] for choline. Moreover, the food patterns recommended by the 2015–2020 Dietary Guidelines for Americans are currently insufficient to meet the AI for choline in most age-sex groups. (Wallace et al., 2018)

Sure, you can supplement with choline to achieve an adequate intake in an attempt to activate the Cholinergic Anti-inflammatory Pathway, but you may be better served by taking the supplement lecithin.

Lecithin, basically, is choline protectively bound to a molecule of fat—which makes it less likely that gut bacteria will be able to reach it to degrade it and lessen its availability for transfer into the bloodstream (Magil et al., 1981). Accordingly, *"lecithin raises blood choline concentrations far more effectively than equimolar doses of choline chloride, causing elevations that persist for more than 8 hours."* (Magil et al., 1981) A good hard look at elevating choline levels, by lecithin supplementation, appears reasonable. Remember, physician approval first.

Smoking/Nicotine

*Nicotine, one agonist of the cholinergic anti-inflammatory pathway, has been demonstrated that has benefit effect on the patients with ulcerative colitis. **The patients with ulcerative colitis who upon cessation of smoking experienced more severe disease progress**, as the reports* *showed, and the disease was ameliorated when the patients returned to smoking. Smoking can also prevent pouchitis in patients with restorative proctocolectomy for ulcerative colitis. However, nicotine administration has side effects as addiction, myocardial infarction and stroke, which limit the clinical use of nicotine.* ~**Bai et al., 2007, emphasis added**

*Nicotine itself has also been tested in clinical trials for IBD, however **its use is jeopardized by its toxicity.*** ~**De Winter and De Man, 2010, emphasis added**

Hard to believe that something so destructive as smoking could be beneficial to the ulcerative colitis patient, but it is. Smoking, as a source of nicotine, can prevent ulcerative colitis (De Jonge and Ulloa, 2007). It can also limit its destructive power (Tracey, 2002). It can promote healing (Seyedabadi et al., 2018). It can even suppress the onset of ulcerative colitis (De Jonge and Ulloa, 2007). But it can also kill, or harm in other ways (Bai et al., 2007; De Winter and De Man, 2010). Nicotine and its impact on ulcerative colitis underscores the power of the Cholinergic Anti-inflammatory Pathway.

Listen to this:

*Ulcerative colitis is a continuous idiopathic inflammation of the colonic or rectal mucosa that is normally associated with loss of tolerance to indigenous enteric flora, abnormal humoral and cell-mediated intestinal immunity, and/or generalized enhanced reactivity against intestinal bacterial antigens. **About 90% of the victims of ulcerative colitis are nonsmokers.** Among sectors, the rates of ulcerative colitis are five times higher among nonsmoking Mormons than in the general population. **Patients with a history of smoking acquire their disease after they have stopped smoking. Patients who smoke intermittently often experience improvement in their colitis symptoms during the periods when smoking. In ex-smokers, onset is nearly always after quitting smoking.** Smoking appears to have a protective effect against the development of this disease and also reduces its severity. This is important because the* *earlier it occurs, and the more extensive it is, the greater is the risk of future colorectal cancer.* (De Jonge and Ulloa, 2007)

If you are a current smoker and considering quitting, you should probably discuss this with your physician before acting. It may not be wise to quit, at least while efforts are ongoing to get a handle on the inflammation you are experiencing. Some people have actually started smoking as therapy for ulcerative colitis. Advisable? Not sure this is wise. Your doctor will advise. Which brings up the question, "How about a nicotine patch?" Consider this:

Seventy-seven patients diagnosed with active ulcerative colitis were treated with either transdermal nicotine or placebo patches for 6 weeks in a randomized, double-blind study. The patients in the nicotine group had a statistically significant greater improvement in the histological and global clinical score of colitis, including lower abdominal pain, stool frequency and fecal urgency. Seventeen of the 30 patients that finished the nicotine treatment had complete remissions, as compared with 9 of the 37 patients in the placebo group. (De Jonge and Ulloa, 2007)

Regarding the risks involved with smoking/nicotine, you should be aware that

Cigarette smoking causes lung cancer and other cancers, is a risk factor for metastatic spread of established cancer, and increases overall mortality in cancer patients. In addition, smokers have increased vulnerability to several infections and are predisposed to allergic airway disease. These studies suggest that by altering host immunity, smoking enables tumor cells and infectious pathogens to evade appropriate immune responses. (Vassallo et al., 2005)

But what about secondhand smoke?

[Secondhand smoking] can engender quantities of nicotine among nonsmokers similar to the amounts obtained during active smoking. (Okoli et al., 2007)

Secondhand smoke contains twice as much tar and nicotine per unit volume as does smoke inhaled from a cigarette. It contains 3x as much cancer-causing benzpyrene, 5x as much carbon monoxide, and 50x as much ammonia. Secondhand smoke from pipes and cigars is equally harmful, if not more so. (University of Minnesota, 2003)

While nicotine works, there is a price to pay. If considering starting smoking or considering quitting, or if you are consistently exposed to second-hand smoking, have a substantive conversation with your physician on the topic of smoking and nicotine. That's what I would do.

Sleep

*Chronic sleep disruption can be regarded as a physiological stressor, as it impairs brain functions, **increases sympathetic tone**, blood pressure and evening cortisol levels, raises the levels of proinflammatory cytokines, and also elevates insulin and blood glucose. Disturbed sleep is not only a symptom of mood disorders, but may also sensitize individuals to the development of depression.* ~**Lucassen et al., 2010, emphasis added**

The Cholinergic Anti-inflammatory Pathway links sleep, or lack thereof, to inflammation. But there is a vicious cycle in play here. *"Inflammatory cytokines such as TNF-α and IL-1 are known to disrupt sleep . . . ."* (Swanson et al., 2011) And here we go . . .

Thus, disturbed sleep and chronic inflammation in IBD could form a self-perpetuating feedback loop with the chronic inflammation of IBD worsening sleep, and decreased sleep exacerbating the production of inflammatory cytokines and the inflammatory milieu. Moreover, it is well known that disrupted sleep can cause fatigue in inflammatory diseases and may be one of the causes of fatigue in IBD patients. It should be noted that fatigue is one of the most common complaints in patients with IBD with a major negative impact on quality of life and this complaint cannot simply be explained by active inflammation alone. Thus, consideration of sleep disruption and attempting to diagnose and treat disrupted sleep in IBD patients is a potential promising therapeutic approach that not only could improve patients' quality of life, but may even modify disease course by preventing disease flare and prolong periods of remission. (Swanson et al., 2011)

You should be aware that there is a form of sleep disruption that can negatively influence the vagus nerve, and hence negatively impact the Cholinergic Anti-inflammatory Pathway. It is the problem of sleep apnea, a disorder that episodically deprives the brain and body of enough oxygen to satisfy its needs and to work properly, and the effects of this translate into physiological problems, such as memory issues, daytime fatigue, increased risk of metabolic disease, and accelerated aging. But it does one more thing. It impairs vagal tone (Hilton et al., 2001). You can discuss sleep apnea with your physician, too. Use the term "vagal tone" in the conversation so you sound pretty smart, and talk about any health issues you have that may be related to any sleep problems you may have.

Melatonin

Ulcerative colitis (UC), an inflammatory bowel disease, affects many people across the globe, and its prevalence is increasing steadily. Inflammation and oxidative stress play a vital role in the perpetuation of inflammatory process and the subsequent DNA damage associated with the development of UC. UC induces not only local but also systemic damage, which involves the perturbation of multiple molecular pathways. Furthermore, UC leads to an increased risk of colorectal cancer, the third most common malignancy in humans. Most of the drugs used for the treatment of UC are unsatisfactory because they are generally mono-targeted, relatively ineffective and unaffordable for many people. Thus, agents that can target multiple molecular pathways and are less expensive have enormous potential to treat UC. **Melatonin has beneficial effects** *against UC in experimental and clinical studies because of its ability to modulate several molecular pathways of inflammation, oxidative stress, fibrosis, and cellular injury.* ~Jena et al., 2013, emphasis added

Interestingly, at any time of the day or night, the gut contains at least 400 times more melatonin than the pineal gland, once again emphasizing the functional importance of melatonin in the gut. ~**Chen et al., 2011**

Melotinin is called the *"darkness hormone"* (Markus et al., 2010). Its elevated production in the evening by the pineal gland serves to promote sleep. It has other benefits other than the promotion of sleep that should be placed under consideration. And surprisingly, *"the gut contains at least 400 times more melatonin than the pineal gland"* *"with the highest levels in the rectum and the colon"* (Chen et al., 2011). In the gut its role is to regulate GI motility as well as regulate inflammation and pain. (Chen et al., 2011). But there is one more thing that melatonin does. It is a *"significant regulator of a7nAChR levels and activity"* (Anderson and Maes, 2016), which places melatonin smack-dab in the middle of the Cholinergic Anti-inflammatory Pathway. How nice! Which means melatonin supplementation may be an appropriate therapy for ulcerative colitis.

And what are the benefits melatonin has to offer the intestine, your intestine?

In the intestine, melatonin influences physiological effects such as regeneration of the epithelium and regulation of its function, modulation of the immune response and reduction in the tone of GI muscles through specific membrane receptors such as melatonin-1 receptor (MT-1), MT-2, and possibly through MT-3.

Melatonin is also reported to act as a potent antioxidant, anti-inflammatory and antigenotoxic agent in all organs. (Jena et al., 2013, emphasis added)

And with that, I have a case report to share:

The first case report of melatonin supplementation for treatment of IBD was in a patient with UC who used melatonin supplementation for jet lag and incidentally noted an improvement in his UC symptoms. (Swanson et al., 2011)

This individual *"observed that his ulcerative colitis (UC) symptoms were virtually absent."* (Chen et al., 2011) This case report was duly noted, and I am certain it prompted much discussion and many studies, including studies in mice, perhaps to include the following study.

So in this following study, instead of punching a hole in a mouse, something a little more kind was offered. Melatonin was given to mice before the induction of experimental colitis. The outcome? Besides getting the best sleep ever, the mice were able to avoid contracting colitis (Swanson et al., 2011).

Specifically, melatonin was able to reverse both the increase in intestinal permeability and influx of bacterial endotoxins, and decrease myeloperoxidase (MPO) and TNF-α activity, which leads to ulcerations. The ability of melatonin to modulate the inflammatory cascade, scavenge reactive oxygen radicals and its ability to prevent and treat animal models of colitis have provided a compelling rationale to study its effectiveness in human IBD. Indeed, melatonin is an attractive therapeutic intervention in human patients with IBD not only for its mechanistic properties, but also because melatonin is readily available, inexpensive and has a low side-effect profile. (Swanson et al., 2011)

However, not everyone is thrilled with melatonin.

One patient decided to take melatonin capsules (3 mg) at bedtime. Two months later, the patient started to experience the symptoms of active UC, including bloody mucous diarrhea. He continued taking melatonin and received corticosteroids orally and rectally. Since the symptoms did not calm down, the patient was hospitalized and stopped consuming melatonin; 48 h later there was a complete remission of the UC symptoms. (Chen et al., 2011)

I sensed that the above accounting did not tell the entire story, so I ordered and read the paper that includes the actual case report, Maldonado and Calvo, 2008. I learned that this patient had ulcerative colitis for approximately 15 years prior to the above-reported incident. The first 5 years with ulcerative colitis did not go smoothly. However, the following ten years was *"satisfactory following basic anti-inflammatory therapy (corticoids and salicylazosulfapyridine) and diet (lactose-free diet and increased fiber intake)."* (Maldonado and Calvo, 2008) The patient did have one reported *"reactivation"* of his disease, related to work stress, approximately 2 years prior to starting melatonin, in 1994.

Again, from the actual case report,

> *In September 2006, the patient decided by himself to take melatonin capsules (3 mg) before going to sleep. Two months later, the patient started to experience the symptoms of active UC, including bloody diarrhea with mucus. He continued taking melatonin and* **the corticosteroids began to be administered at higher dose and rectally (enema).** *On this occasion, the disease did not remit and the patient was hospitalized where gastroenterologist recommended him to stop consuming melatonin; 24–48 hr later there was a complete remission of the UC symptoms.* (Maldonado and Calvo, 2008)

So, the symptoms of ulcerative colitis can vanish in two days, just by stopping melatonin? Possible, but not so fast. Didn't he receive intensified anti-inflammatory therapy? I think there is a strong case for a coincidence occurring in this patient's case. Who knows? It may be that melatonin was behind his disease exacerbation. Who knows?

The two case reports reported here underscore the fact that one therapy may be helpful for one individual but may not be helpful for another. The second report underscores the need to discuss with your doctor any therapeutic measure you are considering or currently using, to see if it is appropriate.

Exercise

*Exercise reduces levels of TNF-α and other cytokines, **increases vagus nerve activity** and protection against cardiovascular disease and type II diabetes.* ~**Wang et al., 2009**

Surprisingly, exercise increases vagal tone. I'm not talking about competitive or strenuous exercise. I'm talking something so simple as a long walk in the park. I'm talking physical activity you find as pleasurable. I'm talking tai chi.

And let me add this:

There are many benefits to exercise, one of which is weight loss. Weight loss, if progressive, leads to the resolution of obesity. Obesity, in the context of the Cholinergic Anti-inflammatory Pathway, should be targeted, as *"obesity is characterized by diminished vagus nerve output and elevated cytokine levels, both of which involve the pathogenesis of insulin resistance and atherosclerosis."* (Wang et al., 2009, emphasis added)

Pretty clear, the vagus nerve can be positively influenced by proper exercise. Proper exercise could help calm things down.

Electrical/mechanical stimulation

Interestingly, it has been shown that stimulation of the vagus nerve can dampen macrophage function. Thus, electrical stimulation of the vagus nerve inhibits the synthesis of TNFalpha in various organs and attenuates the release of TNFalpha and other proinflammatory cytokines. ~**Jönsson et al., 2007**

We ordinarily associate a pacemaker with cardiac patients—a means to electrically stimulate the heart rhythm so life can go on. Imagine, a vagal nerve pacemaker that can electrically stimulate the vagus nerve to reduce inflammation in the gut (so normal life can return). What a concept!

One way to electrically stimulate the vagus nerve is to surgically implant a pacemaker, in addition to implanting a wire that leads to and wraps around portions of the vagus nerve. The pacemaker unit is typically implanted under the skin in the upper chest, with a connecting wire (lead) tunneled under the skin to allow it to reach the vagus nerve in the patient's neck. The latest generation of vagal nerve pacemakers dispense with a separate generator unit and lead, all contained in a small programmable pacemaker that can be placed directly on the vagus nerve (manufactured by **SetPoint Medical**).

Another method to electrically stimulate the vagus nerve is to pace the vagus nerve through the skin, with an electroconductive patch placed on the neck or clipped to the earlobe, connected to an external pacemaker. Such a device is available by prescription from **CES Ultra** and is relatively inexpensive.

Ordinarily, electrical vagal stimulation is reserved for drug-resistant depression or a difficult-to-control seizure disorder (Bonaz, 2018). But that's about to change.

Experimentally, electrical stimulation of the vagus nerve improves colitis in rats (Willemze et al., 2015). According to one such study, *"the course of TNBS-induced colitis was ameliorated, associated with an inhibited nuclear translocation of NF-κB and dampened upregulation of mitogen-activated protein kinase, both important factors in inflammation."* (Willemze et al., 2015) To be fair, although the results of this study were *"intriguing,"* the results were *"mild and only seen at sites surrounding the inflammatory lesion, and not at the lesions themselves."* Perhaps a human will mount a more impressive response to vagal nerve stimulation for IBD.

In a pilot study (Trial identifier: NCT02569503), first of its kind, seven patients with mild to moderate Crohn's disease underwent electrical vagus nerve stimulation via an implanted device (Bonaz et al., 2016). The study period duration was 6 months. In summary,

> *Vagus nerve stimulation was feasible and well-tolerated in all patients. Among the seven patients, two were removed from the study at 3 months for clinical worsening and five evolved toward clinical, biological and endoscopic remission with a restored vagal tone.* (Bonaz et al., 2016)

These results were promising, and to me quite impressive. And follow-up study (Trial identifier: NCT02311660) was even more impressive. In this study, electrical vagal nerve stimulation *"induced clinical and biomarker and endoscopic improvement in a significant proportion of drug refractory CD patients."* (D'H'ens et al., 2018) What is particularly notable in the study is that fact that *"highly refactory patients were included with failure of biologics."* (Bonaz, 2018) And I think I've located a patient involved with this study. Her name is Kelly.

Case report: Kelly

Kelly was 29 years old at the time her story appeared in an article written by Emily Waltz, posted in 2018. She had been ill since age 13— first with inflammatory arthritis in one ankle, then over the course of a few years both ankles became involved as the disease worked its way up to include both arms. Pain was both severe and debilitating. Shortly after the onset of arthritic symptoms, here come the tummy troubles that soon lead to the diagnosis of Crohn's disease. And if that wasn't enough, skin ulcerations showed up from out of nowhere, to add to all the misery. Years of misery.

"*I went very quickly from being an athletic kid to feeling like a 90-year-old woman,*" she recounts. And, like the majority of 90-year-old women, Kelly developed osteoporosis, due to the chronic use of steroids, prescribed to control her disease. "*By her mid 20s, she couldn't walk a* couple of blocks without stopping on a bench to rest. *Each movement was painful. She had to quit her job as a high school English teacher."* (Waltz, 2018) Kelly's life was so vastly different from anything she had in mind. Putting up with this crap (medical term, I think), for well over a decade, would be enough to take the fight out of the best of the best. But not Kelly. She was *determined* to find a way out.

Kelly just happened to run across an on-line interview with Dr. Kevin Tracey, showcasing a revolutionary treatment for inflammatory disorders, based on the discoveries of he and his colleagues. Kelly was more than intrigued, she was <u>convinced</u> that this revolutionary treatment—electrical vagal nerve stimulation—could help her in her battle against Crohn's. She tracked down Dr. Tracey's email address and shared with him her story. At the time (2014), Dr. Tracey did not have a lot to offer Kelly. So, she continued with all the suffering and with all the failure of conventional therapy for another 3 years (Lama, 2019).

But enough is enough, and Kelley once again contacted Dr. Tracey, hoping for a better outcome. From this contact, Kelly learned there was a company based in California, **SetPoint Medical**, that was conducting a clinical trial in Europe using electrical vagal nerve stimulation to treat Crohn's (Lama, 2019). This was all she needed to know. Shortly after contacting SetPoint Medical, Kelly was enrolled in the clinical trial of her dreams.

For Kelly, soon it was off to Europe, wheelchair bound, with her supportive husband at her side, to participate in the clinical trial in question. The rest is history.

A surgeon implanted her device on June 22, 2017, she says. Stimulation started two weeks later. Two weeks after that "I was running from train to train to make my appointments," said Owens in the interview with Spectrum. *"I remember one time my husband and I were late for an appointment at the Academic Medical Center, and I ran up two flights of stairs and got to the top and didn't see my husband anywhere. I looked down to the bottom of the stairs and he's standing there with his mouth open, shocked at what I had just done.*

Now, a year since her surgery, Owens says she runs, does weight training, exercises on the elliptical, and has no more Crohn's symptoms. "It's just gone," she says. "I don't have pain or swelling. I'm able to eat regular foods. A salad used to destroy my stomach and now I live on salad." She still has osteoporosis, but hopes that will improve too with calcium supplements. (Waltz, 2018)

Read Kelly's story yourself. You'll be impressed. Her story is told at the following:

https://spectrum.ieee.org/the-human-os/biomedical/devices/vagus-nerve-stimulation-takes-on-crohns-disease

https://www.brainfacts.org/brain-anatomy-and-function/body-systems/2019/realizing-the-benefits-of-vagus-nerve-stimulation-042419

https://www.newsday.com/news/health/crohns-drugs-feinstein-institute-1.20780533

https://time.com/5709245/bioelectronic-medicine-treatments/

Conclusion

The above case report is a powerful testament to the power of the Cholinergic Anti-inflammatory Pathway. It is anticipated that similar results may be achieved in the patient with ulcerative colitis. We'll find out soon.

Currently, there are two ongoing clinical trials that will eventually report on the efficacy of transcutaneous (through the skin) electrical vagal stimulation in ulcerative colitis. One clinical trial involves adults with ulcerative colitis (Trial identifier: NCT03908073), and the other involves pediatric patients with either Crohn's or ulcerative colitis (Trial identifier: NCT03863704). I am hoping for best here, but my gut feeling tells me that an implantable vagal nerve stimulator is the more effective approach to ulcerative colitis than the transcutaneous approach.

Regardless of the results of any clinical trial, there is little doubt that the Cholinergic Anti-inflammatory Pathway can be targeted in ulcerative colitis, and lives can be changed. And it may be successful simply because

By lowering the inflammation in IBD patients, induction or maintenance of remission may be achieved." (Sharifi et al., 2016)

Not without risk

As with just about everything, there are some risks associated with vagal nerve stimulation. However, treating ulcerative colitis is ordinarily risky business, so the following potential adverse effects may be acceptable risks to take.

So, with respect to implanted vagal nerve stimulators:

VNS as a means of pain treatment has been traditionally administered through invasive procedures, known as invasive VNS (iVNS), which typically involve the surgical implantation of electrodes around the cervical vagus nerve. iVNS has a high risk for adverse events that include voice alteration, paresthesia, cough, headache, dyspnea, pharyngitis, and pain at the site of stimulation. These adverse events often require a decrease in stimulation strength or even permanent deactivation and/or removal of the iVNS device. An effective non-invasive alternative to iVNS is transcutaneous VNS (tVNS). (Paccione and Jacobsen, 2019)

Transcutaneous, "through-the-skin" vagal nerve stimulation also has a few drawbacks that should be brought to our attention.

The tVNS system sends electrical impulses through the skin (transcutaneous) of the outer ear straight into the auricular branch of the vagus nerve. Intensity, pulse duration, and frequency of the tVNS can be adjusted accordingly. Even though a number of studies using high intensity tVNS have not found any major side-effects, tVNS can still be accompanied by slight pain, burning, tingling, or itching sensations near the sight of the electrodes. tVNS devices, like implantable VNS systems, are expensive to obtain, maintain, and have a narrow patient distribution. There is also no scientific consensus regarding the frequency and strength of tVNS stimulation for pain treatment nor is there a clear understanding of how a constant pulse frequency mirrors endogenous vagal nerve activity (it likely does not communicate in consecutive 30 s intervals as most of the tVNS devices do). (Paccione and Jacobsen, 2019)

So, while you are processing all of this, not quite sure if implanted or transcutaneous vagus nerve stimulation is right for you, perhaps you should take a slow, deep breath (and a lot of them).

Breath taking

VN [vagal nerve] activity is modulated by respiration. It is suppressed during inhalation and facilitated during exhalation and slow respiration cycles. ~**Gerritsen and Band, 2018**

That something so normal as breathing could be fashioned into a weapon to fight inflammation, is simply amazing. That you already have a vagal nerve stimulator, built right inside of you and ready to be activated, is equally amazing. Who would have thought?

As it turns out, breathing is under the control of both the sympathetic and parasympathetic nervous systems, in an arrangement whereby **"exhalation is under direct control of VN [vagus nerve]."** (Gerritsen and Band, 2018, emphasis added). And this arrangement is why activities such as meditation, yoga, and tai chi—activities that incorporate *"slow, deep, and diaphragmatic"* patterns of breathing—

can exert a profound effect on vagal nerve activity (Gerritsen and Band, 2018).

For breathing to be an effective vagal nerve stimulator, the following should be placed under consideration:

> *The breathing techniques used . . . include, but not restricted to, slow down respiration cycles, shifting to longer exhalations compared to inhalations, shifting the main locus of respiration from the thorax to the abdomen (diaphragmatic breathing), or paying attention to "natural breathing."*

> *Slow breathing techniques with long exhalation will signal a state of relaxion by VN [vagus nerve], resulting in more VN activity and further relaxation.* (Gerritsen and Band, 2018)

In a nutshell, the principles put forth above by Gerritsen and Band help us know what to look for when searching for a breathing exercise with the power to increase vagal tone and take advantage of the Cholinergic Anti-inflammatory Pathway.

If meditation, yoga, or tai chi is not for you, don't worry, there are many other avenues to pursue. What you are looking for is breathing techniques that emphasize *"slow, deep, and diaphragmatic"* patterns of breathing. No surprisingly, slow, pursed lip exhalation (particularly combined with abdominal breathing), humming, playing a musical instrument that requires slow, controlled exhalation, are all powerful vagal nerve stimulants.

Of course, merely taking a couple of slow, deep, abdominal breaths with slow expiration, a couple of times a day and hoping for results, is clearly not enough. Sessions, perhaps 10 to 20 minutes of duration, and several times a day, are more likely to produce results. Surprisingly, *"performing DB [deep breathing] at a rate around 6 breaths per minute . . . may yield analgesic effects."* (Paccione and Jacobsen, 2019) The nice thing about breathing exercises is that they can be done anytime and anywhere, and in your underwear. And if you recognize that you are in a stressful situation, with slow, deep breathing you can better withstand the negative effects of stress and be better able to maintain a healthy vagal tone.

Reinforcing the mucus layer of the colon

*A new concept for the therapy of UC has been developed based on the observation that **a lack of PC [phosphatidylcholine] in colonic mucus is of key pathogenic relevance.** It is the logical consequence that insufficient PC content requires substitution to maintain the mucosal barrier. Only a delayed release oral PC preparation is able to deliver PC to the distal ileum.* **~Stremmel et al., 2010, emphasis added**

Of special interest was that the low PC content of mucus in UC was also observed when the patients were in remission, as defined by the endoscopic appearance of 'mucosal healing.' This indicates that a lack of mucus PC in UC patients might be an intrinsic feature of UC. **~Stremmel and Gauss, 2013**

Why would you *not* want to reinforce the mucus barrier of defense in a disease such as ulcerative colitis? Of course, you would. Phosphatidylcholine (AKA lecithin) will do this, as it is a principle component of the mucus that covers and protects the surface of the colon.

The problem with oral supplementation with phosphatidylcholine is that it is digested before it can reach the colon where it is needed. So, one team of researchers developed a "delayed" or "retarded-release" formula that allows phosphatidylcholine to reach the colon, then to disperse to become incorporated into the river of mucus that shields the colon from harm. That's the theory, but does it work?

The results of phase II preliminary trials were very encouraging. Using a retarded-release preparation of PC in a randomized double-blind placebo-controlled trial, 90% of patients either reached clinical remission (defined as a clinical activity index (CAI) ≤3) or significantly improved by >50% compared with 10% in the placebo group. (Torres et al., 2013)

But there is more,

> *In a more difficult to treat patient population of steroid-refractory UC, steroid withdrawal with concomitant achievement of a CAI index of ≤3 or CAI improvement of >50% was achieved in 50% (15/30) of the patients treated with PC compared with 10% (3/30) in the placebo group.* (Torres et al., 2013)

I have only been able to find one source for delayed-release phosphatidylcholine (Lecithin). It is available from the German pharmaceutical company named **KliniPharm**. The funny thing, although manufactured in Germany, the product label is in English, so they must be servicing the international community. The product is called **SpongiCol**. It is available in both capsule form and in granular form. The company website is http://www.klinipharm.com/spongicol.html. I must admit, I am impressed with this product. Anything with this degree of success should be actively promoted and made easily available everywhere, not basically ignored. Consider the following:

> *Even in the most difficult-to-treat population of steroid-refactory UC, 80% of the patients [supplementing with delayed-release phosphatidylcholine] could be withdrawn from steroids, and 50% achieved overall clinical remission.* (Stremmel and Gauss, 2013)

~References~

Anderson G, Maes M. **Alpha 7 nicotinic receptor agonist modulatory interactions with melatonin: relevance not only to cognition, but to wider neuropsychiatric and immune inflammatory disorders.** In press. Chap 4. bk: Frontiers in Clinical Drug Research-Central Nervous System. Bentham Press. doi. 2016 Dec 16;10(9781681081892116021):186-202.

Bai A, Guo Y, Lu N. **The effect of the cholinergic anti-inflammatory pathway on experimental colitis.** Scandinavian journal of immunology. 2007 Nov;66(5):538-45.

Bhatia V, Tandon RK. **Stress and the gastrointestinal tract.** Journal of gastroenterology and hepatology. 2005 Mar;20(3):332-9.

Bonaz B. **Is-there a place for vagus nerve stimulation in inflammatory bowel diseases?.** Bioelectronic Medicine. 2018 Dec 1;4(1):4.

Bonaz B, Sinniger V, Hoffmann D, Clarencon D, Mathieu N, Dantzer C, Vercueil L, Picq C, Trocmé C, Faure P, Cracowski JL. **Chronic vagus nerve stimulation in Crohn's disease: a 6-month follow-up pilot study.** Neurogastroenterology & Motility. 2016 Jun;28(6):948-53.

Bonaz B, Sinniger V, Pellissier S. **Vagus nerve stimulation: a new promising therapeutic tool in inflammatory bowel disease.** Journal of internal medicine. 2017 Jul;282(1):46-63.

Bonaz B, Bazin T, Pellissier S. **The vagus nerve at the interface of the microbiota-gut-brain axis.** Frontiers in neuroscience. 2018 Feb 7;12:49.

Breit S, Kupferberg A, Rogler G, Hasler G. **Vagus nerve as modulator of the brain–gut axis in psychiatric and inflammatory disorders.** Frontiers in psychiatry. 2018 Mar 13;9:44.

Chandra R, Liddle RA. **Cholecystokinin.** Current Opinion in Endocrinology, Diabetes and Obesity. 2007 Feb 1;14(1):63-7.

Chen CQ, Fichna J, Bashashati M, Li YY, Storr M. **Distribution, function and physiological role of melatonin in the lower gut.** World journal of gastroenterology: WJG. 2011 Sep 14;17(34):3888.

Chen C, Yu Z, Li Y, Fichna J, Storr M. **Effects of berberine in the gastrointestinal tract—a review of actions and therapeutic implications.** The American journal of Chinese medicine. 2014;42(05):1053-70.

Dawood T, Schlaich M, Brown A, Lambert G. **Depression and blood pressure control: all antidepressants are not the same.** Hypertension. 2009 Jul 1;54(1):e1.

De Jonge WJ, Ulloa L. **The alpha7 nicotinic acetylcholine receptor as a pharmacological target for inflammation.** British journal of pharmacology. 2007 Aug;151(7):915-29.

De Winter BY, De Man JG. **Interplay between inflammation, immune system and neuronal pathways: effect on gastrointestinal motility.** World journal of gastroenterology: WJG. 2010 Nov 28;16(44):5523.

D'H'ens G, Cabrijan Z, Eberhardson M, van den Bergh R, Löwenberg M, Fiorino G, Danese S, Levine Y, Chernoff D. P574 **The effects of vagus nerve stimulation in biologic-refractory Crohn's disease: A prospective clinical trial.** Journal of Crohn's'and Colitis. 2018 Jan 16;12(supplement_1):S397-8.

Furlan R, Ardizzone S, Palazzolo L, Rimoldi A, Perego F, Barbic F, Bevilacqua M, Vago L, Porro GB, Malliani A. **Sympathetic overactivity in active ulcerative colitis: effects of clonidine.** American Journal of Physiology-Regulatory, Integrative and Comparative Physiology. 2006 Jan;290(1):R224-32.

Gerritsen RJ, Band GP. **Breath of life: the respiratory vagal stimulation model of contemplative activity.** Frontiers in human neuroscience. 2018;12:397.

Ghia JE, Blennerhassett P, Collins SM. **Vagus nerve integrity and experimental colitis.** American Journal of Physiology-Gastrointestinal and Liver Physiology. 2007 Sep;293(3):G560-7.

Ghia JE, Blennerhassett P, Collins SM. **Impaired parasympathetic function increases susceptibility to inflammatory bowel disease in a mouse model of depression.** The Journal of clinical investigation. 2008 Jun 2;118(6):2209-18.

Giebelen IA, Leendertse M, Florquin S, van der Poll T. **Stimulation of acetylcholine receptors impairs host defence during pneumococcal pneumonia.** European Respiratory Journal. 2009 Feb 1;33(2):375-81.

Goverse G, Stakenborg M, Matteoli G. **The intestinal cholinergic anti-inflammatory pathway.** The Journal of physiology. 2016 Oct 15;594(20):5771-80.

Grippo AJ, Johnson AK. **Biological mechanisms in the relationship between depression and heart disease.** Neuroscience & Biobehavioral Reviews. 2002 Dec 1;26(8):941-62.

Hilton MF, Chappell MJ, Bartlett WA, Malhotra A, Beattie JM, Cayton RM. **The sleep apnoea/hypopoea syndrome depresses waking vagal tone independent of sympathetic activation.** European Respiratory Journal. 2001 Jun 1;17(6):1258-66.

Hofer S, Eisenbach C, Lukic IK, Schneider L, Bode K, Brueckmann M, Mautner S, Wente MN, Encke J, Werner J, Dalpke AH. **Pharmacologic cholinesterase inhibition improves survival in experimental sepsis.** Critical care medicine. 2008 Feb 1;36(2):404-8.

Hollander D. **Inflammatory bowel diseases and brain-gut axis.** Journal of physiology and pharmacology. 2004;55:183-90.

Huston JM, Tracey KJ. **The pulse of inflammation: heart rate variability, the cholinergic anti-inflammatory pathway and implications for therapy.** Journal of internal medicine. 2011 Jan;269(1):45-53.

Jakob S, Zabielski R, Mosenthin R, Valverde Piedra JL, Evilevitch L, Kuria M, Rippe C, Sörhede Winzell M, Pierzynowski SG. **Influence of intraduodenally infused olive and coconut oil on postprandial exocrine pancreatic secretions of growing pigs.** Journal of animal science. 2001 Feb 1;79(2):477-85.

Ji H, Rabbi MF, Labis B, Pavlov VA, Tracey KJ, Ghia JE. **Central cholinergic activation of a vagus nerve-to-spleen circuit alleviates experimental colitis.** Mucosal immunology. 2014 Mar;7(2):335.

Jena G, Trivedi PP. **A review of the use of melatonin in ulcerative colitis: experimental evidence and new approaches.** Inflammatory Bowel Diseases. 2013 Nov 15;20(3):553-63.

Jönsson M, Norrgård Ö, Forsgren S. **Presence of a marked nonneuronal cholinergic system in human colon: study of normal colon and colon in ulcerative colitis.** Inflammatory bowel diseases. 2007 Jul 30;13(11):1347-56.

Kolgazi M, Uslu U, Yuksel M, Velioglu-Ogunc A, Ercan F, Alican I. The role of cholinergic anti-inflammatory pathway in acetic acid-induced colonic inflammation in the rat. Chemico-biological interactions. 2013 Sep 5;205(1):72-80.

Lama CL, 2019; Apr 24 https://www.brainfacts.org/brain-anatomy-and-function/body-systems/2019/realizing-the-benefits-of-vagus-nerve-stimulation-042419

Lerman-Garber I, Ichazo-Cerro S, Zamora-González J, Cardoso-Saldaña G, Posadas-Romero C. Effect of a high-monounsaturated fat diet enriched with avocado in NIDDM patients. Diabetes care. 1994 Apr 1;17(4):311-5.

Lucassen PJ, Meerlo P, Naylor AS, Van Dam AM, Dayer AG, Fuchs E, Oomen CA, Czeh B. Regulation of adult neurogenesis by stress, sleep disruption, exercise and inflammation: Implications for depression and antidepressant action. European Neuropsychopharmacology. 2010 Jan 1;20(1):1-7.

Luyer MD, Greve JW, Hadfoune MH, Jacobs JA, Dejong CH, Buurman WA. Nutritional stimulation of cholecystokinin receptors inhibits inflammation via the vagus nerve. Journal of Experimental Medicine. 2005 Oct 17;202(8):1023-9.

Magil SG, Zeisel SH, Wurtman RJ. Effects of ingesting soy or egg lecithins on serum choline, brain choline and brain acetylcholine. The Journal of nutrition. 1981 Jan 1;111(1):166-70.

Maldonado MD, Calvo JR. Melatonin usage in ulcerative colitis: a case report. Journal of pineal research. 2008 Oct;45(3):339-40.

Markus RP, Silva CL, Franco DG, Barbosa Jr EM, Ferreira ZS. Is modulation of nicotinic acetylcholine receptors by melatonin relevant for therapy with cholinergic drugs?. Pharmacology & therapeutics. 2010 Jun 1;126(3):251-62.

Maroy B. Dramatic and long-lasting effects of amiodarone in a case of Behçet's'disease. GastroHelp.com; 2009; July 7.

Okoli CT, Kelly T, Hahn EJ. Secondhand smoke and nicotine exposure: a brief review. Addictive behaviors. 2007 Oct 1;32(10):1977-88.

Ondicova K, Tillinger A, Pecenak J, Mravec B. The vagus nerve role in antidepressants action: Efferent vagal pathways participate in peripheral anti-inflammatory effect of fluoxetine. Neurochemistry international. 2019 May 1;125:47-56.

Paccione CE, Jacobsen HB. **Motivational nondirective resonance breathing as a treatment for chronic widespread pain.** Frontiers in Psychology. 2019;10:1207.

Parrish WR, Rosas-Ballina M, Gallowitsch-Puerta M, Ochani M, Ochani K, Yang LH, Hudson L, Lin X, Patel N, Johnson SM, Chavan S. **Modulation of TNF release by choline requires α7 subunit nicotinic acetylcholine receptor-mediated signaling.** Molecular medicine. 2008 Sep 1;14(9-10):567-74.

Pavlov VA, Tracey KJ. **Controlling inflammation: the cholinergic anti-inflammatory pathway.** Biochemical Society transactions. 2006 Dec;34(Pt 6):1037.

Peña G, Cai B, Ramos L, Vida G, Deitch EA, Ulloa L. **Cholinergic regulatory lymphocytes re-establish neuromodulation of innate immune responses in sepsis.** The Journal of Immunology. 2011 Jul 15;187(2):718-25.

Pravda J. **Radical induction theory of ulcerative colitis.** World journal of gastroenterology: WJG. 2005 Apr 28;11(16):2371.

Radek KA. **Antimicrobial anxiety: the impact of stress on antimicrobial immunity.** Journal of leukocyte biology. 2010 Aug;88(2):263-77.

Riber C, Hojgaard L, Madsen JL, Rehfeld JF, Olsen O. **Gallbladder emptying and cholecystokinin response to fish oil and trioleate ingestion.** Digestion. 1996;57(3):161-4.

Seyedabadi M, Rahimian R, Ghia JE. **The role of alpha7 nicotinic acetylcholine receptors in inflammatory bowel disease: involvement of different cellular pathways. Expert opinion on therapeutic targets.** 2018 Feb 1;22(2):161-76.

Sharifi A, Hosseinzadeh-Attar MJ, Vahedi H, Nedjat S. **A randomized controlled trial on the effect of vitamin D3 on inflammation and cathelicidin gene expression in ulcerative colitis patients.** Saudi journal of gastroenterology: official journal of the Saudi Gastroenterology Association. 2016 Jul;22(4):316.

Stremmel W, Gauss A. **Lecithin as a therapeutic agent in ulcerative colitis.** Digestive diseases. 2013;31(3-4):388-90.

Stremmel W, Hanemann A, Ehehalt R, Karner M, Braun A. Phosphatidylcholine (lecithin) and the mucus layer: Evidence of therapeutic efficacy in ulcerative colitis?. Digestive diseases. 2010;28(3):490-6.

Sun R, Yang N, Kong B, Cao B, Feng D, Yu X, Ge C, Huang J, Shen J, Wang P, Feng S. **Orally administered berberine modulates hepatic lipid metabolism by altering microbial bile acid metabolism and the intestinal FXR signaling pathway.** Molecular pharmacology. 2017 Feb 1;91(2):110-22.

Swanson GR, Burgess HJ, Keshavarzian A. **Sleep disturbances and inflammatory bowel disease: a potential trigger for disease flare?.** Expert review of clinical immunology. 2011 Jan 1;7(1):29-36.

Torres J, Danese S, Colombel JF. **New therapeutic avenues in ulcerative colitis: thinking out of the box.** Gut. 2013 Nov 1;62(11):1642-52.Tracey KJ. The inflammatory reflex. Nature. 2002 Dec;420(6917):853.

Tracey KJ. **The inflammatory reflex.** Nature. 2002 Dec;420(6917):853-9.

Tracey KJ. **Fat meets the cholinergic antiinflammatory pathway.** Journal of Experimental Medicine. 2005 Oct 17;202(8):1017-21.

Tracey KJ. **Understanding immunity requires more than immunology.** Nature immunology. 2010 Jul 1;11(7):561.

University of Minnesota 2003 **Secondhand Smoke Facts.** www.umn.edu/perio/tobacco/secondhandsmoke.html

University of Sothern California 2012 **Huperzine A.** www.doctorsofusc.com/condition/document/21761?printstyle=true

Van Der Zanden EP, Boeckxstaens GE, De Jonge WJ. **The vagus nerve as a modulator of intestinal inflammation.** Neurogastroenterology & Motility. 2009 Jan;21(1):6-17.

Van Westerloo DJ, Giebelen IA, Florquin S, Daalhuisen J, Bruno MJ, de Vos AF, Tracey KJ, Van Der Poll T. **The cholinergic anti-inflammatory pathway regulates the host response during septic peritonitis.** Journal of Infectious Diseases. 2005 Jun 15;191(12):2138-48.

Van Westerloo DJ. **The vagal immune reflex: a blessing from above.** Wiener Medizinische Wochenschrift. 2010 Mar 1;160(5-6):112-7.

Vassallo R, Tamada K, Lau JS, Kroening PR, Chen L. **Cigarette smoke extract suppresses human dendritic cell function leading to preferential induction of Th-2 priming.** The Journal of Immunology. 2005 Aug 15;175(4):2684-91.

Wallace TC, Blusztajn JK, Caudill MA, Klatt KC, Natker E, Zeisel SH, Zelman KM. **Choline: The Underconsumed and Underappreciated Essential Nutrient.** Nutrition Today. 2018 Nov;53(6):240.

Waltz E, 2018; Jun 12 https://spectrum.ieee.org/the-human-os/biomedical/devices/vagus-nerve-stimulation-takes-on-crohns-disease

Wang DW, Zhou RB, Yao YM. **Role of cholinergic anti-inflammatory pathway in regulating host response and its interventional strategy for inflammatory diseases.** Chinese Journal of Traumatology (English Edition). 2009 Dec 1;12(6):355-64.

Wang D, Wu Y, Wang A, Chen Y, Zhang T, Hu N. **Electrocardiogram Changes of Donepezil Administration in Elderly Patients with Ischemic Heart Disease.** Cardiology research and practice. 2018;2018.

Wang KF, Chen Q, Wu N, Li Y, Zhang R, Wang J, Gong D, Zou X, Liu C, Chen J. **Berberine ameliorates spatial learning memory impairment and modulates cholinergic anti-inflammatory pathway in diabetic rats.** Frontiers in pharmacology. 2019;10:1003.

Willemze RA, Luyer MD, Buurman WA, De Jonge WJ. **Neural reflex pathways in intestinal inflammation: hypotheses to viable therapy.** Nature Reviews Gastroenterology & Hepatology. 2015 Jun;12(6):353.

Chapter 22
Vitamin D and IBD

VDD [vitamin D deficiency] is <u>highly prevalent</u> among patients with UC. Patients with longer disease duration, more severe symptoms, and pancolitis are likely to have lower vitamin D levels.

We recommend that patients with UC should be assessed for vitamin D levels and appropriately supplemented as part of long-term management. **~Law et al., 2019, emphasis added**

Studies have linked low vitamin D levels with an increased risk of cancer, particularly colon cancer. **~Ananthakrishnan, 2016**

In a vitamin D-deficient state, mucosal barriers are more susceptible to injury that leads to infection and IBD. **~Li, 2008, emphasis added**

We discussed vitamin D before, rather extensively in *Chapter 3*. But there is more you should know. So, we will visit this subject once again. It is that important.

My purpose in writing this chapter is to drive home the message that vitamin D should not be ignored in the battle against ulcerative colitis. Close attention to it should be paid.

To get us off to a good start in understanding vitamin D and its relevance to you the patient with ulcerative colitis, I'll share with you a little piece I wrote a number years ago on the natural history of vitamin D. For me, it's a walk down memory lane. For you (and for me), it will be fun.

Vitamin D: A natural history

In terms of human history, humans were not confronted with vitamin D deficiency until the industrial revolution began. **~Holick, 2003**

Despite evidence of its profound importance to human health, vitamin D inadequacy is not widely recognized as a problem by physicians and patients. **~Holick, 2006**

Calling vitamin D a "vitamin" is something of a misnomer. Although the name is still used for historical reasons, vitamin D is more properly classified as a secosteroid [steroid hormone] because it consists of a cholesterol backbone and exerts steroid-like effects throughout the body, directly affecting the expression of over 1000 genes through the nuclear vitamin D receptor. **~Cekic et al., 2011**

Vitamin D has been around for a very long time; it was perhaps the first true hormone in continuous use on planet earth. And it was free, freely derived from the sun. The single-celled creature created it for personal use in many of its metabolic activities. Then along came a hungry multi-celled creature that ate the single-celled creature. And in this manner, driven by the need of some creatures to eat other creatures in order to survive, vitamin D became a hormone that could be passed along from creature to creature within the food chain, a hormone useful to the metabolic processes of the one who had not yet been eaten.

Somewhere along the way, along came the hungry human. And, as luck would have it, the human saw a fish. And so the human ate the fish that ate other little fishes that ate the multi-celled creatures that ate the single-celled creatures, and in this manner the human was able to obtain an important ingredient, a hormone that somehow became necessary to sustain life. But the food chain was just one way to get this hormone. Nudity was another. So like many other creatures both big and small (and naked), humans were able to obtain vitamin D in abundance by exposure to the sun. Eventually, nudity gave way to clothing (thank God!), and still mankind was able to get plenty of vitamin D, both by diet and by sunlight exposure.

And so, for what seems like forever, the human race obtained plenty of vitamin D to meet its needs. Then came the Industrial Revolution, and boy, did we get into trouble. And then came the dermatologists with truckloads of sunscreen, and boy, did we get into even more trouble.

In this context of reduced exposure to sunlight and alterations in diet, humanity is now faced with a host of diseases that are related, in part, to a lack of vitamin D; related, in part, to an immune system that is compromised; related, in part, to a medical profession that just can't seem to wrap its mind around this simple truth: Vitamin D *must* be in adequate supply or people will show up in droves to get drugs to treat diseases that are related, in part, to vitamin D deficiency. Multitudes will suffer. Many will die. All of this is so very true. This is why I wrote a certain little book on vitamin D.

How vitamin D became so essential to our musculoskeletal system, to our nervous system, to our immune system, even to the hair we grow on our head, is indeed somewhat of a mystery. Many a physician is still waiting for all the details to be worked out before venturing forth and paying very close attention to this vitamin, this hormone, the one we call vitamin D. Fortunately, things are beginning to change. But, be aware, your physician may not be all that into vitamin D, in addition to all the other things he or she is not all that into. I am speaking in generalities, of course. Let's hope that your physician is very knowledgeable in the issues that surround vitamin D and its relationship to the diseases that he or she sees each and every day. But you are clueless, probably, so I will need to get you up to speed.

Let's start with the skin. The skin is really dead. It is the under-the-skin skin that is important to our discussion. Here we find a living tissue containing all sorts of things, including cholesterol. As with so many other hormones, cholesterol is the backbone of the vitamin D molecule.

Sunlight, specifically the UVB wavelength, has the capacity to displace an electron from the cholesterol molecule, and the beginning of a hormone is born. This altered cholesterol molecule no longer "fits in" with its neighbors (it must look kinda different) so it is forcibly evicted to eventually find its way to the liver where it is stored, processed, and sent forth as a prohormone to the kidney or to many other organs, tissues, and cells where it is converted by an enzyme called 1-alpha-hydroxylase into its active form. While in its active form, called calcitriol or $1,25(OH)_2D_3$, vitamin D joins up with a nuclear receptor called the vitamin D receptor (VDR) and the magic happens. Up to 1000 genes or more can respond, orchestrating genetic events that promote health and resistance to disease.

So now you know the natural history of vitamin D. Please keep in mind that you, too, have a natural history, one that is currently in progress. This vitamin, this hormone, may help make the story of you a lengthy one and a relatively smooth ride. ~The end.

Before we move on . . .

The incidence of vitamin D deficiency is rising worldwide, yet in the vast majority of patients, the condition remains undiagnosed and untreated.

Vitamin D deficiency is one of the most common and underdiagnosed medical conditions in the world. Emerging evidence indicates vitamin D deficiency may be pandemic.

Accordingly, approximately 90% of the dark-skinned people in the United States and more than 50% of the white population have vitamin D insufficiency or deficiency. ~**Wimalawansa, 2012**

Before we get to the heart of the chapter, there are a few more vitamin D-related concepts I need to bring to your attention. Listen up!

First, it is so easy to become vitamin D deficient. Diet won't prevent it, as most foods are low in vitamin D unless it is added (Wimalawansa, 2012). You can try to become vitamin D sufficient by diet if you so choose. But are you really prepared to drink 30 to 40 glasses of vitamin D-fortified milk per day? Sunlight exposure, the primary means available to generate substantial quantities of vitamin D, doesn't seem to cut it—if we were obtaining enough vitamin D from the sun, why we would be in the *"pandemic"* of vitamin D deficiency we find ourselves in? (see Wimalawansa, 2012; Holick, 2017) So, to achieve and maintain vitamin D sufficiency, what we're left with is adequate vitamin D supplementation, added to the small amounts we typically receive from dietary sources.

Second, vitamin D sufficiency is not all that easy to achieve and maintain by sun exposure. Due to the angle of the sun with respect to the axis of the earth during mid-fall through late-spring, vitamin D is not created by sunlight exposure during this portion of the year—the UVB rays are completely absorbed by the ozone layer and do not penetrate (Holick, 2017). Furthermore, during the times when vitamin D could be generated by sunlight exposure, such exposure typically needs to occur between the hours of 9 AM to 3 PM (Holick, 2017). Outside of this time frame, no vitamin can be synthesized no matter how much skin is exposed (Holick, 2017). So, if you are relying on diet, or diet plus casual sunlight exposure to achieve and maintain vitamin D sufficiency, you will likely not succeed. But join the club, as most of the inhabitants of Earth are vitamin D deficient due to following this way of life.

Third, vitamin D insufficiency *is* vitamin D deficiency. Why not tell it like it is? Whether your lab value is considered "deficiency" or considered "insufficiency," if you don't have enough vitamin D on board to meet the needs of the cells, you don't have enough. You are deficient . . . period! Of course, when it comes to vitamin D, it is better to have a better lousy level of vitamin D than have a worse lousy level. But say no to both, say I.

Fourth, you may be hearing voices. No, you're not crazy (although some people may not agree with this assessment). It's just that some "voices" (thought leaders and health care professionals) tell us we need only a little vitamin D each day to maintain health and deal with disease, and this is misinformation. Study after study has demonstrated that thousands of IUs/day of vitamin D are required to maintain health and modify a disease process. Yet, a convention of physicians, held in 2010, determined that only small amounts of vitamin D are required to maintain health (Wimalawansa, 2012). The convention in question, called the **Institute of Medicine (IOM)**—charged with developing vitamin D supplementation recommendations for all to follow—decided to primarily evaluate studies related to bone health *and* dismiss a plethora of studies that indicate substantial vitamin D levels are required to prevent or reduce the severity of various diseases (Holick, 2011; Holick, 2017). When their report was released, the vitamin D research community were *"shocked and dismayed"* at what they read (Grant, 2011). I was in the process of writing a book on vitamin D at the time, and when I heard the news I was flabbergasted, and my heart sank. I instinctively knew that those who simply follow others (physicians included), having no time to look things up on their own and come up with their own informed conclusions, will assume that the conclusions of the IOM are sound and we really don't need to be all that concerned about vitamin D. And because of this, people will be harmed, and people will die. This is so true. This is so true.

Fortunately, about the same time the IOM was fooling around, another organization, the **Endocrine Society**, considered a wider range of studies and issued recommendations that called for greater vitamin D supplementation levels than recommended by the IOM, to meet health requirements and to deal with disease (Holick, 2017). But even so, their recommendations may fall short of what it takes to achieve a targeted effect, such as boosting endogenous antimicrobial production or maintaining optimal intestinal epithelial barrier function.

Fifth, it takes thousands, not hundreds of international units of supplemental vitamin D to achieve and maintain vitamin D sufficiency. In the absence of 30-40 glasses of milk per day, or generous UVB exposure, an individual will likely be vitamin D deficient and live a life of compromise.

Finally, UVA exposure actually destroys circulating vitamin D (Carrera-Bastos et al., 2011). This means, suntanning outside of the season and time of day an individual can synthesize vitamin D, the UVA rays which penetrate the skin will reduce circulating vitamin D levels. This also means, using a UVA tanning bed is just another way to become vitamin D deficient.

Now, let's get down to business.

What vitamin D can do for you

Vitamin D has been known to have strong immunomodulatory and anti-inflammatory effects. It regulates both the innate and adaptive arms of the immune system. ~**Ahamed et al., 2019**

Over the 5-year study period, subjects with low mean vitamin D required significantly more steroids, biologicals, narcotics, computed tomography scans, emergency department visits, hospital admissions, and surgery compared with subjects with normal mean vitamin D levels. ~**Kabbani et al., 2016, emphasis added**

With respect to the needs of the ulcerative colitis patient, the benefits of vitamin D sufficiency include:

- Reduction in proinflammatory Th1 and Th17 cell numbers (Hlavaty et al., 2015)

- Promotion of Treg cell numbers and function (recall, Tregs reduce inflammation and promote healing) (Gubatan et al., 2017)

- Promotion of anti-microbial peptide production (Hlavaty et al., 2015)

- Increase in *"the expression of tight junctions in intestinal epithelium"* (Karimi et al., 2019) with reduction in intestinal permeability (Hlavaty et al., 2015)

- Prevention of premature epithelial cell death (apoptosis), thereby acting to maintain intestinal epithelial barrier integrity (Meckel et al., 2016)

- Reduction in relapse risk (Karimi et al., 2019)

- Reduction of colon cancer risk (Ananthakrishnan, 2016)

There is more I could add to the list, but I think you get the point: Vitamin D should not be ignored in the battle against ulcerative colitis. Vitamin D sufficiency could be of benefit to the patient who has had enough of this hideous disease.

Could it happen to you?

*The prevalence of vitamin D deficiency in inflammatory bowel disease (IBD) varies in different studies, but it appears that, at least in some studies, **up to 60% to 70% of people with IBD have insufficient vitamin D levels. Of these, more than half meet the threshold for deficiency,** and the remainder have levels consistent with vitamin D insufficiency.*
~Ananthakrishnan, 2016, emphasis added

In conclusions [sic], vitamin D deficiency is highly prevalent in patients with UC and is related to disease severity, extent, and duration. Patients with UC should be assessed for their serum 25 (OH) vitamin D levels and appropriately supplemented in order to prevent vitamin D–related systemic morbidity and aid in the restoration of the gut mucosal immune homeostasis. ~**Law et al., 2019**

Yes. Of course, it could happen to you. It probably already has. Unless proven otherwise, you are, more likely than not, vitamin D deficient or at best vitamin D insufficient. As we read at the beginning of this section, " . . . *up to 60% to 70% of people with IBD have insufficient vitamin D levels. Of these, more than half meet the threshold for deficiency . . ..*" (Ananthakrishnan, 2016, emphasis added)

While I was preparing this chapter, I asked one of my favorite gastroenterologists the following question: "Are gastroenterologists, today, paying close attention to the vitamin D status of their IBD patients?" He assured me that they were. Boy, I hope he is right. But I have my doubts. Why? **Where are they finding all the vitamin D deficient ulcerative colitis patients they include in their studies?** I think they are easily finding them because vitamin D deficiency is not paid attention to as much as it should. Or it may be that a considerable number of IBD patients are simply non-compliant. **Be compliant!** Vitamin D sufficiency has its rewards.

How to put vitamin D to work for you

Our results indicate that 2000 IU daily dose of vitamin D can increase serum 25-OHD concentration, and quality of life, while it reduces disease activity in UC patients with vitamin D deficiency. **We recommend assessment of the vitamin D status in all patients with UC because they may benefit from vitamin D therapy.** ~Karimi et al., 2019, emphasis added

The dose depends on whether a patient is insufficient or deficient in vitamin D. For patients with mild insufficiency, I recommend approximately 1000 to 2000 units of vitamin D per day. In patients who are more deficient, I tend to recommend higher doses, between 2000 and 4000 units daily, until patients develop sufficient levels, at which time I recommend 1000 units per day for maintenance. For many patients with levels of vitamin D less than 20 ng/mL, and certainly less than 15 ng/mL, I use high-dose weekly vitamin D supplementation. For example, ergocalciferol (50,000 units weekly) can be used for 10 weeks to 3 months to get vitamin D levels back to normal. **~Ananthakrishnan, 2016**

Vitamin D deficiency is so easy to come by. Recognizing this will set you apart from those who just don't get it. And fixing vitamin D deficiency is so easy to do.

Putting vitamin D to work means compliance, plus putting an adequate dose to work. The above recommendations are a start in the right direction. But I take issue with the dose. It may take more than 2,000 IUs/day to achieve an intended outcome and maintain sufficiency. Obviously, vitamin D testing is essential. How else are you going to know? Testing can reveal how deficient an individual is, when enough is enough, and if excessive vitamin D supplementation is occurring.

Importantly, if an individual is tested in the Winter, he or she may require more than 4,000 IU of vitamin D per day to achieve and maintain vitamin D sufficiency. On the other hand, if an individual is tested during the summer—a time when we are or should be generating vitamin D from UVB exposure—this level of supplementation may not be necessary. In my opinion: Testing, retesting, and testing during different seasons of the year, is called for. Such actions will make sure the ulcerative colitis patient is maintaining a respectable level of vitamin D.

And what might be a respectable level of vitamin D?

An optimal vitamin D supplementation protocol for patients with IBD remains undetermined, but targeting serum 25-hydroxy vitamin D [25(OH)D] **levels between 30 and 50 ng/mL appears safe and may have benefits for IBD disease activity.** *Depending on* *baseline vitamin D serum concentration, ileal involvement in CD, body mass index, and perhaps smoking status, **daily vitamin D doses between 1 800–10 000 international units/day are probably necessary.*** (Hlavaty et al., 2015, emphasis added)

In remission, then what?

In this prospective cohort study of 70 patients with ulcerative colitis, we showed that vitamin D levels are associated with baseline endoscopic and histologic inflammation severity during clinical remission, and are associated independently with the longitudinal risk of clinical relapse. These results suggest that vitamin D status is linked not only to current disease severity, but also has an impact on future risk of clinical relapse.

*In conclusion, our study provides **evidence that low vitamin D levels (≤35 ng/mL) correlate with endoscopic and histologic inflammation and are associated with an increased risk of subsequent clinical relapse during periods of clinical remission.** Vitamin D is an affordable, accessible, and relatively nontoxic supplement that may have protective effects in the maintenance of clinical remission in patients with ulcerative colitis.*
~Gubatan et al., 2017, emphasis added

Why even bother to add to the above? The quotation tells you all you need to know about remission and vitamin D. But I can't resist following up with this:

*By lowering the inflammation in IBD patients, induction or maintenance of remission may be achieved. In one study 1200 IU/d Vitamin D supplementation reduced CD relapse rate from 29% to 13% (P < 0.06). Besides these, recent studies have shown an inverse correlation between serum Vitamin D levels and the incidence of polyps and adenomas in the colon that are common complications of UC. **Vitamin D has additional benefits to UC patients including bone health and treating depressive symptoms.**** (Sharifi et al., 2016, emphasis added)

Conclusion

In conclusions [sic], **vitamin D deficiency is highly prevalent in patients with UC and is related to disease severity, extent, and duration.** *Patients with UC should be assessed for their serum 25 (OH) vitamin D levels and appropriately supplemented in order to prevent vitamin D–related systemic morbidity and aid in the restoration of the gut mucosal immune homeostasis.* **~Law et al., 2019, emphasuis added**

A few rules of the road to leave with you before we move on: Work with your physician on all things vitamin D—the dose, the vitamin D form to take, the advisability of sun exposure. Report any negative effects you believe may be related to vitamin D supplementation, particularly if you are taking what may be considered high-dose vitamin D. Some people react negatively to vitamin D supplementation, but not many. Likely, this is a dose-related issue. Testing and adjusting vitamin D dosage, testing again, and adjusting the dosage again as needed, can help prevent some of this. Frequent testing, I believe, is essential. The cost of frequent testing may be brought up as a concern—are you kidding me?!! The cost of a $60 test is *nothing* compared to the extravagant cost of the medicines you may not need in the future, should you achieve and maintain vitamin D sufficiency.

Although important to get a handle on, vitamin D deficiency is not the only deficiency that should be considered when it comes to the patient with ulcerative colitis. We'll take a quick look at other deficiencies of concern in the following gray box.

Other deficiencies to consider

IBD patients are at an increased risk for a number of vitamin and mineral deficiencies. Vitamin D, iron, and vitamin B12 are frequently low in patients with IBD and, in my opinion, are the most clinically relevant deficiencies in these patients; thus, these 3 nutrients should be systematically measured periodically in patients with IBD. Iron, in particular, is important because people with low iron levels have a lower quality of life, as the deficiency impacts their energy levels.

There are also other micronutrients that may be deficient in patients with IBD. For example, zinc seems to be deficient in IBD patients, although we do not fully understand the implications of this deficiency yet. Clinicians should keep an open mind for deficiencies of other vitamins as well.
~Ananthakrishnan, 2016

We'll take things fast paced, one by one. **Vitamin D deficiency.** We've covered that. **Iron deficiency.** Your physician will want to correct this—hopefully, taking care not to give an inappropriate dose and considering the probability that IV iron may be more appropriate than oral iron replacement (see *Chapter 9*, section Iron in excess). **Vitamin B12 deficiency.** Easy to identify and correct. Sublingual B12 is a good option—avoids malabsorption issues. **Folic acid deficiency.** Not mentioned in the above quote but can be a problem for the ulcerative colitis patient. A deficiency of this nutrient can occur from taking the drugs sulfasalazazine and methotrexate. Among other things, correcting folic acid deficiency *"can lower your risk of colon cancer, which is higher in people with ulcerative colitis."* (*Web*MD, 2019) **Zinc deficiency.** Zinc is important to the health of the intestinal epithelial cell and the normal function of the intestinal epithelial barrier. Zinc is required for normal immune cell function. Furthermore, *"Zinc may promote intestinal epithelial wound healing by enhancement of epithelial cell restitution, the initial step of epithelial wound healing. Zinc supplementation may improve epithelial repair; however, excessive amounts of zinc may cause tissue injury and impair epithelial wound healing."* (Cario et al., 2000)

Zinc supplementation is a case-in-point for the need to have your physician guide you every step of the way in dealing with the variety of nutrient deficiencies that may cross your path. You don't want to make a mistake here.

A case for DHEA

There is one hormone deficiency that is likely impacting the patient with ulcerative colitis. Get ready to love the use of abbreviations. The hormone in question is called **dehydroepiandrosterone**. Even the most scholarly of scientists have trouble pronouncing this one, so I'll make it easy on everyone and use the abbreviation DHEA.

DHEA is a hormone derived from the adrenal hormone **pregnenolone**. Subsequently over time, the body transforms DHEA into other hormones like estrogen and testosterone. Unfortunately, DHEA is low in patients with Crohn's disease and ulcerative colitis (Andus et al., 2003). One reason why this is important is that DHEA has anti-inflammatory properties, capable of restraining the release of intracellular NF-κB, the main driver of inflammation, and also capable of inhibiting the secretion of two proinflammatory cytokines, IL-6 and IL-12 (Andus et al., 2003). All this could come in handy in the battle against ulcerative colitis. Will someone *please* put DHEA to the test! Oh! It looks like somebody already has.

Reported in 2003, a study was performed using DHEA, 200 mg daily, to treat both Crohn's and ulcerative colitis patients (Andus et al., 2003). In the ulcerative colitis arm, all 13 patients were refractory to at least one of several different IBD medications. In brief, 8 of 13 ulcerative colitis patients responded to treatment withing the 65-day study period, with 6 of the 8 responders achieving remission. Remission. Boy, does that sound good.

But if DHEA can successfully treat ulcerative colitis, can it also successfully treat pouchitis? It certainly helped the lady I will call Carol.

Carol was a participant in the above study and was one of the responders, indicated by a change in stool from liquid to formed and the cessation of blood in the stool (Klebl et al., 2003). Unfortunately, changes in the appearance of her epithelial cells suggested cancer was just around the corner. Subsequently, due to this finding, a total colectomy was performed to prevent colon cancer from complicating (further) and threatening Carol's life.

Fortunately, under these circumstances, a J-pouch can be created from the terminal ilium, and people like Carol can live a more normal life. With no colon, there can be no colon cancer. Problem solved.

Common to the patient with an ileal pouch is the development of inflammation, called pouchitis, typically responsive to antibiotics and other interventions. Unfortunately, approximately six months after her J-pouch surgery, Carol developed pouchitis. After five months of antibiotics, corticosteroids, and mesalamine without resolution, it was time to turn to an old friend, DHEA.

Recall, Carol was a responder to DHEA in the clinical trial mentioned above. And based on this experience, Carol found herself taking DHEA 200 mg/day, added to her current treatment regimen. And once again, she was a responder.

During DHEA treatment, the number of stools gradually dropped to eight per day, stool consistence improved from liquid/soft to soft solid. At the end of the treatment period, no more mucus or blood was found in her stools. She had been free of abdominal pain for the last 14 days. (Klebl et al., 2003)

Following this success, DHEA treatment ended. But there is more to the story. Unfortuinately, eight weeks later, the suffering returned in the form of 12 to 18 liquid to soft stools per day, along with mild abdominal pain. Looks like someone needs to stay on her DHEA.

Carol's experience should draw attention to DHEA as a useful treatment for IBD—Crohn's disease, ulcerative colitis, and the form of IBD called pouchitis.

~References~

Ahamed Z, Dutta U, Sharma V, Prasad KK, Popli P, Kalsi D, Vaishnavi C, Arora S, Kochhar R. **Oral Nano Vitamin D Supplementation Reduces Disease Activity in Ulcerative Colitis.** Journal of clinical gastroenterology. 2019 Nov 7;53(10):e409-15.

Ananthakrishnan AN. **Vitamin D and inflammatory bowel disease.** Gastroenterology & hepatology. 2016 Aug;12(8):513.

Andus T, Klebl F, Rogler G, Bregenzer N, Schölmerich J, Straub RH. **Patients with refractory Crohn's'disease or ulcerative colitis respond to dehydroepiandrosterone: a pilot study.** Alimentary pharmacology & therapeutics. 2003 Feb;17(3):409-14.

Cario E, Jung S, Harder JD, Schulte C, Sturm A, Wiedenmann B, Goebell H, Dignass AU. **Effects of exogenous zinc supplementation on intestinal epithelial repair in vitro.** European journal of clinical investigation. 2000 May;30(5):419-28.

Carrera-Bastos P, Fontes-Villalba M, O'K'efe JH, Lindeberg S, Cordain L. **The western diet and lifestyle and diseases of civilization.** Research Reports in Clinical Cardiology. 2011 Mar 9;2:15-35.

Cekic M, Cutler SM, VanLandingham JW, Stein DG. **Vitamin D deficiency reduces the benefits of progesterone treatment after brain injury in aged rats.** Neurobiology of aging. 2011 May 1;32(5):864-74.

Grant WB. **The Institute of Medicine did not find the vitamin D–cancer link because it ignored UV-B dose studies.** Public health nutrition. 2011 Apr;14(4):745-6.

Gubatan J, Mitsuhashi S, Zenlea T, Rosenberg L, Robson S, Moss AC. **Low serum vitamin D during remission increases risk of clinical relapse in patients with ulcerative colitis.** Clinical Gastroenterology and Hepatology. 2017 Feb 1;15(2):240-6.

Hlavaty T, Krajcovicova A, Payer J. **Vitamin D therapy in inflammatory bowel diseases: who, in what form, and how much?.** Journal of Crohn's and Colitis. 2015 Feb 1;9(2):198-209.

Holick MF. **Vitamin D: A millennium perspective.** Journal of cellular biochemistry. 2003 Feb 1;88(2):296-307.

Holick MF. **High prevalence of vitamin D inadequacy and implications for health.** InMayo Clinic Proceedings 2006 Mar 1 (Vol. 81, No. 3, pp. 353-373). Elsevier.

Holick M. **The D-batable Institute of Medicine report: a D-lightful perspective.** Endocrine Practice. 2011 Jan 1;17(1):143-9.

Holick MF. **The vitamin D deficiency pandemic: approaches for diagnosis, treatment and prevention.** Reviews in Endocrine and Metabolic Disorders. 2017 Jun 1;18(2):153-65.

Kabbani TA, Koutroubakis IE, Schoen RE, Ramos-Rivers C, Shah N, Swoger J, Regueiro M, Barrie A, Schwartz M, Hashash JG, Baidoo L. **Association of vitamin D level with clinical status in inflammatory bowel disease: a 5-year longitudinal study.** The American journal of gastroenterology. 2016 May;111(5):712.

Karimi S, Tabataba-vakili S, Yari Z, Alborzi F, Hedayati M, Ebrahimi-Daryani N, Hekmatdoost A. **The effects of two vitamin D regimens on ulcerative colitis activity index, quality of life and oxidant/anti-oxidant status.** Nutrition journal. 2019 Dec;18(1):16.

Law AD, Dutta U, Kochhar R, Vaishnavi C, Kumar S, Noor T, Bhadada S, Singh K. **Vitamin D deficiency in adult patients with ulcerative colitis: Prevalence and relationship with disease severity, extent, and duration.** Indian Journal of Gastroenterology. 2019 Feb 14;38(1):6-14.

Li YC. **Investigating the role of vitamin D in IBD pathophysiology and treatment.** Gastroenterology & hepatology. 2008 Jan;4(1):20.

Klebl FH, Bregenzer N, Rogler G, Straub RH, Schölmerich J, Andus T. **Treatment of pouchitis with dehydroepiandrosterone (DHEA)-a case report.** Zeitschrift für Gastroenterologie. 2003 Nov;41(11):1087-90.

Meckel K, Li YC, Lim J, Kocherginsky M, Weber C, Almoghrabi A, Chen X, Kaboff A, Sadiq F, Hanauer SB, Cohen RD. **Serum 25-hydroxyvitamin D concentration is inversely associated with mucosal inflammation in patients with ulcerative colitis.** Clin Nutr. 2016;104:113-20.

Sharifi A, Hosseinzadeh-Attar MJ, Vahedi H, Nedjat S. **A randomized controlled trial on the effect of vitamin D3 on inflammation and cathelicidin gene expression in ulcerative colitis patients.** Saudi journal of gastroenterology: official journal of the Saudi Gastroenterology Association. 2016 Jul;22(4):316.

*Web*MD, 2019 https://www.webmd.com/ibd-crohns-disease/ulcerative-colitis/vitamins-and-supplements-for-ulcerative-colitis#2

Wimalawansa SJ. **Vitamin D in the new millennium.** Current osteoporosis reports. 2012 Mar 1;10(1):4-15.

Chapter 23
Fecal Microbial Transplantation (FMT)

Fecal microbiota transplantation is a therapeutic method via administration of fecal bacteria from a healthy individual into the intestinal tract of a recipient in order to directly change the recipient's gut microbiota composition and confer a health benefit. **~Qin et al., 2017**

The results were spectacular. Patients entered clinical remission immediately, remission was maintained in one case until the writing of this article and for two other cases for 10 to 12 months. **~Laszlo et al., 2016**

O f all the therapies discussed in this book, fecal microbial transplant (FMT) is perhaps the one I am most passionate about. Why? In the medical literature there is case after case of remission in ulcerative colitis using this form of therapy. And if it can happen to them, there's a good chance it can happen to you.

The concept is simple: Stool from one individual, a healthy individual, is transferred to the gut of another individual, a sick individual, an individual like you, to confer a health benefit. No one is chuckling or cracking a joke while performing this procedure. This is serious business! He or she knows they are playing with power. I know they are playing with power. And soon, so will you.

And with that, let's take a few minutes and go back in time.

FMT: Brief historical perspective

The history of fecal microbiota transplantation (FMT) dates back even to ancient China. Recently, scientific studies have been looking into FMT as a promising treatment of various diseases, while in the process teaching us about the interaction between the human host and its resident microbial communities. **~de Groot et al., 2017**

In China, sometime during the 4th century AD, the recorded history of FMT began (de Groot et al., 2017). Why someone thought transferring poop from one individual to another individual would be a good idea, is still a mystery. But a thought is a powerful thing, and a medical therapy was born. And if you believe your doctor knows what he or she is doing, you'll drink just about anything, particularly if your life is on the line. According to the historical record, the Chinese called this early form of FMT "yellow soup." It must have tasted like crap.

Taste buds be damned, the practice caught on and began its march through the pages of history.

By the 16th century, the Chinese had developed a variety of feces-derived products for gastrointestinal complaints as well as systemic symptoms such as fever and pain. (de Groot et al., 2017)

I could go on and on about the "colorful" history of FMT, there are so many interesting things to discuss, but I need to move things along. However, I will add this: Be glad you don't live in a region where camel poop is in generous supply, or it could be offered to you in your hour of need. Astonishingly, and as recently as World War II, German soldiers ate camel poop to prevent infectious gastroenteritis (de Groot et al., 2017). They learned it from the locals. It must have tasted like . . . well, you know.

Fast forward to today. Thanks to the weight of scientific evidence, including an abundance of successful case reports, there is clear justification of the use of FMT in a variety of medical conditions, including ulcerative colitis—conditions where an abnormal intestinal microflora plays a supporting and decisive role. And due to its effectiveness, FMT is currently an FDA-approved treatment for one form of inflammatory bowel disease, pseudomembranous colitis. I should tell you more.

Pseudomembranous colitis is an extremely serious medical condition caused by the bacterium *Clostridium difficile* (*C-diff*). Worldwide, it costs *"over $4.8 billion per year in healthcare costs."* (Winston and Theriot, 2016) It used to kill a lot of people, and still does—to the tune of 29,000 individuals per year in the USA alone (CDC, 2017). But it doesn't have to. FMT can stop it, dead in its tracts, and with a high probability of success.

> *Fecal microbiota transplantation (FMT) is a highly effective therapy of recurrent Clostridium difficile infection (CDI) with consistent disease resolution rates of 85%–90% after 1 treatment and up to 100% after a second treatment, using either fresh or cryopreserved stool from healthy, well-characterized donors.* (Ott et al., 2017)

Antibiotic use in medicine gives rise to the growth of *C-diff*, as antibiotics kill off a lot of beneficial bacteria that ordinarily hold in check the overgrowth of this pathogen (Baktash et al., 2018; Wilson et al., 2019). *C-diff* is a major problem occurring in the general patient population and has apparently become more prevalent in those who suffer from ulcerative colitis (Kariv et al., 2010). And if suffering from ulcerative colitis alone wasn't bad enough, add *C-diff* to the mix to see what happens. This infection can *". . . worsen UC and increase the risk for colectomy or even death . . .."* (Seicean et al., 2014)

"Oh! Let's not get carried away, now," seems to be the attitude of the FDA. Unacceptable to me and disappointing to many others, in 2013 the FDA declared FMT a drug and restricted its use only for the treatment of *C-diff* (Aroniadis and Brandt, 2014). And with that, the FDA put the brakes on the use of FMT as a treatment for ulcerative colitis. They said, in effect, "You can't have it." Have they not heard of your plight? Have you no right to try? Is not your microbiome disturbed way beyond belief?

The microbiome is clearly disturbed in ulcerative colitis. One clear example: *". . . FMT from UC donors to normal recipient rats triggered UC symptoms, UC-prone microbial shift, and host metabolic adaption."* (Yan et al., 2018) As to be expected, once the rats realized what was going on, they demanded FMT from a healthy human (or a healthy rat) to reverse a disease process that was hideous, unacceptable, and destroying their lives. But they were out of luck. Characteristically, the FDA said, in effect, "You can't have it."

And so, we have arrived at a point in history of FMT where you may need it, you may want it, you may be at the end of your rope with nowhere else to turn, but in you hour of need it is placed beyond your reach.

I get it, the thought of FMT may not be appealing to you (I'll work on that), but it is appealing to the vast majority of ulcerative colitis patients who would jump at the chance to take advantage of this therapy (Kahn et al., 2013). To underscore,

> *Our patients showed that they were willing to receive this new method despite its unappealing nature, for its [sic] better to have FMT than to be tortured by the disease.* (Wei et al., 2015)

And the reasons for choosing FMT, the reasons for its success, just keep piling up.

What it can do for you

The aim of FMT is to reintroduce a stable community of GI microbes from a healthy donor to replace the disrupted populations in a diseased individual. **~Guinane and Cotter, 2013**

FMT for Ulcerative colitis has been described in several publications which showed complete resolution of all symptoms even cessation of medications without relapse. **Recent studies** *have confirmed these findings; a meta-analysis of FMT for patients with IBD found that* **63% of patients with UC entered remission, 76% were able to stop taking medications for IBD, and 76% experienced a reduction in gastrointestinal symptoms.** ~Wei et al., 2015, emphasis added

Dealing with inflammation using drug therapy is something quite different than dealing with a disturbed microbiome with FMT. Indeed, FMT challenges the status quo. I'm ok with that. Drug therapy and little else *should* be challenged. Why not throw at ulcerative colitis all the weapons we have at our disposal, particularly the ones most promising? And speaking of promising, FMT has "promising" written all over it. It has "success" written all over it, too.

FMT is, of course, the transfer of healthy microbiome from donor to recipient, but it is so much more. The following is a review of the benefits FMT has to offer:

- FMT stabilizes/balances immune responses (Shen et al., 2018)

- FMT restores numbers of anti-inflammatory bacteria (Shen et al., 2018)

- FMT transfers secondary bile acids to the recipient, correcting a secondary bile acid deficiency and suppressing the growth of unfavorable bacteria (Nie et al., 2015; Baktash et al., 2018)

- FMT transfers antimicrobial peptides from donor to recipient (Baktash et al., 2018)

- FMT induces synthesis of immunoglobins IgA, IgG, IgM— antibodies that recognize and neutralize a variety of pathogens (Shen et al., 2018)

- FMT transfers a stable microbiome, an ecosystem of organisms in balance with each other (Guinane and Cotter, 2013)

- FMT transfers bacteriophages—viruses that attack and kill pathogenic bacteria and suppress their numbers (Bojanova and Bordenstein, 2016; Zuo et al., 2018; Baktash et al., 2018)

- FMT reduces intestinal permeability (Shen et al., 2018)

- FMT increases the production of butyrate (a fatty acid important to the health of the colonocyte and a modulator of immune responses) (Shen et al., 2018)

- FMT increases the acidity of the colonic environment, favoring the growth of beneficial bacteria and inhibiting the growth of pathogenic bacteria (Shen et al., 2018)

- FMT may help resolve extra-intestinal manifestations of IBD (e.g., skin lesions, remote infections) (Cui et al., 2015)

There is no single therapy in existence that offers more than one or a few of the above-mentioned benefits, those ascribed to FMT. With FMT you get it all! No wonder it can induce remission in ulcerative colitis, rapidly and with long-lasting effect. And not a single taste bud need be involved.

A procedure, not a meal

FMT for refractory UC has been described in 3 publications, comprising 9 patients, all of whom had severe, active, long-standing UC . . .. FMT was administered as retention enemas and resulted in the complete resolution of all symptoms with cessation of UC medications within 6 weeks without relapse. Remission was maintained for up to 13 years, and follow-up colonoscopy in 8 of the 9 patients showed no evidence of UC . . . or only mild chronic inflammation . . .. **~Aroniadis and Brandt, 2014**

Fortunately, advances in medical technology allows us to go beyond "yellow soup" and a camel poop energy bar in our quest to transfer gut bacteria from one individual to another. (Camels are individuals, too.) Today, we have colonoscopes, we have electric blenders, we have filters, we have capsules, we have donor screening strategies and technologies, we have successful case reports—we have it all!

FMT is, itself, a rather straight-forward and *"elegantly simple"* procedure (Borody et al., 2014). But before the procedure is performed (in straight-forward, elegant fashion), the FMT donor is carefully screened. I won't go into great detail on donor screening here, but obviously a suitable donor needs to be healthy and living a healthy lifestyle, is someone without recent antibiotic use, and should be an individual without a current or recent medical condition that could potentially transfer a pathogen to a recipient. Blood tests are used to rule out transmissible disease. Finally, a stool sample from the potential donor is screened for gastrointestinal pathogens and parasites before the potential donor receives the seal of approval. All this is exceptionally laid out in DeFilipp et al., 2019.

Although a family member may be the ideal donor, a suitable FMT donor may be a professional. In the crazy world you live in, some people sell their poop to supplement their income, and some people sell that poop to earn a living. Today, stool can be purchased from a stool bank. As to be expected, the donors used are carefully screened and their stool is thoroughly examined to make sure it is disease-free and the best that money can buy.

So, it's a go! The stool has been collected (or purchased), and it's time to perform the procedure. But first, the stool is blinded with saline, filtered, then placed in large syringes to be instilled via a colonoscope or via an enema tube. If the stool is from a stool bank, ordinarily frozen, it must first be thawed; otherwise, the procedure is essentially the same as described above.

As an alternative to the above, FMT can be taken in pill form, with the donor and the donated stool meeting all safety requirements. If there is a happy face on the pill bottle, you know it can be trusted. Unfortunately, the "pill" is awfully big, and many pills need to be taken to constitute a single dose. FMT in pill form is a highly effective approach for *C-diff* (Ramai et al., 2019). And it looks like this approach will work for the ulcerative colitis patient, as well.

In 2017, seven patients suffering from ulcerative colitis were given something else to complain about (Cold et al., 2019). Can you imagine swallowing 25 poop-filled capsules (rather large) each day, taken on an empty stomach, and for a period of *50 days?!!* Just the regimen alone is enough to make one sick. But apparently it doesn't. *"All participants completed the treatment and no serious adverse events were reported throughout the study period."* (Cold et al., 2019) In the study, at two weeks, three of the seven participants were in clinical remission. By week eight, two more participants achieved clinical remission. And at six months, four participants remained in clinical remission. That's pretty impressive. But it better be impressive! The FMT pills cost about $65 each, and a fifty-day supply (1,250 poop-filled pills) will set you back $81,250.

Whether taken in pill form, whether delivered by a tube placed through the nose and into the stomach (NG tube), or administered in liquid form via an enema tube or colonoscope, there is no doubt that FMT can be an effective and relatively safe therapy in the battle against ulcerative colitis. There are stories I could tell.

Stories of success

In January 1989, Bennet and Brinkman published a case of FMT in non-CDI [C-diff infection] UC, documenting reversal of Bennet's own colitis after large-volume retention enemas of healthy donor flora 6 months prior. Before FMT, he reported continuously active, severe UC of 7 years' duration. At 3 months post-FMT, however, the patient was asymptomatic in the absence of UC therapy for the first time in 11 years, with no active inflammation. (Borody and Campbell, 2012)

Historically, the modern use of FMT as a therapy for ulcerative colitis began in 1988 (Bennett and Brinkman, 1989; Fang et al., 2018). Credited as the first ulcerative colitis patient to receive FMT, was a gastroenterologist who personally knew this disease all too well (Borody et al., 2014). Frankly, he hated it! This is his story:

Case report: Dr. Justin D. Bennet

For a period of eleven years prior to his fecal transplant, Dr. Bennet experienced *"continuously active, severe"* ulcerative colitis for seven of the eleven years he was battling this disease. *"The condition was refactory to standard management including steroids and sulphasalazine and every time daily prednisone dosage was reduced below 30 mg severe symptoms . . . recurred."* (Bennet and Brinkman, 1989) Motivated by the belief that gut bacteria were in some way behind a disease that was so unrelenting, he set up an experiment designed to replace his diseased microflora with an infusion of disease-free donor stool. The experiment was performed, and the rest is history. *"At 3 months post-FMT, . . . the patient was asymptomatic in the absence of UC therapy for the first time in 11 years, with no active inflammation."* (Borody and Campbell, 2012)

Case report: Johnathan

Dr. Bennet may not be the first ulcerative colitis patient to receive a fecal transplant, after all. It may be Johnathan. Both individuals received their FMTs in 1988, and both case reports were published in 1989 (Bennet and Brinkman, 1989; Borody et al., 2014) But regardless of who was first, they each have an impressive story to tell. Get used to the word impressive.

Johnathan was 45 years old at the time of his fecal transplant. His ulcerative colitis had only been of 18-month duration but was extensive and totally unacceptable. Current therapy (olsalazine) was inadequate. *"The patient underwent an exchange of bowel flora, and his condition improved sufficiently to cease all treatment within days."* (Borody et al., 1989) At three months post-FMT, his colonoscopy showed a normal looking colon and mucosal biopsies also looked normal (Borody et al., 1989). Twenty-three years later, Johnathan remained *"asymptomatic and in histologic remission."* (Borody et al., 2012). And all this was the result of *only one FMT!*

Case Report: Shelly

Shelly's ulcerative colitis started at age 11. At the time of her FMT, she was *"A 21-year-old patient with a 10-year history of severe UC, uncontrolled with anti-inflammatory agents, steroids, antibiotics, and finally anti–tumor necrosis factor therapy . . . ."* (Borody et al., 2012) Time to act! And there was no fooling around.

> *Pre-FMT symptoms included severe diarrhea with marked urgency and presence of blood and mucus. The patient underwent colonoscopy where the first FMT was administered. After this, daily rectal infusions were performed for 7 days followed by 26 weekly rectal infusions. The patient experienced an immediate reduction in symptoms, passing 2 formed stools daily without blood, urgency, or mucus. Follow-up colonoscopy at 12 months revealed virtually nil inflammation or edema and she remains clinically well at 12 months on no medication.* (Borody et al., 2012)

I'm happy for Shelly. Shelly is happy for Shelly. Her doctor is still smiling.

Case Report: Li Jie

Li Jie lives in China. He was 24 years old at the time of his FMT—presenting with a 7-year history of recurrent ulcerative colitis (Ni et al., 2016). His disease was extensive, involving the entire colon. As a constant reminder of the severity of his disease, Li Jie found himself passing 4-6 mucopurlent, bloody stools per day. I can certainly see why FMT was offered. Aside from the removal of his entire colon, there was nowhere else to go. Interestingly, in his case the route of passage was via a tube placed through the abdominal wall, with the tip of the tube residing in the cecum, the terminal portion of the small intestine which is positioned right above the beginning of the colon. How innovative! Makes sense.

The donor in this case was Li Jie's father, who was carefully screened and certified free of transmissible disease. With the tube in place and the stool produced and processed, it was time to turn things around. But was it too late?

In this case, in addition to the donor stool, 3 grams of mesalazine was also given (route not specified). Additionally, Li Jie was maintained on IV and tube feeding during his hospitalization, with tube feeding supplying his nutritional needs until 1 month post-FMT. After which, a normal diet was resumed. Clearly, Li Jie was very ill and FMT was offered as a last-resort, rescue therapy. Clearly, his physicians were putting FMT to the test. Likely, fingers were crossed.

Well, it worked. But it was not easy. After the initial FMT, it was repeated once a day for one month. This, of course, kept Dad very busy and eating with purpose. Once Li Jei was released from the hospital, the fecal transplants continued twice weekly for another three months. After two months at home, his tube feedings ended and he resumed a normal diet. The fecal transplants ended a month later. Let the historical record show, Dad was all pooped out.

Within a week after his first FMT, Li Jie was symptom-free. At one-month post-FMT, his colonoscopy showed only small scattered ulcers in the rectum, with the rest of the colon looking relatively normal. The use of mesalazine 2 grams daily ended at that point in time. At three months post-FMT the colonoscopy showed no signs of disease in colon or rectum. Twelve months later, Li Jie remained symptom free. His life was back.

Comment: If only I had written this book 10 years earlier, if only it had been translated into Chinese, if only Li Jie had read my book and put into practice at least some of the life-style changes and alternative and complimentary therapies outlined therein, then perhaps he would have achieved remission much earlier and would not have reached the point of requiring such extreme measures to turn things around.

Case Report: Eddie

Eddie was 25 years old at the time of his fecal transplant (Borody et al., 2003). Six years dealing with ulcerative colitis was long enough. His life revolved around passing frequent bloody stools, revolved around diarrhea 6-7 times a day, revolved around abdominal pain, abdominal cramping, fevers, weight loss, nausea, and revolved around misery. The medications used to treat his ulcerative colitis became ineffective. A more potentially dangerous drug, azathioprine (Imuran), was offered to the patient but was refused. Also, at the time of his FMT, Eddie's liver enzymes were elevated indicating substantial liver injury, secondary to sclerosing cholangitis.

Prior to his FMT, *"Colonoscopy confirmed pancolitis with granular mucosa, contact bleeding, microulceration and histologically active chronic colitis."* (Borody et al., 2003)

The donor was his female partner, appropriately screened to rule out transmissible disease.

Before fecal transplant, Eddie took antibiotics for a number of days, as a measure employed to suppress the numbers of specific bacteria.

Rather than via a colonoscopy, the fecal transfer was through an enema tube. Five transplants were given on consecutive days. Eddie's current medications (salazopyrin, prednisone) were continued. At the end of the transplant series, salazopyrin was discontinued and a five-week prednisone taper was initiated. Eddie was on his way to a better life.

At one-week post-transplant, Eddie's symptoms markedly improved, along with reductions in stool frequency. By four months post-fecal transplant, he was asymptomatic without medical treatment and defecating 2-3 times/day without bleeding. Furthermore, his liver enzymes returned to normal. And to put icing on the cake,

*On his most recent review **after 13 years follow-up without other therapy he had no clinical or colonoscopic evidence of UC and histopathology samples from several sites around the colon were normal.*** (Borody et al., 2003, emphasis added)

Case report: Arjun

Arjun was 6 years old at the time of his fecal transplant (Butta et al., 2018). He was facing a life of permanent damage, at the hands of a hideous disease. His ulcerative colitis was advanced; his meds and specialized diet were not up to the task. According the report, Arjun had ulcerative colitis for at least two years prior to his fecal transplant. Imagine, an ulcerative colitis victim at 4 years old! Boy, do I hate this disease.

He presented in clinic *"with history of loose, watery stools with mucus and blood for one year associated with periumbilical pain."* (Butta et al., 2018) His colonoscopy was *"suggestive of pancolitis."* Enough was enough, and his parents requested FMT to save their son from the clutches of this disease. It is safe to say, they are glad they did.

The donor choice was Arjun's father, who was screened and tested and met safety requirements. I don't think the long arm of the FDA reaches all the way to India, so I don't believe the message "You can't have it" got through.

Arjun did not receive antibiotics or bowel prep prior to this fecal transplant, as is often the case. The first transplant was delivered as a small-volume enema every 15 minutes for one hour. This treatment protocol was repeated daily for 5 days. Each small volume enema (60 ml each) was instilled slowly over a 5-minute period, and Arjun was turned 180 degrees, from left side to right side during each transplant session—an effort to disperse the enema to reach areas further up in the colon.

By the end of the 5 days of therapy, Arjun's Paediatric Ulcerative Colitis Disease Activity Index dropped from 35 to 15. Three years later, he was eating a normal diet and his ulcerative colitis meds were being tapered. *"The child is showing improvement in symptoms and has not had any relapse since then."* (Butta et al., 2018)

Although not out or the woods yet, Arjun was clearly improved and may continue to progress to a point where victory can be declared. That being said, I'm still a little worried about him. In the future, Arjun may need a repeat series of FMTs to turn things around and again head him in the right direction. I hope someone doesn't say . . . well, you know.

Case report: Kumar

Kumar was forty-four at the time he received a 2-week series of fecal transplants—presenting with a history of ulcerative colitis extending over a period of 11 years and undergoing a severe relapse (Seth et al., 2016). For the eleven-year period, Kumar reported *"frequent relapse despite daily sulfasalazine 4 g, azathioprine 125 mg, and rectal 5-aminosalicylic acid. Repeated use of corticosteroids led to cataract. At enrollment, he was passing eight stools a day with blood with a Mayo score of 9 (3+1+3+2)."* (Seth et al., 2016)

The donor of choice was Kumar's brother-in-law, who was carefully screened and declared to be one heck of a brother-in-law (and free of transmissible disease).

It all went well. Three sessions of FMT, at 2-week intervals, was all it took. (It also took a colonocope and a blender.) And the results were pleasing:

> Clinical response to FMT was noted within 2 weeks of first session of FMT. Complete remission with Mayo scores improving to 0 for stool frequency, blood in stool, and colonoscopy were noted at weeks 4, 8, and 12, respectively. Significant histological improvement, as determined with Geboes score, was noted at 16 weeks. Azathioprine and 5- ASA were tapered, and he remains in clinical and endoscopic remission 10 months after FMT and 5 months after withdrawal of all medication. Histopathology at 10 months follow up was normal. (Seth et al., 2016)

Case report: Daniel

Daniel (whose story is also told in *Chapter 7*) presented in clinic with worsening ulcerative colitis. Previously, he was successfully treated with corticosteroids, 5 ASA, and Azathioprin for the better part of 12 years (Laszlo and Pascu, 2014). Then, due to a return of symptoms, biological therapy (Infliximab; Remecade) was started and quieted his symptoms and gave Daniel another year of remission. Unfortunately, ulcerative colitis symptoms returned. A decision was made to give FMT a try, and a first degree relative was screened and determined free from transmissible disease.

The fecal transplant procedure was described as "transcolonic," performed using a colonoscope. Post-FMT, the patient was given medications to slow GI mobility, and was instructed to stay in a supine (lying flat on back) position for a non-specified period of time. Obviously, the goal here was to allow the transplanted stool to remain in Daniel's colon as long as reasonably possible, allowing, within the colon, a prolonged exposure time to the transplanted material (before it's time to go).

For Daniel, *"clinical and biological remission was achieved."* (Laszlo and Pascu, 2014). *"Immediately after FMT the biological therapy was stopped."* (Laszlo and Pascu, 2014). At follow-up, 5 months post-FMT, clinical and endoscopic remission was confirmed. Daniel continued on ASA 2g/day. Intriguingly, all this progress from 1 fecal transplant.

But is only one enough? How about 80 FMTs? Will 80 be enough?

Case report: Shawn

Let's let Dr. Borody and colleagues tell Shawn's story.

A 33-year-old male with ulcerative colitis presented with abdominal pain, bloody diarrhea, and mucus discharge. Failing standard antiinflammatory drugs with frequent relapses, fecal microbiota transplantation (FMT) was introduced. FMT was first administered via a transcolonoscopic route followed by daily enemas, reducing to twice weekly, weekly, and then fortnightly. After 80 FMT infusions, he was passing normal stool once per day and was off all drugs for 7 months. He was recolonoscoped, and the difference is shown." (Borody et al., 2013)

If you would like to see Shawn's pre- and post-FMT photos, go online and find the following paper:

Borody TJ, Paramsothy S, Agrawal G. **Fecal microbiota transplantation: indications, methods, evidence, and future directions.** Current gastroenterology reports. 2013 Aug 1;15(8):337.

Case Report: Ethan

Again, let's let Dr. Borody and colleagues tell the story. I go on forever. They know how to be brief and get right to the point. Here is Ethan's story:

A 38-year-old man with a 6-year history of ulcerative colitis, concurrent multiple sclerosis, sacroilitis and sclerosing cholangitis was treated with an initial transcolonoscopic FMT infusion, followed by over 100 FMT enemas during the next 12 months. After 4 weeks of daily FMT enemas, the patient's IBD symptoms had dramatically improved, liver biochemical tests had normalized and sacroilitis pain was absent. (Borody et al., 2014)

We've got pictures! If you would like to see Ethan's pre- and post-FMT photos, go online and find the following paper:

Borody TJ, Brandt LJ, Paramsothy S. **Therapeutic faecal microbiota transplantation: current status and future developments.** Current opinion in gastroenterology. 2014 Jan;30(1):97.

Case Report: Keiko

Keiko is a 11-year old Japanese girl with severe ulcerative colitis, refractory to both steroids and Infliximab (Remicade) (Shimizu et al., 2016). *"Before FMT, she had been hospitalized five times within 6 months because of disease flare and had missed most school days."* (Shimizu et al., 2016) Although she was enjoying a brief period of remission from clinical symptoms, her disease had reached a point where it was recommended that she have her colon removed. Who wants this? Keiko didn't. Mom didn't. Dad didn't. Mom knew what *this* was like! She, too, had a history of ulcerative colitis and her colon was removed because of colon cancer. This is a family who knew, firsthand, what life is like without a colon. Unsurprisingly, the patient and both parents requested a fecal transplant *"to save her colon"* (Shimizu et al., 2016).

Due to Mom's medical history, she was automatically disqualified from being the stool donor. However, Dad was healthy, and careful screening qualified him to be the donor.

The fecal transplants were described as follows:

> The first FMT was performed via colonoscopy to distribute the suspension throughout the colon and observe the colonic mucosa. The patient had undergone bowel preparation with magnesium citrate the day before the first colonoscopic FMT. After the first colonoscopic FMT, FMT by retention enema were performed for the next 4 days. After this 5 day sequential course, 11 additional FMT by retention enema were performed every 2 to 4 weeks over 10 months. FMT by retention enema was performed as described by Kunde et al. with minor modifications. Fecal material was prepared in five–six 50 mL syringes. Each aliquot was infused over 5 min followed by positional change of the recipient in order to move the fecal content proximally. The recipient was asked if she was willing to proceed after each aliquot. She successfully received all fecal material prepared for FMT throughout the treatment course. (Shimizu et al., 2016)

And the results were quite remarkable. And keep in mind, this was the experience of an 11-year old girl who was on the verge of undergoing a colectomy.

> Shortly after the first 5 day course, UC recurred, and scheduled IFX [Infliximab] infusion improved her condition. As the FMT continued, the patient remained in clinical remission with a tapering dose of corticosteroid and scheduled IFX. At week 40, she was in clinical remission with only 1.5 mg corticosteroid. (Shimizu et al., 2016)

Forty weeks post-FMT, Keiko remained in clinical remission. At the time, *". . . endoscopy showed relative improvement in the sigmoid colon and continuous inflammation in the transverse colon while pathology showed active inflammation with crypt abscesses and paucity of crypts."* (Shimizu et al., 2016)

I hope Keiko continues to improve. If things start heading in the wrong direction, it is my hope that there will be another series of FMTs in her future.

Time for one more case report? Of course you do.

Case Report: Olivia

Olivia was 28 at the time she underwent a series of 5 fecal transplants in her battle against ulcerative colitis (Borody et al., 2003). Imagine having one half of your entire life dominated by this dreadful disease. Fourteen years is enough—all the diarrhea, bleeding, cramping, nausea, vomiting, fever and fatigue Olivia had to endure. Her meds—prednisone, olsalazine, mercaptopurine—were no match for the disease.

After Olivia's series of fecal transplants, using stool donated by her brother-in-law, mercaptopurine was immediately stopped, and apparently a taper of her prednisone began. Olsalazine was continued for a further 6 weeks. Post-FMT, *"Immediate improvements included reduced bleeding, urgency, nausea, and vomiting, while abdominal cramping persisted for 1 week."* (Borody et al., 2003)

Unfortunately, *"The patient experienced 1 episode of bleeding 3 weeks post-HPI [post-FMT] and the total withdrawal of prednisone was delayed until week 6."* (Borody et al., 2003) Other than this little "speed bump" on the road to recovery, two months following fecal transplant Olivia was *"well, with no urgency or bleeding."*

I like this story. I like all these stories!

At 2 years follow-up, she had had no more UC relapses despite episodes of stress and continued to be clinically, colonoscopically, and histologically disease-free without treatment. (Borody et al., 2003)

Note: With the exception of Dr. Justin D. Bennet, the names in this section are fictious.

Thoughts on case reports and clinical trials

ClinicalTrials.gov currently lists more than 300 studies evaluating FMT for various indications, primarily gastrointestinal, but also for neurologic, behavioral, and metabolic conditions. **~DeFilipp et al., 2019**

The treatment effects on patients who have undergone FMT to treat UC appear very promising, especially for patients with multiple infusions administered via the lower gastrointestinal tract. **~Fang et al., 2018, emphasis added**

Additionally, FMT provided greater therapeutic benefit in patients whose onset of UC was associated with an alteration in the fecal microbiota from antibiotic use or concomitant colonic infection. Experience with FMT for UC is just beginning, and controlled trials are needed to establish its safety, administration regimen, and therapeutic role, if any. **~Aroniadis and Brandt, 2014**

Impressive care reports are one thing, clinical trials composed of groups of individuals (who are all basically treated the same), are quite another. But taken together, they teach us several valuable lessons. And with respect to FMT, we have learned the following:

First, not everybody responds to FMT. **Second**, one FMT session, or even a few, may not be enough. In fact, as the case reports previously discussed confirm, many, many sessions may be necessary. A relentless effort is often required to defeat a relentless disease. **Third**, the continuation of ulcerative colitis medications may be necessary—helpful in association with FMT to achieve and maintain remission. **Fourth,** complications from FMT are rare. **Fifth,** FMT is often used as a rescue therapy rather than used as a front-line treatment, offered earlier in the course of the disease and at a time when FMT, combined with medication, may be more effective. **Finally,** not everything FMT goes smoothly. There can be initial symptoms such as nausea and abdominal pain. The patient may also experience a flare in symptoms. Furthermore, serious complications, although extremely rare, may occur and may result in death (more later).

Studies evaluating FMT in groups of individuals report many cases of success as well as many cases of failure—sounds like what happens with standard drug therapy! By way of example, if a study only shows, say a 38% success rate, that means 62% did not respond to therapy. However, 38% means welcome relief to one in three. Not too bad! But in ulcerative colitis, the FMT response rate appears to be much higher.

> *Recent studies have confirmed these findings; a meta-analysis of FMT for patients with IBD found that **63% of patients with UC entered remission, 76% were able to stop taking medications for IBD, and 76% experienced a reduction in gastrointestinal symptoms.*** (Wei et al., 2015, emphasis added)

Published a year later from the above report, an analysis of twenty-five studies, comprising of 234 ulcerative colitis patients, found that FMT induced **remission in 41% of study subjects and demonstrated a clinical response rate of 65%** (Shi et al., 2016). Not quite as good as the above report, but still impressive. Of note: *"Most adverse events were slight and self-resolving."* (Shi et al., 2016)

Most recently, a meta-analysis found only **26%** of adults and only **10%** of pediatric ulcerative colitis patients achieved clinical remission from FMT (Fang et al., 2019). I would say "Goodbye" to this meta-analysis and show it to the door. The study subjects involved were treated so differently in the various studies analyzed, that it can only muddy the waters. Some subjects were given fresh stool; some were given frozen then thawed stool. Some fecal transplants were given by colonoscopy; some by enema. Some subjects were given 2 fecal transplants; some were given 40. **Now, is this any way to judge the effectiveness of a therapy?** I think not. If it takes 40 FMTs for some subjects to achieve and sustain remission, why would two or three FMTs tell us anything of value regarding the percentage of effectiveness of this therapy? Should FMT be denied to the ulcerative colitis patient based on this kind of foolishness? I think not.

From case reports and research studies, it seems clear: FMT can be a very effective therapy to achieve remission, but likely it will take many transplant sessions to turn things around. There is a great case to be made for FMT to be offered to the patient in need, particularly so if nothing else is working.

What's up with that?

Fortunately, advances in medical technology allow us to go beyond "yellow soup" and a camel poop energy bar in our quest to transfer gut bacteria from one individual to another. (Camels are individuals, too.)
~The Author, 2020

With a therapy as truly bizarre as FMT, there is bound to be a few strange things about this therapy that show up unannounced, pop up from out of the blue, things no one would *ever* expect to see. I'll point out a few.

Surprisingly, at least with respect to *C-diff*, filtered donor stool, filtered to remove all bacteria, works just as well as normal, bacteria-replete FMT (Ott et al., 2017; Zuo et al., 2018). Incredible! So unexpected. When it comes to the effectiveness of FMT, it may not be the bacteria after all! Apparently, the other things that are found in stool, such as bile acids, bacteria-killing viruses, or factors that promote healing, are what make FMT an effective therapy. (see Bojananova and Bordenstein, 2016; Baktash et al., 2018).

Even more surprising, you, the ulcerative colitis patient, can actually donate your own stool, have it processed, return it to the very colon from whence it came, and remission can be achieved (Costello et al., 2019). Placebo response? Some cases, maybe. But in every case? Maybe not. **It should be pointed out that stool, once processed in typical FMT-fashion, is modified in a substantial way.** It is not the same coming back as it was coming out. The reason? When you blend stool you aerate it, and by doing so, the oxygen kills perhaps a majority of the good bacteria you were counting on to come to the aid of the FMT recipient. Therefore, the bacteria that are not killed by oxygen, those capable of thriving in the presence of oxygen, are selected to dominate. An aerated stool is a modified stool—but, amazingly, it still works! However, it is suggested by some investigators that aerated stool may have reduced effectiveness in FMT (Rogers and Bruce, 2013; Costello et al., 2019).

The promise and success of FMT has given rise to a few variations of the theme. It has been suggested that an ulcerative colitis patient could donate stool when his or her disease is in remission, to be frozen, banked, then later returned as a FMT in the event that relapse occurs.

> *For those patients with mild IBD, it may be good that the fecal samples can be collected and stored in the remission stage and offered to the same patients when they come into the active stage of IBD.* (Wang et al., 2014)

Think of it! You are both the donor and recipient! No screening required! You come to your own rescue, and you do it with your own poop! This is a very novel concept when it comes to FMT. Might work! I can't wait to see this thing really put to the test.

Related to the above, is a study that demonstrated the feasibility of banking stool from a patient before antibiotic therapy, to be returned later, to the same patient, to restore microbiota diversity post-antibiotic use (Taur et al., 2018). It worked!

Another strange thing we have learned along the way is that obesity, long linked to a person's fecal microbiome, can be transferred to the FMT recipient (Alang and Kelly, 2015). *"We report a case of a woman successfully treated with FMT who developed new-onset obesity after receiving stool from a healthy but overweight donor."* (Alang and Kelly, 2015) And that brings us up to this: The choice of a donor may make a *big* difference when it comes to success.

Apparently, although certified as healthy and free of transmissible disease, not all donors are created equal. Observations that some donors produce better results than do other donors, has given rise to the concept of a *"super donor"* (Wilson et al., 2019). Donor diet may be a factor. My belief is, a vegetarian or semi-vegetarian (and free of transmissible disease) would be an excellent choice, a "super donor" if you will. These two dietary practices promote an exceptional healthy bowel microflora, as previously discussed.

A final, related strange thing to consider, and I've mentioned this before, but it bears repeating: A fecal transplant from an ulcerative colitis patent given to a healthy rat, transfers ulcerative to the rat. *". . . FMT from UC donors to normal recipient rats triggered UC symptoms, UC-prone microbial shift, and host metabolic adaption."* (Yan et al., 2018) My firm belief is, if you hate a rat so much that you would intentionally give it ulcerative colitis, you need to get a hold of yourself and seek professional help. You are really messed up.

Not without risk, not without danger

FMT is generally of safety and tolerance with few serious adverse events. As many patients need to receive more than one FMT therapy, more procedural complications will probably be reported due to the invasion of procedure. Despite rigorous donor selection and screening for infectious agents, known and unknown risks still remain a major problem for widely application of FMT in UC. ~**Shi et al., 2016**

Although no serious adverse events were reported, some patients experienced fever, chills, bloating, flatulence, vomiting, diarrhea, and abdominal tenderness. The adverse events were more likely with nasogastric route of administration for FMT. Flares of UC following FMT were also described. ~**Seth et al., 2016**

Medicine poses risks, but generally acceptable risks. But for a few, the ultimate price may be paid. (Oh, the stories I could tell.) This is true with drug therapy; this is true with FMT.

In the modern day, there are at least three individuals who have lost their life as a result of complications from FMT. As horrifying as this sounds, FMT is still regarded as generally safe. Keep in mind, there is always a risk to be assumed when on the receiving end of medical care.

Despite my little disagreement with the "You can't have it" FDA, I will cut the FDA (and other regulators) some slack. Clearly, they are committed to safety. They want every therapy to be safe, as safe as possible. Clearly, they have your best interests in mind.

The regulators have a formidable task to develop policies that optimize access to important therapies, ensure their safety and efficacy, and allow innovation so that next-generation products can benefit future patients even more. It is clear that FMT opened a new frontier of medicine and demonstrated the healing powers within our own bodies. It is important that we are guided by up-to-date science on this journey. At the same time we need to be careful not to allow limited scientific knowledge turn into arrogance. We are still taking only the initial steps, even though they have already saved thousands of lives. (Khoruts, 2017)

Back to the three deaths associated with FMT, I should tell you more. One death was from fecal aspiration (fecal material entering the lungs) which accidently occurred during the procedure (Aroniadis and Brandt,

2014). I can't begin to tell you how dreadful fecal aspiration is. Another reported death was due to fecal material entering the abdominal cavity due to a dislodged transabdominal gastric tube, the route used for the fecal transfer to treat the patient's *C-diff* (Solari et al., 2014). Under such circumstances an overwhelming infection results, which can lead to death. And tragically, in this case, death occurred. The third recorded death occurred quite recently and was related to an unanticipated transfer of an antibiotic-resistant *E. Coli* bacterium from donor to recipient using FMT in pill form, resulting in an overwhelming blood infection called sepsis (DeFilipp et al., 2019). Importantly, this unfortunate patient was concurrently being treated by chemotherapy drugs that profoundly suppress the immune system. Is this case report an appropriate example to be used to justify withholding FMT . . . from you?

Clearly, with respect to FMT, care should be taken. *Clearly!* Care to comprehensively screen the health of the potential donor. Care to adequately screen the stool of the potential donor, and to the latest standards. Care to administer the stool with care—with tubes and devices carefully evaluated to ensure a safe procedure will occur. Care to exclude patients who are profoundly immunosuppressed. Such are the lessons of the three patients whose fecal transplants ended in disaster.

FMT is often perceived as "natural" remedy by many patients and physicians. However, considering the fact that the transfer of complex microbiota can modify the host phenotype with unknown long-term effects, it is preferable to exclude certain categories of patients in which the delivery of FMT may worsen their condition, or it may even be fatal. For example, patients with severe bowel disease cannot undergo colonoscopy, while those with severe immunosuppression and decompensated liver cirrhosis are excluded considering the potential risk of enteric microbe transmission from donor's stool. (Sunkara et al., 2018)

Meeting safety requirements is *so* important. With respect to fecal transplants destined to be delivered through a nasogastric (NG) tube, it is necessary for the correctness of tube position to be *"verified with x-ray before transplant"* (Shi et al., 2016).

Of course, there is always a risk of bowel perforation anytime instrumentation is performed (Ramai et al., 2019). Furthermore, there are risks associated with anesthesia, required for procedures involving a a colonoscope, the instrument typically used in clinic to perform the fecal transplant (Ramai et al., 2019).

In Medicine, there are risks everywhere! But, by and large, these are acceptable risks both physician and patient are willing to take.

Maybe you can have it (after all)

People are going the do-it-yourself route to relieve everything from a child's autism to male pattern baldness to bad breath, according to Catherine Duff, executive director of The Fecal Transplant Foundation, a nonprofit that is advocating for safer, more widespread access to the treatment. Based on telephone and Internet inquires to her site, she estimates that about 10,000 people do at-home fecal transplants in the U.S. each year. **~Web**MD**, 2015**

Experts Fear FDA Crackdown on FMT Could Backfire **~Blair, 2019**

There is precedent for physician-approved DIY fecal transplantation (Silverman et al., 2010). In the treatment of *C-diff*, multiple relapses can occur and require prompt treatment, which can be readily accomplished in the home setting—no waiting list, no appointment necessary. In the Silverman et al study, seven patients each received a DIY fecal transplant at home, with the donor stool obtained from a carefully screened relative. The results: No adverse effects occurred, and with 100% success, which persisted at 14-month follow-up. A conclusion was reached:

Fecal transplantation by low volume enema is an effective and safe option for patients with chronic relapsing CDI, refractory to other therapies. Making this approach available in health care settings has the potential to dramatically increase the number of patients who could benefit from this therapy. (Silverman et al., 2010)

These are the instructions given to both donor and recipient:

- *Equipment needed: (1) bottle of normal saline (200 mL); (2) standard 2 quart enema bag kit available at a drug store (Life Brand Hot Water Bottle and Syringe kit; Shoppers Drug Mart, Toronto, ON, Canada); and (3) standard kitchen blender (1 L capacity) with markings for volume on side, available at any department store.*

- *Stop vancomycin/metronidazole 24–48 hours before procedure.*

- *Continue S boulardii during transplant and for 60 days afterwards.*

- *Add 50 mL of stool (volume occupied by solid stool) from donor obtained immediately prior to administration (less than 30 minutes) to 200 mL normal saline in the blender.*

- *Mix in the blender until liquefied to 'milkshake' consistency.*

- *Pour mixture (approximately 250 mL) into the enema bag.*

- *Administer enema to patient using instructions provided with enema bag kit. Patient should hold the infusate as long as possible and lie still as long as possible on his or her left side so that the urge to defecate is prevented. Ideally perform the procedure after the first bowel movement of the day (usually in the morning).*

- *If diarrhea recurs within 1 hour, the procedure may be immediately repeated.* (Silverman et al., 2010)

With respect to ulcerative colitis, home FMT is perhaps the only realistic approach, as many follow-up fecal transplant therapy sessions are likely necessary. Recall, some patients require forty, even eighty fecal transplants before victory can be declared. The cost of FMT in clinic, as well as the cost of handful after handful of FMT capsules for home use, are cost prohibitive. Apart from the initial costs of donor screening, which may be as high as $3,600 (Blair, 2019), home FMT is very inexpensive.

This takes us to the question of who the ideal donor would be. In view of the literature, someone who is relative, close friend, or committed neighbor would be the ideal donor, due to the possible need of continuous donor availability and the possibility that many stool donations will be required before victory can be declared. Obviously, such an individual should be living a healthy lifestyle (including diet?), will need to be carefully screened for transmissible disease, and should probably be someone who is not obese, as this can be transmitted.

The bottom line: If you can find a willing physician to approve and guide you in your efforts to treat your ulcerative colitis (or recurrent *C-diff*) with FMT, maybe you can have it after all. Of course, donor selection and screening to the latest standards is essential. FMT is certainly one of the therapies you should *not* undertake all on your own.

My fear—and I share this fear with others (see Kahn et al., 2013)—is that you will go out on your own, FMT yourself without physician approval or guidance, make a mistake with screening or technique, have a negative outcome, and give FMT a bad name. I don't want you to make a mistake. I want you to be safe.

There is a legitimate concern that the strict requirements of the FDA will lead to a backlash—people will be pushed in the direction of doing it themselves regardless of the warnings and restrictions imposed by the FDA, perhaps doing so without proper donor screening and without the direction and guidance of a physician (Blair, 2019). Although unwise, who can blame them? In FMT, there is a readily available, generally safe therapy that can rescue even severe cases of ulcerative colitis, yet someone in the background is saying "You can't have it."

But what if there was a way around this roadblock?

This just might work

Despite these hurdles, compassionate drug use does happen. The FDA receives over 1,000 individual use applications per year, and approves over 99% of those requests. ~**American Cancer Society, 2019**

So, you are convinced. FMT is the route you wish to take. There is a strategy for obtaining approval that just might work. Hasn't the FDA declared FMT to be a drug? Investigational drugs can be allowed on the basis of compassion, regardless of their investigational classification (American Cancer Society, 2019). Perhaps you can get a "Yes" by appealing to the FDA to approve FMT for you on compassionate grounds. If willing, your doctor can assist you in this effort.

Alternatively, perhaps you can enroll in a new clinical study, or be somehow tacked on to a clinical study in progress, with the FMT to be performed locally by your physician in clinic or even performed at home.

People who aren't in clinical trials might be able to get access to an unapproved drug from the company that makes it in 2 ways:
- *Through* ***expanded access programs (EAPs)***
- *Through* ***"Right to Try"*** (American Cancer Society, 2019, emphasis added)

Of the two pathways mentioned above, your physician can help you decide the best path to take and can help you navigate through all the paperwork. Get used to the word "paperwork" and the phrase "Try, try again."

The following sources can help you understand it all—compassionate use qualifications, expanded access program inclusion parameters, and "Right to Try" qualifications:

Compassionate Drug Use. American Cancer Society; November 19, 2019
https://www.cancer.org/treatment/treatments-and-side-effects/clinical-trials/compassionate-drug-use.html

Compassionate use Navigator | Information for Patients. kidsvcancer.org; Accessed 01-30-2020
http://www.kidsvcancer.org/wp-content/uploads/2016/01/Navigator-One-Document.pdf

Expanded Access | Information for Patients. U.S. Food & Drug Administration; May 20, 2019
https://www.fda.gov/news-events/expanded-access/expanded-access-information-patients

FDA Fact Sheet | Right to Try. U.S. Food & Drug Administration; 01-14-2020
https://www.fda.gov/patients/learn-about-expanded-access-and-other-treatment-options/right-try

Emergency Use and Compassionate Use of Experimental Drugs and Devices. University of California San Francisco; Last update: 06-06-2019
https://www.google.com/url?sa=t&rct=j&q=&esrc=s&source=web&cd=11&ved=2ahUKEwiV3efKrqznAhUWr54KHT3HBRMQFjAKegQIAhAB&url=https%3A%2F%2Firb.ucsf.edu%2Fprintpdf%2F736&usg=AOvVaw1Gyn6DF7gYQmeEzdcIwiGF

In your quest to obtain FMT therapy, when it comes to seeking compassionate care or "Right to Try," *sell yourself!* Be rentless in advocating on your behalf. It's your bowel. It's your life. Get your physician on board. Resubmit approval applications, as needed, should the answer come back "You can't have it." Call whomever you think may be of help. Call the Surgeon General. Call the Governor. Call your Representative. Call research centers involved in active FMT studies. Ask them if there is some way they can help. Let everyone know you mean business. Search out every lead. Keep in mind, many patients have declared victory over ulcerative colitis with FMT. And keep in mind, if it can happen to them, there is a good chance it can happen to you.

Loose ends

There are a few more things to discuss before we wrap things up.

First, one drawback to FMT is the cost of donor screening, but there is a nifty way to cut donor screening costs. Find an existing blood donor, or one who is willing to donate blood, to be your prospective stool donor. To qualify to be a blood donor, an individual will first be asked important health screening questions, and their blood will be screened for several transmissible diseases. And as far as transitioning from blood donor to an acceptable stool donor, other relevant laboratory tests can be conducted elsewhere to complete the process of certifying that a person is free from transmissible disease and good to go. As a blood donor, he or she can help other people by donating blood and help you out by pooping for your benefit.

Second, when it comes to FMT, there is reason to believe "the earlier the better." Why wait for ulcerative colitis to get way out of hand? Consider this:

> FMT may be more efficacious in patients with a recent diagnosis of UC, and this is biologically plausible, as a perturbation in the microbiome _might be more easily restored early in the course of the disease_. The efficacy of this approach may also be donor dependent and this may explain why some case series have shown promise, and others have had disappointing results. (Moayyedi et al., 2015, emphasis added)

Third, and for future reference, you should be aware that there is a push for a name change. Instead of Fecal Microbial Transplantation

(FMT), in the future it many go by the name, Intestinal Microbiota Transplantation (IMT) (Blair, 2019). Whatever. Just keep in mind, regardless of the name, it is still the same old . . . well you know.

Finally, there is an alternative to FMT, at least with respect to *C diff.* You should probably have an interest in this, as *C-diff* can happen to you, the ulcerative colitis patient. And this alternative may be a substitute for FMT to treat ulcerative colitis and other diseases as well. We'll take up this discussion in the following gray box.

An alternative to FMT

*These results support the idea that **intra-colonic bile acids play a key mechanistic role in the success of FMT**, and suggests that novel therapeutic alternatives for treatment of R-CDI [recurrent-C-Diff] may be developed by targeted manipulation of bile acid composition in the colon.* ~**Weingarden et al., 2016A, emphasis added**

*Although FMT may combat C. difficile [CDI] by multiple mechanisms, including competitive niche exclusion, elaboration of targeted bacteriocins, and upregulation of host immunity, more recent investigations have **built a compelling case** for a **central role** of secondary bile acid metabolism in curing CDI.* ~**Weingarden et al., 2016B, emphasis added**

*Indeed, the potential for orally administered bile acids as an alternative to FMT is supported by a recent study demonstrating that **UDCA inhibits the germination of C. difficile spores** in vitro [in laboratory setting] and effectively induced and maintained remission from recurrent CDI in a human subject.* ~**Hegyi et al., 2018, emphasis added**

Surprisingly, bile acids—specifically secondary bile acids—can come to the rescue of the person with *C-diff*, serving as an alternative to FMT. Likely, secondary bile acids can successfully treat *C-diff* in the ulcerative colitis patient, as well. With respect to *C-diff*, bile acid therapy has been put to the test.

We have successfully treated a patient with refractory, recurrent C. difficile pouchitis with ursodeoxycholic acid (UDCA) after demonstrating that this minor secondary bile acid was inhibitory to her C. difficile isolate. Unfortunately, UDCA is efficiently absorbed into the enterohepatic circulation and might not be applicable to the majority of patients with CDI [C. difficile infection] in the colon. However, certain modified bile analogues can be made resistant to intestinal uptake and achieve high intracolonic concentrations." (Khoruts and Sadowsky, 2016)

So, here is the scoop (FMT term): It has been discovered that patients who have recurrent *C-diff* have a high concentration of primary bile acids in their stool, *"whereas, **secondary bile acids are nearly non-existant."*** (Aroniadis and Brandt, 2014, emphasis added) Notably, the fecal bile acid profile of the FMT recipient transitions to resemble the fecal bile acid profile of the donor. Problem solved.

*We had previously demonstrated that **patients with RCDI [recurrent C-diff] completely lack secondary bile acids in their feces**, but have increased levels of taurocholic acid. Within days following FMT, however, the fecal levels of secondary bile acids increase and primary bile acids drop to levels found in the donors.* (Weingarden et al., 2016B)

So clearly, measures that increase secondary bile acids are justified in the battle against *C-diff*. *"The spore germination of C. difficile can be stimulated by some primary bile acids"* whereas, *C. diff "can be inhibited by secondary acids."* (Nie et al., 2015) And one of the secondary bile acids that inhibit *C-diff* growth is **UDCA** (Nie et al., 2015).

If you will recall from *Chapter 18, Bile acid advantage*, both *"**TUDCA and UDCA are essentially identical molecules."*** (Vang et al., 2015, emphasis added). The exception being, with TUDCA, there is a taurine molecule attached to the UDCA molecule. In the scheme of things, after TUDCA is ingested, a bacterium in the small intestine will remove the taurine and turn it immediately into UDCA. TUDCA is now UDCA. I don't want to get lost in the weeds here, but one should expect that TUDCA is at least as good as UDCA in the treatment of *C-diff*. And may be better as there seems to be a little problem with UDCA.

> *A major limitation of UDCA for this indication is its rapid uptake into the enterohepatic circulation in the small intestine, resulting in low achievable intracolonic concentrations.* (Weingarden et al., 2016B, emphasis added)

Aside from the above, UDCA still seems to be effective. But TUDCA may even work better because *"TUDCA requires active absorption in the terminal ileum whereas UDCA may be absorbed passively throughout the small intestine . . .."* (Rudolph et al., 2002) It is likely, due to increased hang-around time, TUDCA is more capable of being carried by fecal material into the colon than would be the more easily absorbed and removed UDCA.

Evidence points to both UDCA and TUDCA as viable alternatives to FMT for the treatment of *C-diff*. These two secondary bile acids appear to compensate for the *"nearly non-existent"* secondary bile acids in the stool of the *C-diff* patient. Of note: *"When UDCA or TUDCA was administered, total fecal bile acid excretion increased markedly . . .."* (Invernizzi et al., 1999)

As we have learned in *Chapter 18*, IBD patients have reduced microbial diversity leading to an impaired bacterial conversion of primary to secondary bile acids (Heinken et al., 2017; Van den Bossche et al., 2017). Reduced microbial diversity (as found in ulcerative colitis) leads to *"reduced production of secondary bile acids and decreased levels of sulfated bile acids"* (Joyce and Gahan 2017, emphasis added). So, addressing this issue using UDCA or TUDCA, seems to be warranted. It may save an individual from *C-diff*, even in the context of ulcerative colitis, and prevent the need for a fecal transplant.

What about AS?

*The presence of a wide variety of bacterial species in both RA [rheumatoid arthritis] and other forms of chronic arthritis was an unexpected and novel discovery and indicates that **arthritic joints are not sterile, as thought previously.** ~Kempsell et al., 2000, emphasis added*

There is another disease that may benefit from FMT, the arthritic disease known as ankylosing spondylitis (AS). As if having one hideous disease wasn't enough, it is reported that 8–12 out or every 100 IBD patients also contract AS (Salem et al., 2019). Let's take a look.

AS is a disease in which genetics play a pivotal role in determining who contracts this disease and who does not, but not every time. Only 5% of those with the marker for this disease, HLA B27, will develop this form of arthritis (Tam et al., 2010). But with ulcerative colitis, there is a distinct disadvantage that makes contracting AS more likely; for this disease is one where bacterial translocation from the gut is a way of life . . . because dysbiosis is a way of life. And one problem with dysbiosis is this:

> ***Dysbiosis can be considered an important pathogenetic factor with advancement of growth of invasive bacteria. It can also facilitate bacterial translocation through the mucosal barrier to the mesenteric lymph nodes.*** (Comito and Romano, 2012, emphasis added)

Unfortunately, bacteria don't just arrive and stay in the lymph nodes of the gut. They somehow show up in the joints, unannounced, or they find themselves carried to the joints by immune cells that circulate from gut to joint.

Microbes or their components may enter the joints via blood vessels either as whole organisms that may circulate in the blood or within the cells or as a part of immune complexes. Peripheral blood mononuclear cells [monocytes and macrophages] that contain intracellular bacterial fragments are especially prone to bind to synovial high endothelial venules and transmigrate through the endothelial cell monolayer. (Colmegna et al., 2004)

Is it any wonder that inflammation in the joints occurs under such circumstances? Inflammation is, of course, how we deal with threats. Bacteria in joints are certainly a threat, one that is bound to provoke an inflammatory response.

But there is an out:

*A tight relationship between gut and joint inflammation has been revealed in prospective follow-up studies of patients with SpA [spondyloarthritis, e.g., AS]: **clinical remission of joint inflammation was associated with resolution of gut inflammation, whereas the presence of gut inflammation was associated with persistent joint inflammation.*** (Van Praet et al., 2012, emphasis added)

And there is a very good way to resolve gut inflammation and perhaps eliminate this driver of joint inflammation. We call it FMT.

*Clarifying the pathogenesis of ankylosing spondylitis will undoubtedly have therapeutic implications. If innate immunity is primarily responsible for its pathogenesis, it makes sense that the inhibition of tumor necrosis factor alpha would be an effective therapeutic. But the inhibition of TNF alpha could also itself have an effect on bacterial flora and this effect could potentially be counter therapeutic. **We have entered an era in which some have begun to explore the benefit of fecal transplantation to alter endogenous flora. The reduction of arthritogenic flora or the induction of non-arthritogenic flora are potential avenues of therapy which might be efficacious with fewer risks and even a safety profile that would justify their use for prophylaxis.** Perhaps, nearly forty years after*

*HLA B27's impact on susceptibility to spondyloarthropathy was discovered, **we at last have the tools to elucidate the mechanism for this remarkable association.*** (Rosenbaum and Davey, 2011, emphasis added).

FMT may be a means to bring AS to an end, as well as bring to an end an associated ulcerative colitis, in those who are now being told "You can't have it."

For more on this, I have written a post called *Ankyosing Spondylitis: The Story Not Being Told.* You can access this post at www.impactofvitamind.com

And then we have the unexpected

Detailed fecal microbiome analysis has revealed that MS had [a] distinct microbial community profile compared to healthy controls. **~Chen et al., 2016**

Let me assure you, what I am about to share occurred quite unexpectedly, and at a time when little was known about the role gut bacteria play in multiple sclerosis (MS). This is quite a story.

In 2001, Borody et al. reported three wheelchair-bound patients with MS treated with FMT [fecal microbiota transplantation] for constipation. Bowel symptoms resolved following FMT; however, in all cases, there was also a progressive and dramatic improvement in neurological symptoms, with all three patients regaining the ability to walk unassisted. Two of the patients with prior indwelling urinary catheters experienced restoration of urinary function. In one patient of the three, follow-up MRI 15 years after FMT showed a halting of disease progression and 'no evidence of active disease. (Borody et al., 2014, emphasis added)

And why would FMT come to the aid of the patient with MS?

A growing body of evidence in animal models of MS implicates the gut microbiota in the induction of central nervous system (CNS) autoimmunity. (Berer and Krishnamoorthy, 2012)

In brief: There is growing suspicion that gut bacteria play a pivotal role in initiating and perpetuating neuroinflammatory disease, MS included. That bacteria within the gut could influence a disease process occurring in the brain and spinal cord is, indeed, quite surprising. In the not too distant past, to even consider such a thing would have been crazy. But not now. We have learned so much! Suspicions are giving way to conclusions.

In a laboratory model of MS, known as experimental autoimmune encephalomyelitis (EAE), the administration of non-absorbing antibiotics *"beginning 1 week prior to sensitization, altered the composition of gut flora and, intriguingly, also ameliorated the development of EAE."* (Yokote et al., 2008) And astonishingly, **FMT, using the stool from a MS patient and transplanted into an undeserving mouse, will transfer the disease from human to mouse** (Berer et al., 2017).

Furthermore,

Certain populations of commensal [normally found] bacteria are capable of attenuating CNS inflammation. The gut microbiota has the capacity to affect the development of autoimmune central nervous system (CNS) disorders. (Kamada et al., 2013)

Combined, . . . data indicate that early dysregulation in MS involves an increase in pro-inflammatory and a decrease in anti-inflammatory gut microbiota milieu. (Tremlett at al., 2016, emphasis added)

FMT normalizes gut bacteria. That's what it does. In view of the experiences of the three wheelchair-bound MS patients mentioned above, and in view of emerging data, the time has come to allow MS patients to choose FMT—or at the very least allow FMT as a compassionate therapy, but perhaps also as an approved alternative to drug therapy, which so often fails to induce and/or sustain remission in MS.

I have a great little post on this on my website, entitled *Multiple Sclerosis: The Next Frontier.* You can access this at www.impactofvitamind.com

Let me conclude with this: If I had MS, hearing the words "You can't have it" would not be acceptable. No, not in the least.

~*References*~

Alang N, Kelly CR. **Weight gain after fecal microbiota transplantation.** InOpen forum infectious diseases 2015 Jan 1 (Vol. 2, No. 1). Oxford University Press.

American Cancer Society. **Compassionate Drug Use.** 2019 Nov 19 https://www.cancer.org/treatment/treatments-and-side-effects/clinical-trials/compassionate-drug-use.html

Aroniadis OC, Brandt LJ. **Intestinal microbiota and the efficacy of fecal microbiota transplantation in gastrointestinal disease.** Gastroenterology & hepatology. 2014 Apr;10(4):230.

Baktash A, Terveer EM, Zwittink RD, Hornung BV, Corver J, Kuijper J, Smits WK. **Mechanistic insights in the success of fecal microbiota transplants for the treatment of Clostridium difficile infections.** Frontiers in microbiology. 2018;9.

Bennet J, Brinkman M. **Treatment of ulcerative colitis by implantation of normal colonic flora.** The Lancet. 1989 Jan 21;333(8630):164.

Berer K, Krishnamoorthy G. **Commensal gut flora and brain autoimmunity: a love or hate affair?.** Acta neuropathologica. 2012 May 1;123(5):639-51.

Berer K, Gerdes LA, Cekanaviciute E, Jia X, Xiao L, Xia Z, Liu C, Klotz L, Stauffer U, Baranzini SE, Kümpfel T. **Gut microbiota from multiple sclerosis patients enables spontaneous autoimmune encephalomyelitis in mice.** Proceedings of the National Academy of Sciences. 2017 Oct 3;114(40):10719-24.

Blair J. **Experts fear FDA crackdown on FMT could backfire.** Gastroenterology & Endoscopy News 2019 Aug 14

Bojanova DP, Bordenstein SR. **Fecal transplants: what is being transferred?.** Plos biology. 2016 Jul 12;14(7):e1002503.

Borody TJ, George L, Andrews P, Brandl S, Noonan S, Cole P, Hyland L, Morgan A, Maysey J, Moore-Jones D. **Bowel-flora alteration: a potential cure for inflammatory bowel disease and irritable bowel syndrome?.** Medical Journal of Australia. 1989 May;150(10):604-.

Borody TJ, Warren EF, Leis S, Surace R, Ashman O. **Treatment of ulcerative colitis using fecal bacteriotherapy.** Journal of clinical gastroenterology. 2003 Jul 1;37(1):42-7.

Borody TJ, Campbell J. **Fecal microbiota transplantation: techniques, applications, and issues.** Gastroenterology Clinics. 2012 Dec 1;41(4):781-803.

Borody TJ, Paramsothy S, Agrawal G. **Fecal microbiota transplantation: indications, methods, evidence, and future directions.** Current gastroenterology reports. 2013 Aug 1;15(8):337.

Borody TJ, Brandt LJ, Paramsothy S. **Therapeutic faecal microbiota transplantation: current status and future developments.** Current opinion in gastroenterology. 2014 Jan;30(1):97.

Butta H, Kapoor A, Sibal A, Sardana R, Bhatia V, Mendiratta L. **Fecal Microbial Transplant-A New Hope of Treatment for Ulcerative Colitis.** International Journal of Medicine and Public Health. 2018;8(1).

CDC **Nearly half a million Americans suffered from Clostridium difficile infections in a single year.** 2017; https://www.cdc.gov/media/releases/2015/p0225-clostridium-difficile.html

Chen J, Chia N, Kalari KR, Yao JZ, Novotna M, Soldan MM, Luckey DH, Marietta EV, Jeraldo PR, Chen X, Weinshenker BG. **Multiple sclerosis patients have a distinct gut microbiota compared to healthy controls.** Scientific reports. 2016 Jun 27;6(1):1-0.

Cold F, Browne PD, Günther S, Halkjaer SI, Petersen AM, Al-Gibouri Z, Hansen LH, Christensen AH. **Multidonor FMT capsules improve symptoms and decrease fecal calprotectin in ulcerative colitis patients while treated–an open-label pilot study.** Scandinavian Journal of Gastroenterology. 2019 Mar 4;54(3):289-96.

Colmegna I, Cuchacovich R, Espinoza LR. **HLA-B27-associated reactive arthritis: pathogenetic and clinical considerations.** Clinical microbiology reviews. 2004 Apr 1;17(2):348-69.

Comito D, Romano C. **Dysbiosis in the pathogenesis of pediatric inflammatory bowel diseases.** International journal of inflammation. 2012;2012.

Costello SP, Hughes PA, Waters O, Bryant RV, Vincent AD, Blatchford P, Katsikeros R, Makanyanga J, Campaniello MA, Mavrangelos C, Rosewarne CP.

Effect of fecal microbiota transplantation on 8-week remission in patients with ulcerative colitis: a randomized clinical trial. Jama. 2019 Jan 15;321(2):156-64.

Cui B, Li P, Xu L, Peng Z, Zhao Y, Wang H, He Z, Zhang T, Ji G, Wu K, Fan D. **Fecal microbiota transplantation is an effective rescue therapy for refractory inflammatory bowel disease.** Inflammation and Cell Signaling. 2015 Nov 20;2.

DeFilipp Z, Bloom PP, Torres Soto M, Mansour MK, Sater MR, Huntley MH, Turbett S, Chung RT, Chen YB, Hohmann EL. **Drug-resistant E. coli bacteremia transmitted by fecal microbiota transplant.** New England Journal of Medicine. 2019 Nov 21;381(21):2043-50.

de Groot PF, Frissen MN, De Clercq NC, Nieuwdorp M. **Fecal microbiota transplantation in metabolic syndrome: history, present and future.** Gut microbes. 2017 May 4;8(3):253-67.

Fang H, Fu L, Wang J. **Protocol for fecal microbiota transplantation in inflammatory bowel disease: a systematic review and meta-analysis.** BioMed research international. 2018;2018.

Guinane CM, Cotter PD. **Role of the gut microbiota in health and chronic gastrointestinal disease: understanding a hidden metabolic organ.** Therapeutic advances in gastroenterology. 2013 Jul;6(4):295-308.

Hegyi P, Maléth J, Walters JR, Hofmann AF, Keely SJ. **Guts and gall: bile acids in regulation of intestinal epithelial function in health and disease.** Physiological reviews. 2018 Oct 1;98(4):1983-2023.

Heinken A, Ravcheev DA, Baldini F, Heirendt L, Fleming RM, Thiele I. **Personalized modeling of the human gut microbiome reveals distinct bile acid deconjugation and biotransformation potential in healthy and IBD individuals.** BioRxiv. 2017 Jan 1:229138.

Invernizzi P, Setchell KD, Crosignani A, Battezzati PM, Larghi A, O'C'nnell NC, Podda M. **Differences in the metabolism and disposition of ursodeoxycholic acid and of its taurine-conjugated species in patients with primary biliary cirrhosis.** Hepatology. 1999 Feb;29(2):320-7.

Joyce SA, Gahan CG. **Disease-associated changes in bile acid profiles and links to altered gut microbiota.** Digestive Diseases. 2017;35(3):169-77.

Kahn SA, Vachon A, Rodriquez D, Goeppinger SR, Surma B, Marks J, Rubin DT. **Patient perceptions of fecal microbiota transplantation for ulcerative colitis.** Inflammatory bowel diseases. 2013 Apr 24;19(7):1506-13.

Kamada N, Seo SU, Chen GY, Núñez G. **Role of the gut microbiota in immunity and inflammatory disease.** Nature Reviews Immunology. 2013 May;13(5):321-35.

Kariv R, Navaneethan U, Venkatesh PG, Lopez R, Shen B. **Impact of Clostridium difficile infection in patients with ulcerative colitis.** Journal of Crohn's and Colitis. 2011 Feb 1;5(1):34-40.

Kempsell KE, Cox CJ, Hurle M, Wong A, Wilkie S, Zanders ED, Gaston JH, Crowe JS. **Reverse transcriptase-PCR analysis of bacterial rRNA for detection and characterization of bacterial species in arthritis synovial tissue.** Infection and immunity. 2000 Oct 1;68(10):6012-26.

Khoruts A. **Fecal microbiota transplantation–early steps on a long journey ahead.** 2017: 199-204.

Khoruts A, Sadowsky MJ. **Understanding the mechanisms of faecal microbiota transplantation.** Nature reviews Gastroenterology & hepatology. 2016 Sep;13(9):508.

Laszlo M, Pascu O. **Full Clinical and Endoscopic Remission Following Fecal Microbiota Transplant with Moderate-Severe Treatment-Resistant Ulcerative Colitis.** J Gastroint Dig Syst. 2014;2:183.

Laszlo M, Ciobanu L, Andreica V, Pascu O. **Fecal transplantation indications in ulcerative colitis.** Preliminary study. Clujul Medical. 2016;89(2):224.

Moayyedi P, Surette MG, Kim PT, Libertucci J, Wolfe M, Onischi C, Armstrong D, Marshall JK, Kassam Z, Reinisch W, Lee CH. **Fecal microbiota transplantation induces remission in patients with active ulcerative colitis in a randomized controlled trial.** Gastroenterology. 2015 Jul 1;149(1):102-9.

Ni X, Fan S, Zhang Y, Wang Z, Ding L, Li Y, Li J. **Coordinated hospital-home fecal microbiota transplantation via percutaneous endoscopic cecostomy for recurrent steroid-dependent ulcerative colitis.** Gut and liver. 2016 Nov;10(6):975.

Nie YF, Hu J, Yan XH. **Cross-talk between bile acids and intestinal microbiota in host metabolism and health.** Journal of Zhejiang University-Science B. 2015 Jun 1;16(6):436-46.

Ott SJ, Waetzig GH, Rehman A, Moltzau-Anderson J, Bharti R, Grasis JA, Cassidy L, Tholey A, Fickenscher H, Seegert D, Rosenstiel P. **Efficacy of sterile fecal filtrate transfer for treating patients with Clostridium difficile infection.** Gastroenterology. 2017 Mar 1;152(4):799-811.

Qin C, Zhang H, Zhao L, Zeng M, Huang W, Fu G, Zhou W, Wang H, Yan H. **Microbiota transplantation reveals beneficial impact of berberine on hepatotoxicity by improving gut homeostasis.** Science China Life Sciences. 2017 Nov 29:1-8.

Ramai D, Zakhia K, Ofosu A, Ofori E, Reddy M. **Fecal microbiota transplantation: donor relation, fresh or frozen, delivery methods, cost-effectiveness.** Annals of gastroenterology. 2019 Jan;32(1):30.

Rogers GB, Bruce KD. **Challenges and opportunities for faecal microbiota transplantation therapy.** Epidemiology & Infection. 2013 Nov;141(11):2235-42.

Rosenbaum JT, Davey MP. **Time for a gut check: Evidence for the hypothesis that HLA–B27 predisposes to ankylosing spondylitis by altering the microbiome.** Arthritis & Rheumatism. 2011 Nov;63(11):3195-8.

Rudolph G, Kloeters-Plachky P, Sauer P, Stiehl A. **Intestinal absorption and biliary secretion of ursodeoxycholic acid and its taurine conjugate.** European journal of clinical investigation. 2002 Aug;32(8):575-80.

Salem M, Malaty H, Criner K, Caplan L, Hou J. **The Prevalence and Characterization of Axial Spondyloarthritis Among Veterans with Inflammatory Bowel Disease.** Crohn's'& Colitis 360. 2019 May;1(1):otz005.

Seicean A, Moldovan-Pop A, Seicean R. **Ulcerative colitis worsened after Clostridium difficile infection: efficacy of infliximab.** World Journal of Gastroenterology: WJG. 2014 May 7;20(17):5135.

Seth AK, Rawal P, Bagga R, Jain P. **Successful colonoscopic fecal microbiota transplantation for active ulcerative colitis: first report from India.** Indian Journal of Gastroenterology. 2016 Sep 1;35(5):393-5.

Shen ZH, Zhu CX, Quan YS, Yang ZY, Wu S, Luo WW, Tan B, Wang XY. **Relationship between intestinal microbiota and ulcerative colitis:**

Mechanisms and clinical application of probiotics and fecal microbiota transplantation. World journal of gastroenterology. 2018 Jan 7;24(1):5.

Shi Y, Dong Y, Huang W, Zhu D, Mao H, Su P. **Fecal microbiota transplantation for ulcerative colitis: a systematic review and meta-analysis.** PLos One. 2016;11(6).

Shimizu H, Arai K, Abe J, Nakabayashi K, Yoshioka T, Hosoi K, Kuroda M. **Repeated fecal microbiota transplantation in a child with ulcerative colitis.** Pediatrics International. 2016 Aug;58(8):781-5.

Silverman MS, Davis I, Pillai DR. **Success of self-administered home fecal transplantation for chronic Clostridium difficile infection.** Clinical Gastroenterology and Hepatology. 2010 May 1;8(5):471-3.

Solari PR, Fairchild PG, Noa LJ, Wallace MR. **Tempered enthusiasm for fecal transplant.** Clinical Infectious Diseases. 2014 Jul 15;59(2):319-.

Sunkara T, Rawla P, Ofosu A, Gaduputi V. **Fecal microbiota transplant–a new frontier in inflammatory bowel disease.** Journal of inflammation research. 2018;11:321.

Tam LS, Gu J, Yu D. **Pathogenesis of ankylosing spondylitis.** Nature Reviews Rheumatology. 2010 Jul;6(7):399.

Taur Y, Coyte K, Schluter J, Robilotti E, Figueroa C, Gjonbalaj M, Littmann ER, Ling L, Miller L, Gyaltshen Y, Fontana E. **Reconstitution of the gut microbiota of antibiotic-treated patients by autologous fecal microbiota transplant.** Science translational medicine. 2018 Sep 26;10(460).

Tremlett H, Fadrosh DW, Faruqi AA, Zhu F, Hart J, Roalstad S, Graves J, Lynch S, Waubant E, US Network of Pediatric MS Centers, Aaen G. **Gut microbiota in early pediatric multiple sclerosis: a case–control study.** European journal of neurology. 2016 Aug;23(8):1308-21.

Van den Bossche L, Hindryckx P, Devisscher L, Devriese S, Van Welden S, Holvoet T, Vilchez-Vargas R, Vital M, Pieper DH, Bussche JV, Vanhaecke L. **Ursodeoxycholic acid and its taurine/glycine conjugated species reduce colitogenic dysbiosis and equally suppress experimental colitis in mice.** Applied and environmental microbiology. 2017 Jan 23:AEM-02766.

Vang S, Longley K, Steer CJ, Low WC. **The unexpected uses of urso-and tauroursodeoxycholic acid in the treatment of non-liver diseases.** Global advances in health and medicine. 2014 May;3(3):58-69.

Van Praet L, Jacques P, Van den Bosch F, Elewaut D. **The transition of acute to chronic bowel inflammation in spondyloarthritis.** Nature Reviews Rheumatology. 2012 May;8(5):288.

Wang ZK, Yang YS, Chen Y, Yuan J, Sun G, Peng LH. **Intestinal microbiota pathogenesis and fecal microbiota transplantation for inflammatory bowel disease.** World journal of gastroenterology: WJG. 2014 Oct 28;20(40):14805.

*Web*MD, **The rise of the do-it-yourself fecal transplant.** 2015 https://www.webmd.com/digestive-disorders/news/20151209/diy-fecal-transplant#1

Wei Y, Zhu W, Gong J, Guo D, Gu L, Li N, Li J. **Fecal microbiota transplantation improves the quality of life in patients with inflammatory bowel disease.** Gastroenterology research and practice. 2015;2015.

Weingarden AR, Dosa PI, DeWinter E, Steer CJ, Shaughnessy MK, Johnson JR, Khoruts A, Sadowsky MJ. **Changes in colonic bile acid composition following fecal microbiota transplantation are sufficient to control Clostridium difficile germination and growth.** PloS one. 2016A;11(1).

Weingarden AR, Chen C, Zhang N, Graiziger CT, Dosa PI, Steer CJ, Shaughnessy MK, Johnson JR, Sadowsky MJ, Khoruts A. **Ursodeoxycholic acid inhibits Clostridium difficile spore germination and vegetative growth, and prevents recurrence of ileal pouchitis associated with the infection.** Journal of clinical gastroenterology. 2016B;Sep;50(8):624.

Wilson BC, Vatanen T, Cutfield WS, O'S'llivan JM. **The super-donor phenomenon in fecal microbiota transplantation.** Frontiers in cellular and infection microbiology. 2019;9:2.

Winston JA, Theriot CM. **Impact of microbial derived secondary bile acids on colonization resistance against Clostridium difficile in the gastrointestinal tract.** Anaerobe. 2016 Oct 1;41:44-50.

Yan ZX, Gao XJ, Li T, Wei B, Wang PP, Yang Y, Yan R. **Fecal microbiota transplantation in experimental ulcerative colitis reveals associated gut** microbial and host metabolic reprogramming. Appl. Environ. Microbiol.. 2018 Jul 15;84(14):e00434-18.

Yokote H, Miyake S, Croxford JL, Oki S, Mizusawa H, Yamamura T. **NKT cell-dependent amelioration of a mouse model of multiple sclerosis by altering gut flora.** The American journal of pathology. 2008 Dec 1;173(6):1714-23.

Zuo T, Wong SH, Lam K, Lui R, Cheung K, Tang W, Ching JY, Chan PK, Chan MC, Wu JC, Chan FK. **Bacteriophage transfer during faecal microbiota transplantation in Clostridium difficile infection is associated with treatment outcome.** Gut. 2018 Apr 1;67(4):634-43.

Conclusion

*Treatments for IBD in clinic cause big side effects. Their aims are
ambiguous and they are costly. Their curative effects are not satisfying.*
~Jian et al., 2005

*A significant proportion of patients do not tolerate existing treatments
because of their adverse effects and **about 20% to 30% of patients fail to
respond to the drugs given for induction of remission.** Consequently, new
alternatives for the treatment of UC constantly are being sought.* **~Sood
et al., 2009, emphasis added**

W e have a real problem on our hands. We call it ulcerative colitis.
Likely, you know this disease all too well. You want a way out. I
want to help. This book is what I have to offer. It is my best effort to help
you understand the nature of the disease you have and to share with you
(and the physician) the alternative and complementary therapies
available for its treatment.

It would be nice to say that we are doing well in our battle against
ulcerative colitis—we have the most sophisticated of drugs, and we have
the old standbys. "What more do we need?" I'll tell you what we need.
We need success and we need more of it. Listen carefully:

*IBD affects an estimated 1.4 million people in the USA, and is
associated with high morbidity and decreased quality of life.
Corticosteroids are often used in the short term to achieve
symptomatic relief and decreased inflammation, yet are ineffective
in mucosal healing and not appropriate for long-term maintenance
therapy. Over the past two decades, **monoclonal antibodies
[biologics]** against TNF have revolutionized the treatment and
management of IBD. However, more than one-third of patients*

show no response to induction therapy and, for up to 50% of responders, anti-TNF therapy becomes ineffective over time. Additionally, anti-TNF therapy has multiple concerning side effects including increased risk of infection, anaphylaxis, and increased incidence of malignancies. **Therefore, the development of a novel therapeutic approach, with minimal side effects, for the long-term treatment of IBD represents a significant unmet medical need.** (MacManus et al., 2017, emphasis added)

The *"novel therapeutic approach"* mentioned above is already here. It is found in the medical literature for all to see. It is found in this book for all to read. To be clear, the author is not at all opposed to the use of drug therapy in the treatment of ulcerative colitis, but obviously is no fan of the use of drugs *and little else* in the battle against this disease. With the present-day emphasis on drugs (and little else), so much is set aside, so much is left behind. I believe this is a tragedy, as useful things lay hidden in the shadows and patients are denied the benefits of proven therapies and strategies and perhaps better outcomes. Furthermore, patients are excessively exposed to the side effects of drugs that are not as successful as we had hoped. In all this, it may be up to you to take the initiative in order to achieve and maintain remission.

So much of this book is diet-related—should be easy for your physician to support you in your efforts to follow dietary practices reported to be effective. The first alternative therapy discussed in the book, EnteraGam®, shows great promise, but may be a little more challenging to get your physician on board. But you can do it! If you believe EnteraGam® is right for you, being persistent may just pay off. Other therapies discussed—probiotics, prebiotics, polyphenols, vitamin D—should be easy to obtain approval and guidance. Bile acid therapy for ulcerative colitis is largely unknown (my impression), but I believe worthwhile pursuing. Finally, FMT will likely be the hardest therapy to obtain, but if FMT is on your bucket list, you have your work cut out for you. Be persistent and strategic in your efforts to make it a reality, and let's see what happens. Possibly, should you put into practice other promising therapies and the dietary practices outlined in this book, a FMT will not be necessary.

And for those whose ulcerative colitis is currently in remission, I have an important message: Although victory has been declared, the danger has not passed.

> *Even when routine colonoscopy suggests remission [in UC] and a normal mucosal appearance, **microscopic abnormalities may persist.*** (Ando et al., 2011, emphasis added)

> ***Endoscopic mucosal heading does not necessarily reflect quiescent microscopic disease.** Persistent microscopic **inflammation**, both acute and chronic, in patients with ulcerative colitis (UC) has been **associated with increased relapse rates**, hospitalization, colectomy, and risk of colorectal neoplasia [cancer].* (Bryant et al., 2014, emphasis added)

Therefore, even in remission, ongoing efforts are likely necessary to hold this disease in check. Strategies with the power to do this are found within the pages of this book. **Hint:** Pay close attention to the diets and the dietary dos and don'ts we have previously discussed.

My hope is that by shining a spotlight on the promising alternative and complementary therapies available in the treatment of ulcerative colitis, this book will lead to a greater degree of success in our battle against the disease, one individual at a time.

~*Eugene L. Heyden, RN*

~References~

Ando T, Watanabe O, Nishio Y, Ishiguro K, Maeda O, Nakamura M, Miyahara R, Ohmiya N, Goto H. **Novel Techniques in Endoscopy Are Useful in Evaluating Patients with Ulcerative Colitis.** Ulcers. 2011 Jun 22;2011.

Bryant RV, Winer SS, Travis SP, Riddell RH. **Systematic review: Histological remission in inflammatory bowel disease. Is 'complete' remission the new treatment paradigm? An IOIBD initiative.** Journal of Crohn's and Colitis. 2014 Dec 1;8(12):1582-97.

Jian YT, Mai GF, Wang JD, Zhang YL, Luo RC, Fang YX. **Preventive and therapeutic effects of NF-kappaB inhibitor curcumin in rats colitis induced by trinitrobenzene sulfonic acid.** World journal of gastroenterology: WJG. 2005 Mar 28;11(12):1747.

MacManus CF, Collins CB, Nguyen TT, Alfano RW, Jedlicka P, de Zoeten EF. **VEN-120, a recombinant human lactoferrin, promotes a regulatory T cell [Treg] phenotype and drives resolution of inflammation in distinct murine models of inflammatory bowel disease.** Journal of Crohn's and Colitis. 2017 Sep 1;11(9):1101-12.

Sharifi A, Hosseinzadeh-Attar MJ, Vahedi H, Nedjat S. **A randomized controlled trial on the effect of vitamin D3 on inflammation and cathelicidin gene expression in ulcerative colitis patients.** Saudi journal of gastroenterology: official journal of the Saudi Gastroenterology Association. 2016 Jul;22(4):316.

Sood A, Midha V, Makharia GK, Ahuja V, Singal D, Goswami P, Tandon RK. **The probiotic preparation, VSL# 3 induces remission in patients with mild-to-moderately active ulcerative colitis.** Clinical Gastroenterology and Hepatology. 2009 Nov 1;7(11):1202-9.

~ *Acknowledgments* ~

I wish to thank the following individuals who helped make this book possible: First and foremost, my dear wife Toni, for her encouragement and support in this lengthy endeavor. I extend a special thanks to Dr. Beth Hill at Providence Sacred Heart Medical Center, Spokane, WA, for her efforts to obtain numerous research papers critical to the writing of this book. I also wish to acknowledge the exceptional editing work of Barbara Hollace.